PRACTICAL GUIDE TO ANORECTAL TESTING, 2ND EDITION

PRACTICAL GUIDE TO ANORECTAL TESTING, 2ND EDITION

Edited by Lee E. Smith, M.D.
Professor of Surgery
Director, Division of Colon and Rectal Surgery
The George Washington University School of Medicine
Washington, DC

IGAKU-SHOIN NEW YORK • TOKYO

Published and distributed by

IGAKU-SHOIN Medical Publishers, Inc.
One Madison Avenue, New York, New York 10010

IGAKU-SHOIN Ltd.,
5-24-3 Hongo, Bunkyo-ku, Tokyo 113-91

Library of Congress Cataloging-in-Publication Data

Practical guide to anorectal testing/edited by Lee E. Smith.—2nd ed.
p. cm.
Includes bibliographical references and index.
ISBN 0-89640-278-9 (New York). —ISBN 4-260-14278-X (Tokyo)
1. Defecation disorders—Diagnosis. 2. Anorectal function tests.
I. Smith, Lee E.
[DNLM: 1. Anus—pathophysiology 2. Anus Diseases—diagnosis.
3. Rectal Diseases—diagnosis. 4. Rectum—pathophysiology WI 600 P895 1995]
RC866.D43P73 1995
616.3'5075—dc20
DNLM/DLC
for Library of Congress 95-1315
CIP

ISBN: 0-89640-278-9 (New York)
ISBN: 4-260-14278-X (Tokyo)

Printed and bound in the U.S.A.
10 9 8 7 6 5 4 3 2 1

DEDICATION

I dedicate this book to my children Alexander Smith, Justine and Gregory Barton, Tara Vogt and Brandon Vogt, and especially my wife, Carole, who supported me in this effort and spent hours helping with the work of writing and editing both editions.

PREFACE

In the 5-year interval since the first edition of this text was published, new tests have been developed, others have been refined, and many new laboratories for the study of defecation disorders have emerged. This is gratifying for those of us who have been involved in the evolution of physiological testing. However, our search for the mechanism and parameters of normal continence and normal defecation still is incomplete. More and more frequently, constipation and incontinence of varying degrees are presenting complaints. Hence, there is need to continue our efforts. In this edition most chapters have been rewritten, and many new authors provide different approaches and viewpoints. For example, the new chapter on "Digital Subraction Defecography" takes a fresh look at a dynamic study for defecation disorders. A chapter is devoted to another important new test, anal muscle ultrasound. This is likely the most important test in the study of incontinence.

The purpose of the new edition is to provide a reference source and to describe in detail how to perform the tests. The guidelines presented serve as a practical guide in the laboratory. Our final and most important goal is to define specific diagnoses which may direct a specific therapy; thus, we serve our patients better.

Lee E. Smith, M.D.

CONTRIBUTORS

Pierre Arhan, M.D.
Professor of Physiology
University of Caen
Caen, France

Guy Bédard
Sherbrooke University Hospital Centre
Sherbrooke, Quebec
Canada

Paul Belliveau, M.D.
Associate Professor of Surgery
McGill University
Montreal, Quebec
Canada

Hélèn Bouchard
Sherbrooke University Hospital Centre
Sherbrooke, Quebec
Canada

Patrick Brilliant, M.D.
Fellow, Colon and Rectal Surgery
Mayo Medical School
Mayo Clinic
Rochester, Minnesota

Jeffrey L. Cole, M.D., FAAPMR
Chairman, Department of Physical Medicine and Rehabilitation
Director, Neuromuscular Electrodiagnostic Services
The New York Hospital Medical Center of Queens
Flushing, New York

John A. Coller, M.D.
Clinical Assistant in Surgery
Harvard University Medical School
Department of Colon and Rectal Surgery
Lahey Clinic
Burlington, Massachusetts

Ghislain Devroede, M.D.
Professor of Surgery
Sherbrooke University Hospital Centre
Sherbrooke, Quebec
Canada

Ridzuan Farouk, MBChB, FRCSED, FRCSGlasg
Lecturer in Surgery
University of Hull
Academic Surgical Unit
Department of Colorectal Surgery
Castle Hill Hospital
Hull, England

James W. Fleshman, M.D.
Associate Professor of Surgery
Washington University Medical Center and Program Director of Colon and Rectal Surgery
Jewish Hospital of St. Louis
St. Louis, Missouri

Leonard M. Glassman, M.D., F.A.C.R.
Chief of Radiology
Columbia Hospital for Women Medical Center
Clinical Professor of Radiology
The George Washington University School of Medicine
Washington, DC

Lester Gottesman, M.D.
Assistant Professor of Clinical Surgery
Columbia University College of Physicians and Surgeons
Director, Anorectal Physiology Laboratory
St. Luke's/Roosevelt Hospital Center
Division of Colon-Rectal Surgery
New York, New York

Monique Hémond
Sherbrooke University Hospital Centre
Sherbrooke, Quebec
Canada

Michael M. Henry
Consultant Surgeon
Central Middlesex Hospital NHS Trust
Park Royal, London
England

Steve Heymen
Director, Biofeedback Services
Departments of Psychiatry and Colorectal Surgery
Cleveland Clinic Foundation
Ft. Lauderdale, Florida

Linda L. Jensen, R.N., BCIAC
Clinical Research Director
Colon and Rectal Surgery Associates
Division of Colon and Rectal Surgery
Department of Surgery
University of Minnesota
St. Paul, Minnesota

Lindsay Kerr, M.D.
Assistant Professor of Urology
Director, Incontinence and Urodynamic Study
The George Washington University Medical Center
Washington, D.C.

Davinder Kumar, Ph.D., F.R.C.S.
Consultant General And Colorectal Surgeon
St. George's Hospital
Tooting, London
England

Luc P.A. Lesaffer, M.D.
Department of Radiology
A.S.Z. Hospital
Aalst, Belgium

Amanda M. Metcalf, M.D.
Associate Professor of Surgery
University of Iowa
Iowa City, Iowa

Jeffrey W. Milsom, M.D.
Head, Section of Colorectal Surgery Research
Department of Colorectal Surgery
The Cleveland Clinic Foundation
Cleveland, Ohio

Gregory C. Oliver, M.D.
Clinical Associate Professor of Surgery
Division of Colon and Rectal Surgery
UMDNJ/Robert Wood Johnson Medical School
New Brunswick, New Jersey

Bruce A. Orkin, M.D.
Director, Colorectal Physiology Laboratory
Division of Colon and Rectal Surgery
The George Washington University Medical Center
Washington, DC

Russell K. Pearl, M.D.
Associate Professor of Surgery
University of Illinois
Chicago, Illinois

John H. Pemberton, M.D.
Professor of Surgery
Mayo Medical School
Consultant–Colon, Rectal and General Surgery
Mayo Clinic
Rochester, Minnesota

Yash P. Sangwan, M.D., M.S. (Surg)
Clinical Research Fellow
Pelvic Floor Laboratory
Department of Colon and Rectal Surgery
Lahey Clinic
Burlington, Massachusetts

Marvin M. Schuster, M.D.
Professor of Medicine with Joint appointment in Psychiatry
The Johns Hopkins University School of Medicine
Director, Division of Digestive Diseases
The Johns Hopkins Bay View Medical Center
Baltimore, Maryland

Lee E. Smith, M.D.
Professor of Surgery
Department of Surgery
George Washington University Medical Center
Washington, DC

Alan E. Timmcke, M.D.
Department of Colon and Rectal Surgery
Oschner Clinic
New Orleans, Louisiana

Alain Watier, M.D.
Professor of Gastroenterology
Sherbrooke University Hospital Centre
Sherbrooke, Quebec
Canada

Steven D. Wexner, M.D.
Chairman, Department of Colorectal Surgery
Cleveland Clinic Florida
Fort Lauderdale, Florida

CONTENTS

CHAPTER 1

Anatomy of the Pelvic Floor, Rectum, and Anal Canal

Russell K. Pearl

INTRODUCTION

The anatomical configuration of the pelvic floor, rectum, and anal canal is complex and not well understood. Many of the more traditional concepts based on cadaver dissections are currently being challenged by manometric and other in vivo data that have recently become available. Examples of these anatomical controversies include whether the puborectalis is part of the external sphincter complex or belongs to the levator ani muscles and whether the external sphincter is one continuous circumferential mass or is actually composed of three distinct loops. It is not the aim of this review to answer these questions definitively. Rather, it is to present a current, reasonable model of the muscular, nervous, and vascular system of the anorectum.

THE PELVIC FLOOR

The pelvic floor is formed by overlapping paired musculotendinous sheets of predominantly striated fibers known as the levator ani muscles. The major components of this pelvic diaphragm are the pubococcygeus and the iliococcygeus muscles, although the posteriorly situated coccygeus muscles are sometimes included in this group. Recent evidence suggests that the puborectalis sling, which functions to angulate the anorectal junction anteriorly, is actually an integral part of both the levator ani and external anal sphincter complexes. The levator ani is innervated from branches of the fourth sacral nerves on its pelvic surface and by the perineal branch of the pudendal nerve on its underside. The puborectalis receives additional innervation from below through the inferior rectal nerves (Figs. 1.1 and 1.2).

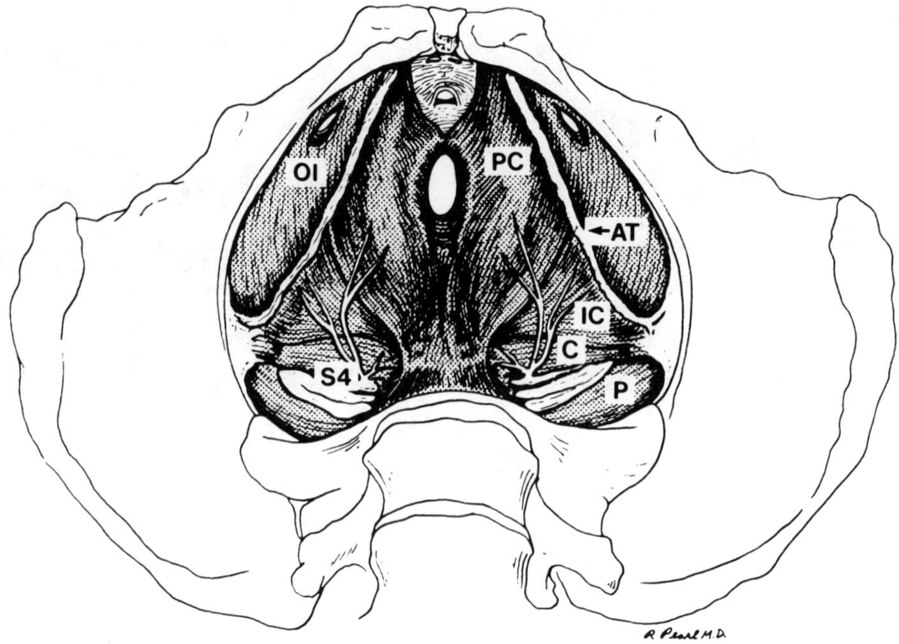

FIGURE 1.1 View of the pelvic floor from above. *OI* = obturator internus muscle; *PC* = pubococcygeus muscle; *AT* = arcus tendineus; *IC* = iliococcygeus muscle; *C* = coccygeus muscle; *P* = piriformis muscle; S4 = branches of the fourth sacral nerve to the coccygeus, iliococcygeus, and pubococcygeus.

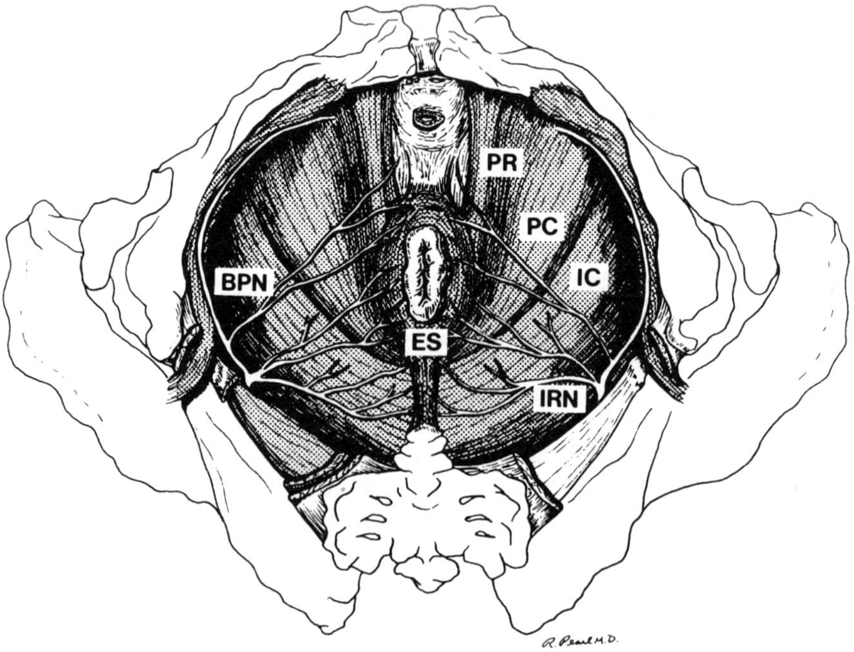

FIGURE 1.2 View of the pelvic floor from below. *PR* = puborectalis muscle; *PC* = pubococcygeus muscle; *IC* = iliococcygeus muscle; *ES* = external anal sphincter muscles; *IRN* = inferior rectal nerve; *BPN* = branches of the perineal nerve.

The pubococcygeus originates from the posterior inferior aspect of the pubis and the inner anterior surface of the obturator fascia, including a portion of the arcus tendineus of the levator ani. Its anterior fibers insert medially into the central tendon of the perineum (hiatal ligament), where they fuse with the musculature of the prostate, vagina, and perineal body to form the levator prostatae, pubovaginalis, and pubourethralis muscles. Some of these intermediate fibers also travel caudally along the intersphincteric plane and contribute to the conjoined longitudinal coat of the anal canal. The muscular fibers of the pubococcygeus merge posteriorly into the broad fibrous band that inserts into the anococcygeal ligament, anterior sacrococcygeal ligament, and coccyx.

The iliococcygeus arises from the arcus tendineus of the fascia of the internal obturator muscle posterior and caudal to the origin of the pubococcygeus. The fibers run posteromedially, where they merge and insert into the anococcygeal ligament and the last two segments of the sacrum.

The puborectalis is the most caudal and controversial component of the levator ani complex. It arises from the posterior aspects of the body of the pubis, the inferior pubic ramus, the superior fascia of the urogenital diaphragm, and the adjacent obturator internus fascia and loops around the rectum posteriorly to form a strong U-shaped sling. Medial fibers of the puborectalis fan out and insert into the central tendon of the perineum. Here they intermingle with fibers from the pubococcygeus and contribute to the conjoined longitudinal muscle of the anal canal. The puborectalis sling, together with the upper borders of the internal and external sphincters, form the anorectal ring, which delineates the anal canal from the rectum.

RECTUM AND ANAL CANAL

The rectum begins at the level of the third sacral vertebra and in general follows along the curvature of the sacrum and coccyx for its entire length of 12 to 15 cm. In addition, it has three lateral curves; the upper and lower ones are convex to the right, the middle one convex to the left. The inner aspects of these three transverse infoldings correspond to the rectal valves of Houston. At the rectosigmoid junction, the fibers of the taenia spread out to form the longitudinal muscle layer of the rectum, which surrounds the inner circular muscle layer. The outer muscle coat is slightly thicker on the anterior and posterior rectal walls than on its lateral surfaces, contributing to the formation of three lateral curves.

The upper third of the rectum is covered by the peritoneum on its anterior and lateral surfaces. The middle third is covered on its anterior surface only, and the lower third is entirely below the peritoneal reflection. The middle valve of Houston is approximately at the level of the anterior peritoneal reflection.

The posterior wall of the rectum is covered with a thick layer of pelvic fascia (fascia propria). A strong sheet of fascia (Waldeyer's or rectosacral fascia) arises from the fourth sacral segment, tracks forward and downward, and attaches to the fascia propria on the posterior surface of the rectal wall at the anorectal junction. The lower portion of the rectum is supported on each side by reflections of endopelvic fascia known as the lateral stalks of the rectum. The anterior extraperitoneal surface of the rectum is covered by Denonvilliers' visceral pelvic fascia which extends to the urogenital diaphragm running between the rectum and prostate or vagina.

As the rectum passes through the pelvic diaphragm at the level of the anorectal ring, it changes its name, shape, and direction. The anal canal begins at this point and extends for approximately 4 cm to the anal verge (surgical anal canal) Fig. 1.3). The circular lumen of the rectum flattens into an anteroposterior slit because of its attachment to the perineal body and coccyx along with the medial pressure exerted by the ischiorectal fat pads. The puborectalis sling in its normal contracted state angulates the anorectal junction forward to create an 80° bend, the perineal flexure, which assists the external sphincter mechanism in maintaining fecal continence.

The internal sphincter is a continuation of the involuntary layer of circular smooth muscle of the rectum that begins at the level of the anorectal ring. As it proceeds distally, it becomes appreciably thicker, and its rounded lower margin can usually be palpated about 1 to 2 cm below the dentate line. The internal sphincter, like the puborectalis, is tonically contracted "at rest."

The conjoined longitudinal muscle coat that surrounds the internal sphincter arises from medial fibers of the pubococcygeus and puborectalis. These striated voluntary fibers course along the intersphincteric plane, fan out through the subcutaneous portion of the external sphincter, and attach to the anoderm and perianal skin, constituting the corrugator cutis ani muscle.

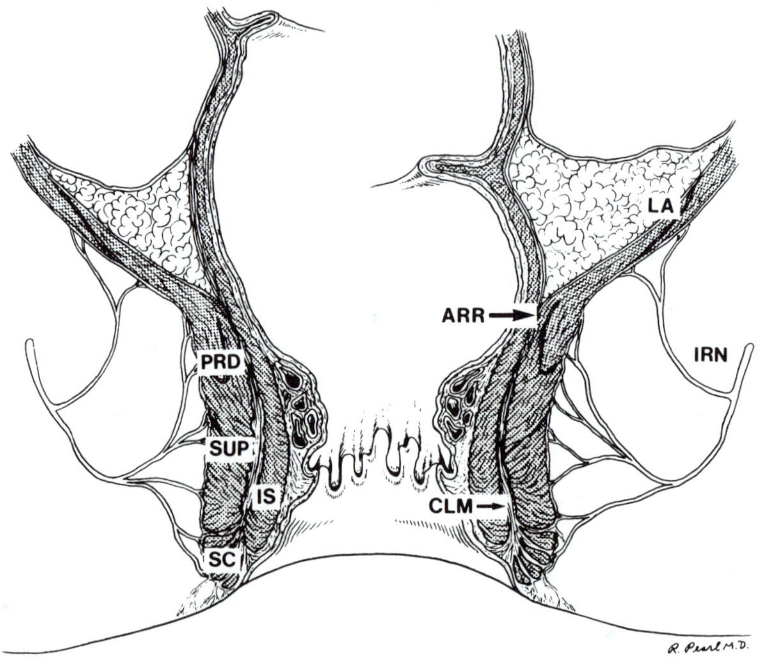

FIGURE 1.3 Coronal section of the anal canal and lower rectum. *LA* = levator ani muscles; *ARR* = level of anorectal ring; *SUP* = superficial external sphincter; *PRD* = puborectalis/deep external sphincter complex; *SC* = subcutaneous external sphincter; *CLM* = conjoined longitudinal muscle; *IRN* = inferior rectal nerve.

Several versions of the musculature of the external sphincter have been proposed, ranging from the single continuous muscle sheet model of Goligher to the three distinct loop theory of Shafik. The inconsistencies of these various descriptions are most likely based on differences in age, sex, and individual variation among the subjects, as well as on differences in points of orientation among investigators (anatomists, physiologists, clinical surgeons). For example, a clinical surgeon repairing a sphincter injury with an overlapping sphincteroplasty generally does not appreciate several subdivisions of the external sphincter. In addition, the external sphincter complex acts as a single functional unit, as demonstrated by electromyography.

Perhaps all that can be stated definitively with respect to structure is that the external anal sphincter is an elliptical cylinder of striated muscle that surrounds the anal canal, and at least the large central portion (superficial component) is firmly tethered to the coccyx, forming the anococcygeal ligament.

Of particular interest is the historical configuration of the fibers of the external sphincter. These consist of two different types of striated muscle, red and white, which function independently, even though they are fully integrated with each other. The red muscle fibers, although voluntary in appearance, behave as involuntary smooth muscle by maintaining a state of tonic contraction in much the same manner as the internal sphincter. The white muscle mass is capable of powerful contractions far exceeding the baseline level of the red fibers. However, these white fibers can only maintain this maximal level of contraction for a short time before they become fatigued.

The configuration of the anal sphincter complex can be clearly depicted in vivo by magnetic resonance imaging (MRI) (Fig. 1.4). However, measurement of the thickness of the internal and external sphincters is more accurately assessed by anal canal endosonography.

The model of the external sphincter mechanism illustrated is a composite of many versions, incorporating features that at least theoretically seem reasonable (Fig. 1.5). In this description, the puborectalis is presented as being intimately related to both the deep external sphincter and the levator ani.

The mucosa of the upper portion of the anal canal is lined primarily by columnar epithelium. The lower portion or anatomical anal canal extends from the dentate line to the anal verge and is lined with anoderm, a thin layer of stratified squamous epithelium that lacks sweat glands and hair follicles. Interspersed between the mucosa of the proximal anal canal and the serrated margin of the dentate line is a narrow indistinct band of cuboidal epithelium known as the transitional zone, which represents the embryological remnants of the (cloacal) membrane.

Several longitudinal mucosal folds, the columns of Morgagni, arise in the proximal anal canal and terminate at the dentate line, where they surround the anal crypts. The majority of the branched tubular anal glands that originate from the depths of these crypts are located in the posterior quadrant of the anal canal. In addition, the normally pink mucosa of the upper anal canal appears purple where it overlies the three vascular anal cushions often referred to as the internal hemorrhoids.

The mucosa proximal to the dentate line lacks somatic innervation. In contrast, the anoderm is richly endowed with cutaneous sensory nerve endings.

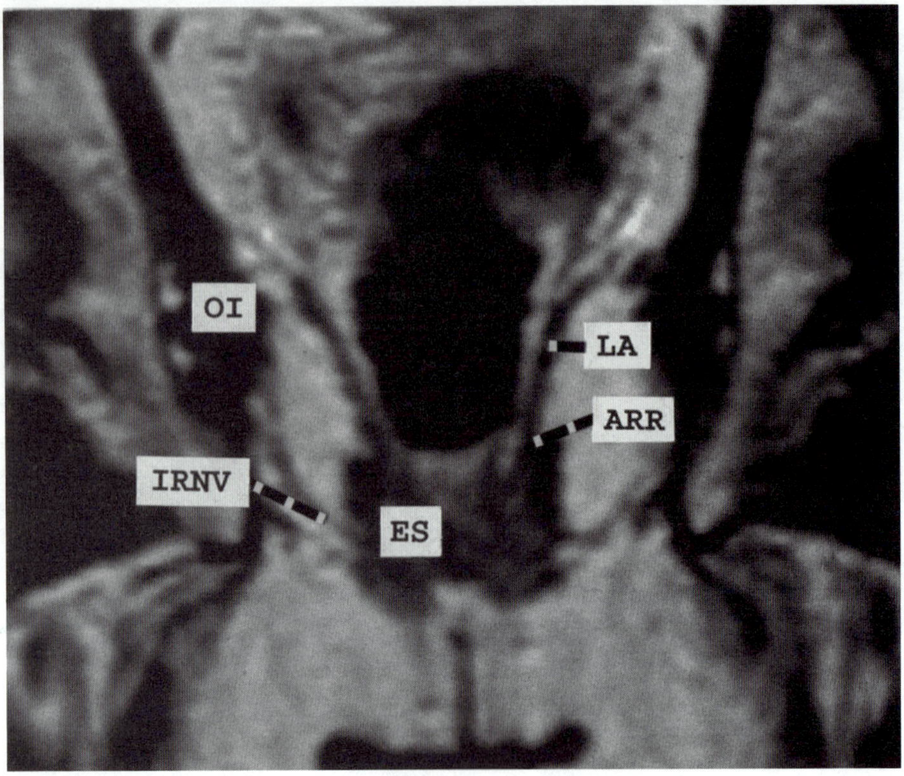

FIGURE 1.4 Magnetic Resonance Image *(MRI)* of the pelvis in the coronal plane highlighting the anal spinchter complex. *OI* = obturator internus; *LA* = levator ani; *ARR* = anorectal ring; *ES* = external sphincter; *IRNV* = inferior rectal nerve and vessels.

The blood supply to the rectum and anal canal originates at three levels (Fig. 1.6). The superior rectal artery, the principal blood supply to the upper and middle portion of the rectum, begins as the terminal branch of the inferior mesenteric artery, where it crosses over the left common iliac vessels. As it descends within the sigmoid mesocolon, it bifurcates at the level of the third sacral vertebra into right and left branches that course along and within either side of the rectal wall. Each vessel divides further so that an average of five small mucosal arteries terminate at the level of the anal valves. There appears to be a paucity of anastomoses on the anterior and posterior surfaces of the rectum between the two collateral branches of the superior rectal artery.

The middle rectal arteries usually arise from the internal iliac arteries, travel along the anterolateral surface of the lower rectum, traversing Denonvilliers' fascia, and enter the rectal wall at the level of the anorectal ring. Although the middle rectal arteries do not run within the lateral stalks, accessory branches may occasionally be found coursing through these ligaments.

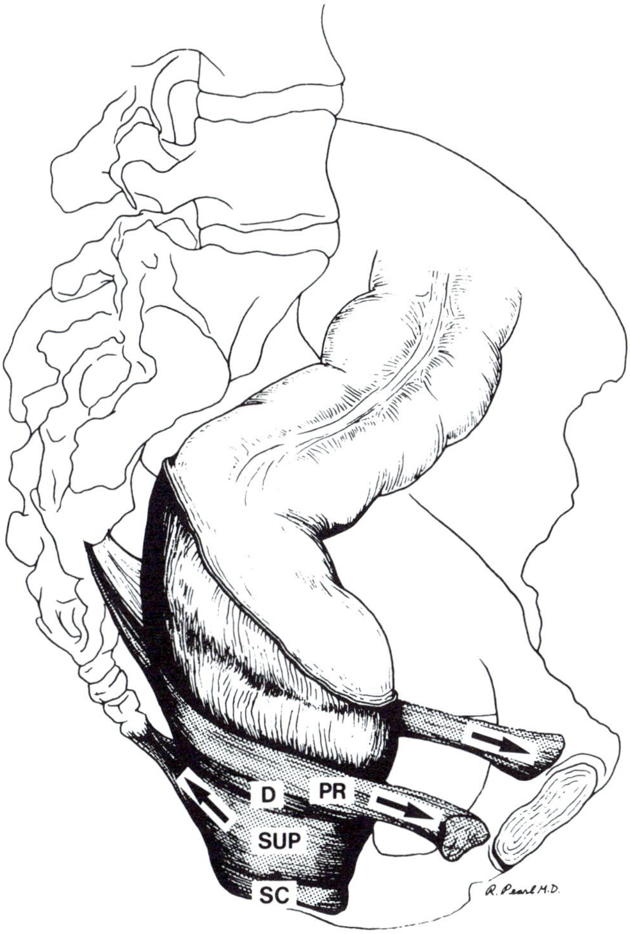

FIGURE 1.5 Model of the external sphincter/puborectalis complex. *PR* = puborectalis sling; *D* = deep external sphincter; *SUP* = superficial external sphincter; *SC* = subcutaneous external sphincter. *Arrows* indicate direction of muscle contraction.

The inferior rectal arteries enter the posterolateral aspects of the ischiorectal fossae as offshoots of the internal pudendal arteries, which run in Alcock's canals. Each of these arteries divides further into two to four vessels that supply the external and internal sphincter, as well as the lining of the anal canal.

Although the degree of confluence between the vessels supplying the rectum and anal canal is controversial, it appears that all three vascular systems are interconnected by a rich intramural plexus. The contribution of the middle sacral artery to this network is at best small and variable.

The venous drainage of the rectum and anal canal parallels the arterial supply. Therefore, blood from the rectum and upper part of the anal canal returns through the superior rectal vein into the portal system, whereas the middle and inferior rectal veins empty into the caval circulation. The submucosal veins of the distal

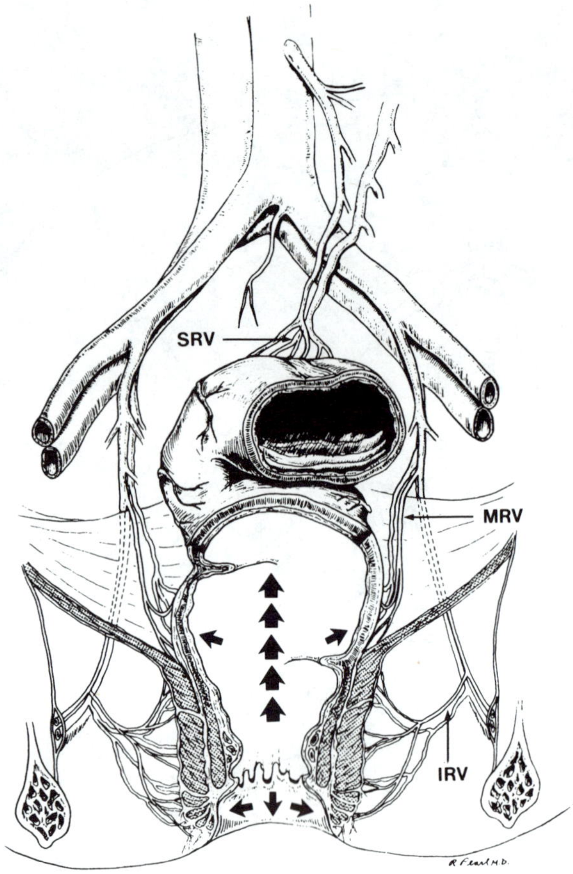

FIGURE 1.6 Blood supply and venous drainage of the rectum and anus. *SRV* = superior rectal vessels; *MRV* = middle rectal vessels; *IRV* = inferior rectal vessels. *Arrows* indicate direction of lymphatic drainage.

anal canal do not have a special connection with the portal circulation. Contrary to earlier beliefs, there is no significant increase in the incidence of symptomatic hemorrhoids in patients with portal hypertension.

The lymphatic system of rectum and anal canal follows the course of the regional blood supply. Lymphatic drainage from the anal canal proximal to the dentate line courses cephalad along the superior rectal vessels and laterally by way of the middle rectal lymphatics to the internal iliac nodes. Lymph from the anal canal below the dentate line usually drains to the inguinal lymph nodes.

The rectum, upper portion of the anal canal, bladder, and genitals are innervated by fibers of the autonomic nervous system. The external sphincter and anoderm are supplied by somatic nerves.

The sympathetic nerves to these pelvic structures originate from the lower thoracic and upper lumbar spinal segments as preganglionic sympathetic fibers that synapse with postganglionic fibers in the preaortic plexus and lumbar sympathetic chains. They then course the pelvis adjacent to the iliac vessels, ureters, and lateral pelvic walls (Fig. 1.7). The preaortic plexus is adherent to the anterior wall

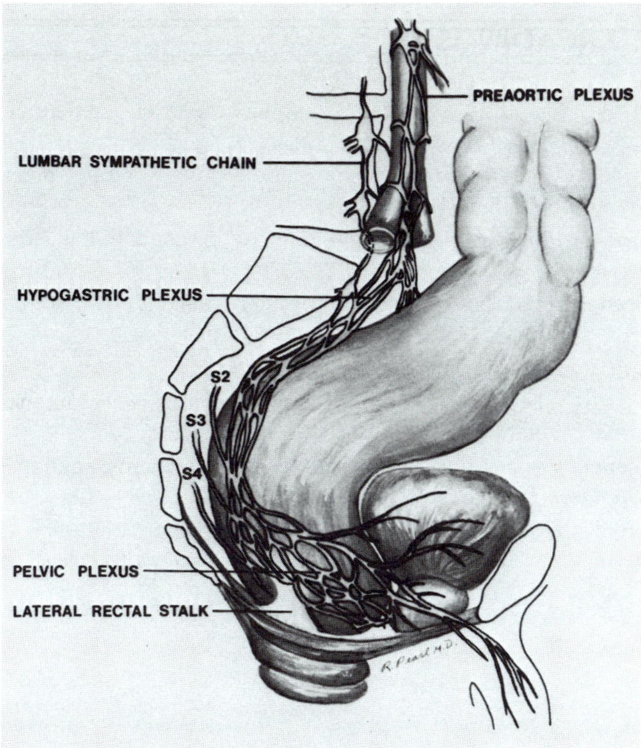

FIGURE 1.7 Lateral view of the rectum and adjacent pelvic structures. Note the proximity of the pelvic plexus to the lower third of the rectum. Pearl RK, et al: Surgical anatomy of the pelvic autonomic nerves, a practical approach. *Am Surg* 52:236–237, 1986.

of the aorta and the common iliac arteries. The lumbar sympathetic chains pass underneath the common iliac vessels and join the fibers from the preaortic plexus to form the left and right hypogastric plexuses just distal to the bifurcation of the aorta. These plexuses are covered by pelvic peritoneum and are generally adherent to the posterolateral pelvic walls.

Preganglionic parasympathetic nerves that arise from the second, third, and fourth sacral segments (nervi erigentes) descend into the pelvis and intermingle with the sympathetic fibers from the hypogastric nerves to form the pelvic plexuses. The pelvic plexuses are at the level of the lower third of the rectum just above the levator ani muscles and are situated well lateral to the pararectal reflections of the endopelvic fascia known as the lateral stalks of the rectum. This dense reticulum of sympathetic and parasympathetic nerves continues anteriolaterally around the bladder and into the prostate and penis.

Sensation to the perianal region and anal canal distal to the dentate line is conveyed by afferent fibers of the inferior rectal nerves. The mucosa of the rectum and proximal anal canal lacks somatic sensory innervation so that mucosal injury caused by cauterization, polypectomy, or rubber band ligation is not perceived as painful. The dull, aching sensation sometimes experienced in this region during transanal procedures is probably mediated via the pelvic parasympathetic nerves.

SUGGESTED READINGS

Boxall TA, Smart PJG, Griffiths JD: The blood supply of the distal segment of the rectum in anterior resection. *Br J Surg* 50:399–404, 1962.

Dalley AF: The riddle of the sphincters, the morphophysiology of the anorectal mechanism reviewed. *Am Surg* 53:298–306, 1987.

Goligher J: *Surgery of the Anus, Rectum, and Colon,* ed 5. London, Bailliere-Tindall, 1984, p 10.

Nivatvongs S, Stern HS, Fryd DS: The length of the anal canal. *Dis Colon Rectum* 24:600–601, 1981.

Oh C, Kark AE: Anatomy of the external anal sphincter. *Br J Surg* 59:717–723, 1972.

Pearl RK, Monsen H, Abcarian H: Surgical anatomy of the pelvic autonomic nerves, a practical approach. *Am Surg* 52:236–237, 1986.

Shafik A: A concept of the anatomy of the anal sphincter mechanism and the physiology of defecation. *Dis Colon Rectum* 30:970–982, 1987.

Wood BA: Anatomy of the anal sphincters and pelvic floor. In Henry MM, Swash M: *Coloproctology and the Pelvic Floor, Pathophysiology and Management.* London, Butterworths, 1985, pp 3–21.

CHAPTER 2

Clinical Examination

Gregory C. Oliver

An accurate history and a careful physical examination will enable a skilled clinician to correctly diagnose the vast majority of anorectal conditions. Until laboratory measures were applied to the study of the lower intestinal tract over the last three decades, these were the clinician's only guideposts to successful treatment. Whenever new technology becomes available, its usefulness must be assessed. The initial skepticism with which anorectal laboratory assessment was greeted has given way to wider applications and futuristic technology. The danger exists that technological advances will obscure the reasons for their initial applications. We have seen physicians refuse to assess a traumatized patient because the CAT scan had not yet been performed. If we are to serve the needs of our patients and determine the proper role of these new technologies in clarifying complex pelvic interrelationships, we must continue to finely hone our most basic of technical skills, the history and physical exam.

HISTORY

This discussion will be limited to aspects of the history that are pertinent to diseases of the hindgut and pelvic floor.

Pain is the complaint to which most patients respond promptly. The *timing of its occurrence* in relation to bowel function and activity help to define its etiology. Does it occur independent of bowel movements, prior to or subsequent to movements? The *character* can also define this complaint. For example, is it sharp or lancinating after movements (as with a fissure) or is it deep, aching and constant as in an abscess? In levator syndrome, pain is aching, deep, but episodic and self-limited. *Duration* of the complaint as well as *location* of the pain will cue the examiner to look for appropriate causes. Experienced clinicians readily note that pain in the anal and perineal area is principally due to (1) infection; (2) fissure; (3) prolapse; (4) inflammation; (5) muscular spasm; and (6) tumor invasion.

Bleeding is another complaint that usually brings patients to a physician without significant delay. Its *color* (bright red or darkened), *duration* (hours, days, weeks),

TABLE 2.1 ETIOLOGICAL FACTORS WHEN ASSESSING ANAL INCONTINENCE

1. Previous anal surgery
   a. Procedures on sphincter muscles
   b. Anal canal surgery, i.e., hemorrhoidectomy
   c. Distal rectal anastomosis
2. Obstetrical injury
   a. Iatrogenic, i.e., episiotomy with inadequate repair
   b. Trauma, i.e., unrecognized tears
3. Aging
   a. Nerve degeneration
   b. Collapse of pelvic support structures, including "cele" and frank prolapse
4. Anorectal trauma
5. Radiation-induced nerve/muscle injury
6. Neurological disorders—central or peripheral
7. Congenital abnormalities
8. Dietary abnormalities
9. Anorectal Crohn's disease
10. Enterocutaneous fistuli to perianal region

and *relationship to bowel movements* allow one to focus the exam. The association of systemic signs with bleeding per anus (tachycardia, hypotension) suggests rapidity of blood loss and volume of loss. The passage of dark blood per rectum is rarely due to hindgut disease.

Discharge per anus suggests distal bowel or pelvic floor disease. Discharge unrelated to bowel movements may suggest some degree of incontinence or leakage of bowel contents that bypasses the sphincter mechanism. Purulent discharge may be secondary to abscess, fistula, or infectious proctitis. Bloody discharge suggests an inflammatory or traumatic component. Evaluation of the perianal skin, anorectal ring, and distal bowel become mandatory.

Continence (Table 2.1) complaints focus the examiner's attention on the sphincter mechanism as well as on processes in the bowel that contribute to abnormal bowel consistency. A history of trauma (i.e., childbirth or previous surgery) will focus attention on muscular defects. Explosive loose movements with frequency and urgency may be related to inflammatory diseases of the bowel. Age is a factor that may relate to incontinence with the sphincter mechanism weakening with advancing years. Laboratory methods to evaluate this complaint, including electromyography (EMG), defecography, manometry, and intra-anal ultrasound are discussed later in this manual.

Irregularity (Table 2.2) of bowel function suggests that an obstructive lesion be ruled out. Intermittent diarrhea and constipation suggest irritable bowel syndrome. Bouts of diarrhea suggest a rapid bowel transit secondary to parasites, infectious agents, small bowel absorption disease, or colonic inflammatory disease.

TABLE 2.2 ETIOLOGICAL FACTORS FOR CONSIDERATION IN CONSTIPATION

Deficient diet
1. Inadequate indigestion fiber
2. Inadequate fluid intake

Poor bowel habits
1. Environmentally induced, i.e., confinement
2. Socially induced

Drugs
1. Laxative abuse
2. Side effects of medications
3. Over-the-counter antimotility drugs

Structural abnormalities of the large bowel/anus
1. Anal disease
2. Obstructing lesion—benign or malignant
3. Rectocele or enterocele
4. Pelvic floor dysfunction
5. Term pregnancy—compressive
6. Congenital or postoperative adhesions

Motility disorders
1. Slow transit syndromes
2. Diverticular disease
3. Irritable bowel syndrome
4. Idiopathic pseudoobstruction

Psychiatric disorders
1. Depression
2. Mental retardation
3. Psychosis
4. Anorexia nervosa

Iatrogenic
1. Side effects of prescription drugs, i.e., iron, narcotics, antidepressants, anticholinergics, some antacids
2. Patient immobilization, i.e., major fractures, significant illness

Neurological
1. Congenital Hirschsprung's disease. or acquired aganglionosis Chagas' disease.
2. Denervation injury—peripheral
3. Spinal cord injury
4. Cerebral injury

Endocrine—uncontrolled
1. Diabetes—uncontrolled
2. Hypothyroidism
3. Hypercalcemia, hypokalemia, hypomagnesemia
4. Hypopituitarism

Perianal swelling focuses the clinician on two major causes: (1) neoplasm and (2) abscess. The presence of pain suggests the latter unless nerve root invasion is present. Large-bore needle aspiration will provide the correct diagnosis.

Protrusion of tissue transanally suggests rectal prolapse, Grade 3 or 4 hemorrhoids, hypertrophic anal papillae, or prolapsing rectal/colonic polyps. Straining at stools to demonstrate the protrusion while in the physician's office will generally suggest the correct diagnosis.

Pruritus ani is a complaint that is often difficult to clearly delineate. Soilage of the perianal area is frequently associated with pruritus, and it is compounded by liquid stools or compromised sphincter function. Diet, oral or topical medicaments, soaps, and scents have been implicated as contributing factors. Correctable abnormalities must also be searched for, such as fissures, fistulas, prolapsing hemorrhoids, rectal prolapse, and inflammatory bowel disease. Diseases of the perianal skin such as psoriasis or cancer should be suspected.

Exposure to risk factors must be defined. Anal sexual practices may result in sphincter injury or infection. Travel to foreign lands prompts concern for infectious etiologies of bowel complaints.

Associated medical conditions should be sought to explain bowel complaints. Uncontrolled diabetics may experience constipation and hard stools secondary to dysmotility patterns and osmotic diuresis and dehydration. Low-flow cardiac conditions may precipitate ischemic conditions or pseudoobstructions of the colon. A history of pelvic irradiation for urological or gynecological malignancy may explain tenesmus, sphincter dysfunction, blood loss per anus and diarrhea. In the geriatric or disabled patient, immobility contributes to bowel complaints.

An accurate *medication history* is essential in evaluating constipation, diarrhea, and bleeding. While a complete list is beyond the scope of this section, frequent problems are encountered with patients taking: (1) colchicine (diarrhea); (2) antacids (constipation or diarrhea); (3) narcotics (constipation); (4) anticoagulants (aspirin, heparin, coumadin, and nonsteroidal antiinflammatory agents) as well as (5) over-the-counter preparations such as Pepto Bismol. History alone may define complaints related to bowel changes and drug ingestion.

Family history suggests diagnoses such as inherited polyposis syndrome, familial cancer syndrome,Crohn's disease, and ulcerative colitis. *Previous pelvic or anorectal surgery* may suggest etiologies of incontinence, constipation, diarrhea, or soilage. *Bleeding disorders* such as hereditary telangiectasia, von Willebrand's disease, and factor VIII deficiency should be inquired for.

PHYSICAL EXAM

Inspection of the anus and perineum can provide insights into disorders of this region. The examiner must look for dynamic abnormalities as well as static ones; having the patient bear down, strain, or squeeze may suggest prolapse, muscular disorder, neurological deficit, and regional associated pathology such as cystocele or rectocele. The shape and location of the anus should be noted. Elongation and displacement anteriorly suggest posterior muscular disruption or anterior muscular injury. Perianal wetness of fecal soilage reflect some degree of sphincter incontinence. Scars relate to the history of trauma, surgery, or infection. Swollen or protruding tissues should be noted to direct the endoscopic elements of the physical exam. Skin lesions may suggest deeper infection, or neoplastic conditions.

Palpation in the perianal area should include the vaginal introitus, perineal body, ischiorectal fossa, and the postanal space. Areas of induration, fluctuance, or crepitance may be discerned. Muscular defects in the anorectal ring may be noted by bidigitally palpating the external sphincter and the aggregate sphincter mechanism. Mucosal and extramucosal masses should be noted for definitive diagnostic evaluation later. The potential perirectal spaces should be palpated to assess for abscess or tumors of mesodermal origin. The adequacy of sphincter mass and function can be reasonably assessed by palpation of the sphincter mechanism while the patient is asked to strain and squeeze.

Neurological assessment of muscle function and local reflux mechanism will be discussed later, under sections on EMG, manometry, and defecography. In the initial exam, however, clues to denervation problems can be discerned by techniques to elicit the "anal wink." Scratching the anal skin margin with a sharp object on each side should result in a local contraction. Innervation of the striated muscular components of the sphincter mechanism and pelvic floor can be assessed by palpation during commands to squeeze, tighten, or strain. Resting anal canal tone reflects the function of the internal sphincter, which is normally contracted.

Endoscopic assessment is here confined to anoscopy and rigid proctosigmoidoscopy. Anoscropy permits assessment of the tissues of the anal canal and distal rectum. Hemorrhoidal prolapse and fissure disease are easily demonstrated. Proctoscopy demonstrates rectal mucosal disease, such as neoplasm, inflammation, infection, and bleeding. In addition, rigid examination may demonstrate the solitary rectal ulcer associated with internal or complete rectal prolapse. In the prolapse situation, the mucosa bulges and follows the scope out on its withdrawal.

Last, stool should be checked for the presence of occult blood. This may be done on digital examination or endocopy. The presence of occult blood in stools obtained by digital rectal examination may indicate a distal rectal source if heme-negative stools are obtained endoscopically from the more proximal rectum. In any event, the presence of blood in the stool necessitates further diagnostic assessment.

SUGGESTED READINGS

Corman ML: Evaluation and diagnostic techniques. In Corman ML: *Colon and Rectal Surgery*. Philadelphia, Lippincott, 1984.

Goldberg SM, Gordon PH, Nivatvongs S: Diagnosis of anorectal disease. In Goldberg SM, Gordon PH, Nivatvongs S: *Essentials of Anorectal Surgery*. Philadelphia, Lippincott, 1980.

Todd IP: Clinical evaluation of the pelvic floor. In Henry NM, Swash M: *Coloproctology and the Pelvic Floor*. London, Butterworth, 1985.

CHAPTER 3

Transit Time

Amanda M. Metcalf

GENERAL CONSIDERATIONS

A technique for measuring total and segmental colonic transit time is a useful tool in the evaluation of patients with complaints of severe constipation. Patient reports of stool frequency are usually inaccurate, and even when accurate, do not correlate well with either total or segmental colonic transit time. Furthermore, it has become apparent that patients with similar complaints may have abnormalities of transit that are localized to different segments of the colon. While the efficacy of various treatments of colonic motility disorders remains relatively unproven, objective measurements of total and segmental colonic transit provide a portion of the information necessary to pursue a logical form of treatment and monitor outcome.

INDICATIONS

1. To measure total and segmental colonic transit times in patients with clinical complaints of constipation.
2. To evaluate the results of surgical or medical therapy of colonic motility disorders.

CONTRAINDICATIONS

1. Pregnancy (radiation may be harmful to the fetus).
2. Bowel obstruction (obstruction invalidates results).

PATIENT EVALUATION AND PREPARATION

Patients with complaints of constipation or diarrhea should undergo a general history and physical examination to rule out obvious etiologies of their complaints. Most patients will require radiographic or endoscopic evaluation of the gastrointestinal tract. Additional tests such as anorectal manometry, balloon and saline defecation, external sphincter EMGs, and defecography will usually be required. Evaluation of the remainder of the gastrointestinal tract for motility disorders is reasonable in patients who prove to have significant colonic transit delay.

Preparation

Radiopaque Markers

Radiopaque markers can be obtained commercially or can be prepared. The advantage of preparing markers, other than decreased expense, is that multiple distinguishable shapes can be fashioned that allow one to gauge factors such as the variability in day-to-day transit and patient compliance.

Markers can be cut in circular (2 mm × 6 mm) or semicylindrical shapes (6 mm × 6 mm) from 16F radiopaque Levine tubes (Tomac 19947-9616 K10R, American Hospital Supply, Evanston, IL), or cylindrical shapes (1 mm × 6 mm) can be cut from radiopaque pediatric tubing. If neither of these are readily available, alternate radiopaque markers can be constructed from Salem sump tubes, although the degree of radiopacity will need to be checked. Markers of the size described can be placed in 00 gelatin capsules. Depending on the study technique used, either 20 or 60 radiopaque markers will be needed.

Commercially prepared markers (sitzmarks™) can be obtained from Lafayette Pharmaceuticals, Forth Worth, TX.

Patients

All contrast material from previous studies should be cleared from the colon prior to the onset of the test, and no contrast studies should be scheduled for the duration of the test. Patients should be instructed to consume their usual diet, continue usual activities, and omit the use of laxatives, enemas or other medications known to affect GI motility. Patients should be on supplemental fiber (1 T of psyllium b.i.d.) for the duration of the study.

Study Technique

Single Marker Bolus

CONSTIPATED PATIENTS. Subjects are asked to ingest 20 radiopaque markers at a specific time (usually 8 a.m.). Abdominal x-rays are then taken at 24-hr intervals thereafter until all markers are passed. Most normal subjects will have passed all markers within 4 to 5 days following ingestion, whereas patients with severe constipation may not have passed all the markers by 10 days after the study onset.

Abdominal x-rays should include the diaphragms and the pubis to ensure that all markers in the colon are visualized.

Multiple Marker Bolus Technique

CONSTIPATED PATIENTS. Patients are asked to ingest 20 markers each day at a specific time for 3 sequential days. An abdominal x-ray should be obtained on the fourth study day and then at 3-day intervals (i.e., 7, 10, 13 days after study onset) until all markers are passed.

INTERPRETATION OF ABDOMINAL FILMS

The localization of markers within the various segments of the colon relies on the identification of bony landmarks and gaseous outlines. Previously obtained barium enemas can also be helpful in determining location. In the absence of clear outlines of the bowel, markers located to the right of the vertebral spinous processes above a line from the fifth lumbar vertebrae to the pelvic outlet are assigned to the right colon. Markers to the left of the vertebral spinous processes and above an imaginary line from the fifth lumbar vertebrae to the anterior superior iliac crest are assigned to the left colon. Markers inferior to a line from the pelvic brim on the right and the superior iliac crest on the left are judged to be in the rectosigmoid and rectum (Fig. 3.1). If bowel outlines clearly show a pelvic cecum or transverse colon, markers are assigned to be in the anatomical segments based on the gaseous outlines.

CALCULATIONS

All calculations are based on modifications or simplification of the formula described by Arhan et al. for use with a single marker technique.

$$\text{Mean transit} = 1/N \sum_{i=1}^{j} \frac{n_i\,(i+1) - t\,(i-1)}{2}$$

where N = the number of markers given, n = number of markers present on a film taken at time t_i, $t(i + 1) - (i - 1)/2$ = the time interval between successive films, and j = the number of abdominal films taken.

Constipation Studies

If a single bolus technique is used and 20 individual markers are given and films are all taken at 24-hr intervals, the above formula can be simplified to:

$$\text{Mean transit} = 1.2\,(n_1 + n_2 + n_3 \ldots n_j)$$

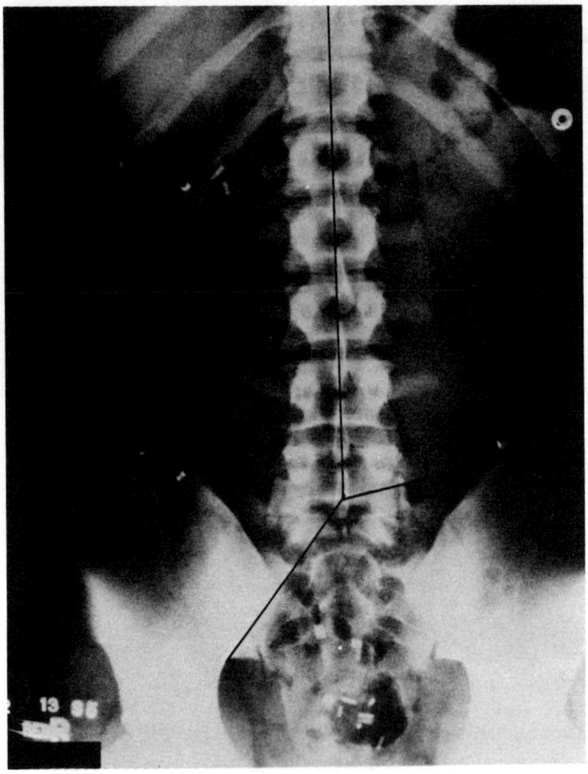

FIGURE 3.1 Segments of the colon as determined by bony landmarks.

where n = the number of markers present on each film, and j = the number of films.

If total colonic transit times are calculated, all markers in the colon are tabulated for each abdominal film and used in the calculations. In calculating segmental transit times, the number of markers in a particular segment of the colon in each film is tabulated and substituted in the formula.

Example:

	Number of Markers Present			
Film	**Right Colon**	**Left Colon**	**Rectosigmoid**	**Colon**
1st	10	6	4	20
2nd	2	4	6	12
3rd	1	2	2	5
4th	0	0	1	1
5th	0	0	0	0
	13	12	13	38

Mean right colon transit = 1.2 × 13 = 15.6 hr
Mean left colon transit = 1.2 × 12 = 14.4 hr
Mean rectosigmoid transit = 1.2 × 13 = 15.6 hr
Mean colonic transit = 1.2 × 38 = 45.6 hr

If a multiple market technique is used, the same formula can be used as long as 20 of each kind of marker is given, and markers are given at 24-hr intervals.

Again, in this situation, the total number of markers in each segment is used in the formula regardless of type.

Example:

	Number of Markers Present			
	Right Colon	Left Colon	Rectosigmoid	Colon
4th day	10	12	12	34
7th day	0	0	1	1
	10	12	13	35

Right colon transit = 1.2 × 10 = 12 hr
Left colon transit = 1.2 × 12 = 14.4 hr
Rectosigmoid = 1.2 × 13 = 15.6 hr
Colon = 1.2 × 35 = 42 hr

INTERPRETATION OF RESULTS

Patients should be asked if their stool patterns and frequency during the study period were representative of their usual habits. If not, the study may need to be repeated.

Other factors need to be considered in the interpretation of results. There can be a moderate variation in transit times from day to day in segments of the colon and, therefore, prolongation of transit in any one segment of the colon can only be considered abnormal if the total colonic transit is also prolonged.

In addition, if markers are still present on the last film taken, then the transit time calculated will be lower than the "real" transit time. This can be a problem, especially in the rectosigmoid colon if transit in the remainder of the colon is extremely prolonged. In this situation additional x-rays are useful in determining whether transit in the rectosigmoid is delayed.

SUGGESTED READINGS

Arhan P, Devroede G, Jehannu B, et al: Segmental colonic transit time. *Dis Colon Rectum* 24: 625–962, 1981.

Metcalf AM, Phillips SF, Zinsmeister AR, et al: Simplified assessment of segmental colonic transic. *Gastroenterology* 92: 40–47, 1987.

CHAPTER 4

Balloon Expulsion

James W. Fleshman

The diagnosis of pelvic floor outlet obstruction is a relatively recent addition to the problems affecting the pelvic floor. The usual patient is a woman with a long history of constipation or extreme straining at defecation. The underlying cause is a failure of the external sphincter puborectalis to relax or even a paradoxical contraction during efforts to empty the rectum. This results in occlusion of the pelvic floor outlet. The persistent bulge of the puborectalis muscle into the posterior aspect of the rectal vault gives a characteristic shadow on the lateral view of the rectum during a defecating barium enema. The posterior bulge with anterior directed motion can be detected during digital rectal exam when the patient is instructed to attempt to expel the examining finger. However, both of these methods are not diagnostic/pathognomonic for the condition. A simple test utilizing balloon expulsion can document the condition and identify individuals who may benefit from biofeedback to retrain the pelvic floor to relax. The patient is also retaught the feeling of rectal distension and the relaxation of the sphincter since this is often forgotten.

EQUIPMENT

A soft latex balloon such as the ones used for determining the presence of the rectoanal inhibitory reflex during anal manometry may be used. The balloon must accommodate 60 cc of water or air. The balloon should be attached to a flexible plastic catheter at least 100 cm long to facilitate retrieval after expulsion. If the catheter has a lumen, the balloon is attached to the end with suture. A stopcock can be used to allow filling and continued inflation of the balloon if necessary. Cidex for balloon and catheter sterilization is essential.

PERSONNEL

The person responsible for performing anal manometry (either a nurse, technician or physician) should be able to explain the procedure to the patient, insert the balloon and fill it with 60 cc of water, assist the patient to the bathroom, retrieve the balloon and sterilize the balloon for the next exam.

SETTING

An exam room with a standard table and an adjoining private bathroom is needed. A standard toilet is adequate.

POSITION

The balloon is inserted with the patient in the left lateral or knee-chest position. The patient evacuates the balloon while sitting comfortably on a toilet in the private bathroom.

METHOD

After completion of the standard anal manometry testing, the balloon-tipped polyvinyl catheter is left in place with the balloon in the rectal vault above the sphincter mechanism. The balloon is then gently inflated with a maximum of 60 cc of water, and the stopcock at the distal end occluded. The patient is questioned regarding first sensation and then feeling of the need to evacuate. The patient is then escorted to the restroom where instructions for expulsion of the balloon are given. The patient is asked to push with abdominal and diaphragm muscles while relaxing the pelvic floor. A maximum of 8 min may be needed to expel the balloon. If the patient complains of pain or the balloon is retained after 8 min of maximal straining, the balloon is deflated and removed, and the exam is terminated.

INTERPRETATION OF RESULTS

Failure to expel the balloon indicates pelvic floor outlet obstruction and nonrelaxing puborectalis muscle.

SUGGESTED READINGS

Fleshman JW, Dreznik Z, Cohen E, et al. Balloon expulsion test facilitates diagnosis of pelvic floor outlet obstruction due to nonrelaxing puborectalis muscle. *Dis Colon Rectum* 35:1019–1025, 1992.

Fleshman JW, Dreznik Z, Meyer K, et al. Outpatient protocol for biofeedback therapy of pelvic floor outlet obstruction. *Dis Colon Rectum* 35:1–7, 1992.

Kodner IJ, Fry RD, Fleshman JW. Rectal prolapse and other pelvic floor abnormalities. *Surg Ann* 24:157–190, 1992.

Kuijpers HC, Bleijenberg G. The spastic pelvic floor syndrome: a cause of constipation. *Dis Colon Rectum* 28:669–672, 1985.

Wexner SD, Cheape JD, Jorge JMN, et al. Prospective assessment of biofeedback for the treatment of paradoxical puborectalis contraction. *Dis Colon Rectum* 35:145–150, 1992.

CHAPTER 5

Methodology and Applications of Water Perfusion Anal Manometry

Alan E. Timmcke

DEFINITION

Anorectal manometry is an objective means of assessing the resistance to spontaneous defecation provided by the anorectal sphincter mechanism and the sensory capabilities of the rectum to provide a feeling of imminent defecation. The information provided by manometry can be useful in determining the causes of anorectal sphincter dysfunction.

INTRODUCTION

Many factors contribute to the ability of the anorectum to retain colonic contents. These include:

1. the tonic and voluntary contraction of the sphincter musculature;
2. the angle between the longitudinal axis of the rectum and that of the anus;
3. the capacity and compliance of the rectum;
4. the impedance to rectal filling provided by the poorly compliant, narrow diameter, high-pressure sigmoid colon;
5. the anterior-to-posterior slit-like nature of the anal opening and the medially directed forces exerted on the anus by surrounding soft tissues;
6. the consistency of the colonic contents presented to the sphincter mechanism.

The ability to limit the passage of stool or flatus to a socially acceptable time and place is by definition a learned behavior. Learned voluntary control is primarily the responsibility of the external anal sphincter and puborectalis muscles. Contraction of these muscles produces a transient increase in anal canal pressure and, by elevating the pelvic floor, a more acute anorectal angle. Both of these effects result in increased resistance to the passage of stool or flatus.

Voluntary efforts are required only when the involuntary sphincter resistance is threatened. Involuntary sphincter resistance, indirectly measured as pressure within the anal canal at rest, is primarily the result of tonic contraction of the smooth muscle internal anal sphincter (IAS). When the rectum is filled, the IAS relaxes; this is the rectosphincteric reflex, sometimes referred to as the "sampling reflex." The amplitude and duration of relaxation are at low volumes directly proportional to the volume filling the rectum. In a normal continent patient, the minimum volume necessary to produce a sensation of rectal fullness also correlates closely with the minimum volume necessary to elicit detectable sphincter relaxation.

It is obvious that reflex receptive relaxation of the internal anal sphincter is antithetical to the maintenance of fecal continence. Continence may be maintained only when a voluntary effort is exerted to counterbalance reflex sphincter relaxation. As the volume within the rectum increases and the amplitude and duration of internal anal sphincter relaxation increase, the capacity for forceful sustained contraction of the striated sphincter muscles may be exceeded, and defecation occurs.

Superimposed on this process is the contribution of the abdominal and diaphragmatic muscles, which control intra-abdominal pressure. Intra-abdominal pressure varies directly with intrarectal pressure. As long as the pressure within the anal canal exceeds that within the rectum, continence is maintained.

Anal manometry provides a means of quantitating these neural and physiological mechanisms contributing to fecal continence. This process of data acquisition and analysis is the bulwark of our advancing scientific understanding.

INDICATIONS

Anal manometry is indicated for the following purposes:

1. To assess the contribution of the neural and muscular components required for fecal continence, in order to determine the most effective treatment for incontinence;
2. To locate and quantify a sphincter defect following injury, whether obstetrical, surgical, or traumatic;
3. To document the level of sphincter function prior to procedures affecting continence or requiring perfect continence;
4. To evaluate chronic constipation, particularly in children and young adults.

EQUIPMENT

Many different catheters and probes have been employed to perform anorectal manometry. Because of this variability of equipment and technique, the data cannot be compared. The system described here was adapted directly from that used to assess esophageal motility and lower esophageal sphincter competence. The equipment used is generally readily available in most large hospitals and clinics (Fig. 5.1).

Catheters (Fig. 5.1A)

These are custom-constructed extruded polyvinyl chloride (PVC) with four channels for measurement (Fig. 5.2). The measurement orifices are concentrically and circumferentially arranged at 90° angles to one another. The catheter without a balloon tip is 3.6 mm in diameter, and the measurement orifices are located 5 cm from the tip. The balloon catheter is 4.8 mm in diameter and has a 150-ml capacity balloon at the tip that is filled via a central catheter lumen. The measurement orifices are located 10 cm from the catheter tip. These catheters cost from $95.00 to $200.00 (Arndorfer, Inc., Greendale, WI).

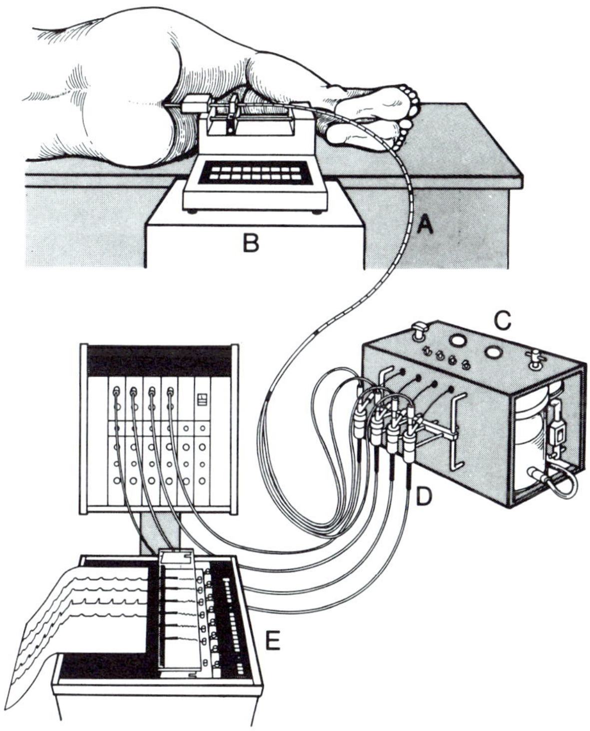

FIGURE 5.1 Anorectal manometry apparatus. **A:** catheter; **B:** withdrawal motor; **C:** perfusion apparatus; **D:** transducers; **E:** multichannel recorder.

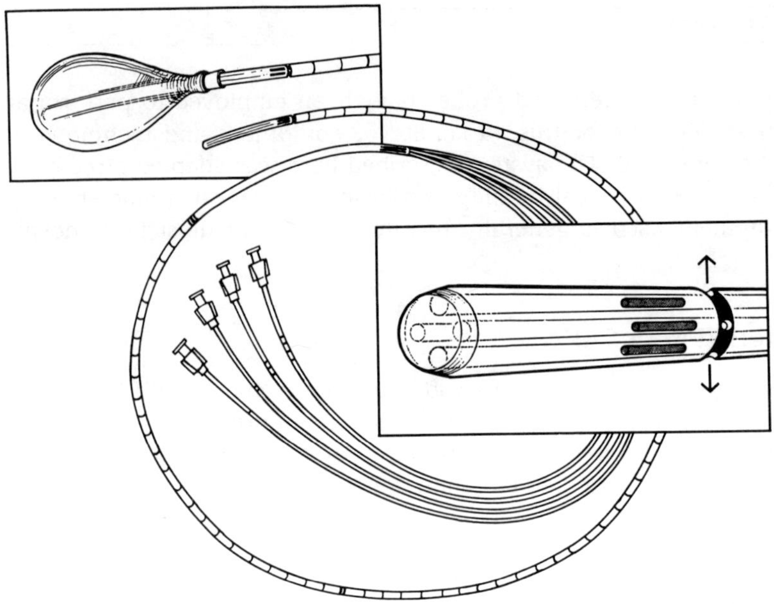

FIGURE 5.2 Four-channel catheters with side viewing measurement orifices.

Withdrawal Motor (Fig. 5.1B)

The withdrawal motor is a Harvard Apparatus model No. 22 syringe infusion pump (Harvard Apparatus, South Natick, MA) with its pulleys reversed during manufacturing to allow for greater speed. In addition, a slotted, hinged plexiglas plate has been mounted to steady the catheter during withdrawal. A clamp has been placed on the pusher block to attach the catheter. The pump is equipped with a RS 232 serial computer interface to enable computer-controlled function. Approximate cost of the withdrawal motor is $1200.

Perfusion Apparatus (Fig. 5.1C)

The perfusion apparatus is a hydraulic capillary infusion system. Water from a reservoir is forced under nitrogen gas pressure through small wire capillary tubes, allowing perfusion of each transducer and catheter channel without interference from the others. The infusion rate can be varied from 0.25 ml/channel/min to 0.5 ml/channel/min. The perfusion apparatus costs approximately $2900 and may be purchased from Arndorfer, Inc.

Transducers (Fig. 5.1D)

Four strain-gauge transducers (Gould Instrument Systems, Inc., Valley View, OH) are connected to the catheter channels. These transducers have a range of from −50 mm Hg to 300 mm Hg and a volume displacement of 0.04 cu mm per 100 mm Hg pressure. They cost approximately $995 each.

Recorder (Fig. 5.1E)

The recorder is a Sensor Medics Corporation model No. R611 rectilinear pen and ink system with a capability to record four, six, or eight channels. Approximate cost, complete with transducer couplers, is $24,250. This particular recorder is currently no longer sold. Less elaborate and less expensive recorders can be obtained such as model R53400 from Gould Instrument Systems, Inc., which records four channels. Complete with signal conditioners, the unit costs approximately $16,500.

TECHNIQUE

Patients are examined in the left lateral decubitus position with hips and knees flexed at 90° Incontinent patients generally require no preparation and, indeed, find it impossible to retain an enema. Constipated patients can be examined several hours after a small prepackaged enema is administered at home.

Profilimetry

A 4-directional anal sphincter profile (Fig. 5.3) is obtained using a slow, constant-speed catheter withdrawal. The 3.6-mm catheter is lubricated lightly with water-soluble gel and inserted through the anus to a point 3 to 6 cm beyond the measurement orifices. A longitudinal marking of the catheter's posterior channel is aligned with the gluteal crease to maintain consistent orientation within the anal canal. After a 60-sec delay the catheter is removed with the withdrawal motor at a speed of 1 mm/sec. By simultaneously recording at a paper speed of 1 mm/sec, a real-time recording of pressures and their distribution within the anal canal is generated. This allows for determination of the length of the anal canal in each of four quadrants. The pressure results are reported as the *maximal resting pressure* obtained during three consecutive pull-throughs. Maximal resting pressure is normally in the range of 40 to 120 mm Hg. The technique or profilimetry has enabled demonstration of asymmetry within the normal anal canal. A short anterior anal sphincter length, particularly in women, highlights the necessity for a more cautious approach to anteriorly located fistulae.

Station Manometry

The remaining examinations are performed with the catheter located at stationary positions within the anal canal. Using either the graduations on the catheters or a small plastic ruler placed on the withdrawal motor adjacent to the pusher block, the catheter is withdrawn in 0.5 to 1 cm increments. After each increment, a 25-sec equilibration period is observed to allow for sphincter stimulation and fatigue.

Voluntary Squeeze

At each of several stations within the sphincter, the patient is asked to voluntarily contract the pelvic floor musculature. It is best to first attempt this maneuver

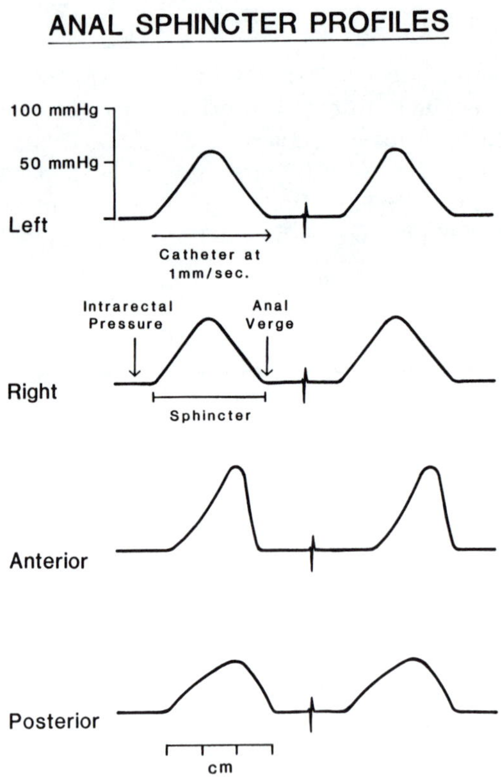

FIGURE 5.3 Representation of repeated anal sphincter profiles.

during the digital examination performed prior to manometry to determine whether the patient indeed understands what has been requested. At each catheter location, three brief squeezes are recorded with a 25-sec delay between squeezes to allow for recovery from fatigue. The catheter is advanced in 0.5 cm increments beginning in the proximal high pressure zone in order to compensate for perineal motion. The results are expressed as the *maximal squeeze pressure,* which should be approximately twice the resting pressure or greater.

Sustained squeezes may be examined, but fatigue is rapid and exponential. It is normally difficult for patients to maintain any increase over resting pressure for longer than 60 sec. In addition, the length of time a given percentage of maximal squeeze can be maintained in normal subjects is not well defined. Therefore, sustained squeeze data are currently of limited clinical usefulness.

Anocutaneous Reflex

With the catheter stationary within the high-pressure area of the sphincter, the perineum is gently stroked or lightly pricked to elicit reflex contraction of the external anal sphincter. Absence of the anocutaneous reflex confirms apparent denervation of the external sphincter suggested by an absent voluntary squeeze. An additional confirmatory maneuver is absence of reflex involuntary contraction when the patient coughs or performs Valsalva's maneuver.

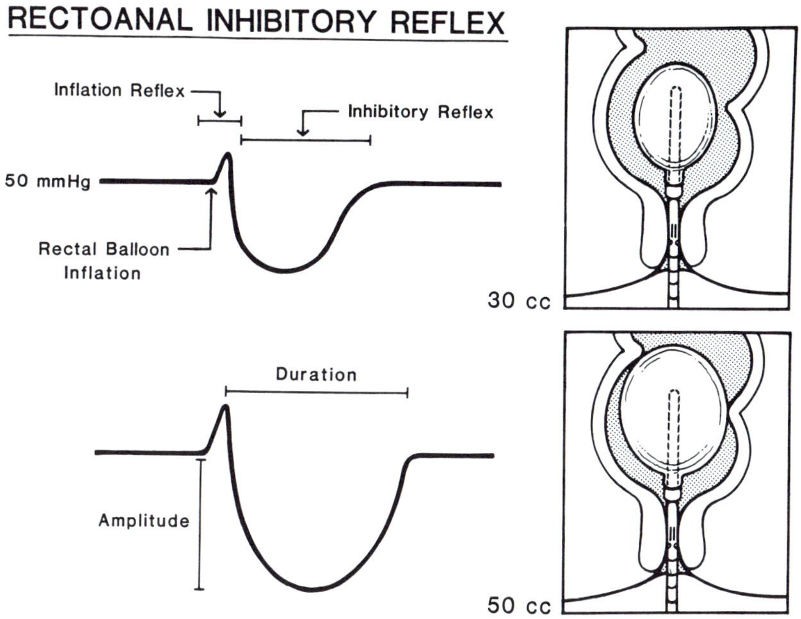

FIGURE 5.4 Rectoanal inhibitory reflex. Note various components and effect of increasing volume.

Rectoanal Inhibitory Reflex

Using a 1 mm/sec pull-through, the balloon-tip catheter is positioned with its measurement orifices within the anal canal. Volumes of air beginning with 60 cc are rapidly inflated in the rectal balloon and removed (inflation time 0.5 to 1 sec). The balloon inflation technique is as described below for determination of the minimum sensory volume. The characteristic normal response consisting of a brief contraction of the external sphincter (inflation reflex) followed by a prolonged relaxation of the internal sphincter (inhibitory reflex) is depicted in Fig. 5.4. The reflex can generally be elicited by inflation volumes of 20 cc or greater but may be absent at lower volumes. In Hirschsprung's disease the reflex is absent.

Minimum Sensory Volume

During the course of testing the rectoanal inhibitory reflex, the sensibility of the rectum can be ascertained. When 60 cc of air is inflated in the balloon catheter the patient is instructed to note the sensation. If no sensation is perceived, the volume is increased in 5-cc increments until balloon inflation is sensed or 150 cc of inflation volume is reached. If 60 cc produces sensation, the volume is decreased to 5 cc. Inflation and deflation are repeated at 25-sec intervals as the volume in the balloon is increased in 5-cc increments. The patient is instructed to respond each time a similar sensation is perceived, no matter how faintly. The smallest volume to which the patient responds is recorded as the minimum sensory volume. One must be careful to record the volume at which the balloon is perceived and not the delayed sensation of anal relaxation.

Maximal Tolerable Volume

A balloon catheter with a 500-cc capacity balloon is inserted in the rectum and gradually inflated with air. The volume at which the patient perceives that additional inflation would be intolerable or at which the balloon is involuntarily expelled is considered the *maximal tolerable volume.* This volume constitutes a rough measure of rectal capacity. Also, by simultaneously determining the pressure within the rectal balloon and subtracting from that the pressure produced by a similar volume when the balloon is not within the rectum, a crude compliance curve is generated. Determination of the maximal tolerable volume is necessary only in those circumstances when decreased rectal volume or compliance is thought to be the cause of incontinence or in those situations when an ileorectostomy is contemplated, as in Crohn's disease. A volume of <150 cc is abnormal.

Table 5.1 indicates the mean and range values for the maximal resting pressure, maximal squeeze pressure, minimum rectal sensory volume, and the minimum volume for reflex relaxation as determined for groups of patients examined in the Ochsner Clinic Anorectal Physiology Laboratory. These values are intended as guidelines, but the considerable overlap in range when the groups are compared should be noted.

CONCLUSION

Anal manometry provides an objective method for determining the intraanal pressure at rest, with various volumes within the rectum and during forceful voluntary contraction. In addition, rectal capacity, compliance, and sensibility can be examined. Thus, many of the factors contributing to fecal continence may be quantitatively evaluated using anal manometry, providing data enabling advancement of our understanding of the physiological and psychological mechanisms of fecal continence.

SUGGESTED READINGS

Dalley AF II: The riddle of the sphincters: the morphophysiology of the anorectal mechanism reviewed. *Am Surg* 53:298–306, 1987.

Duthie HL, Watts JM: Contribution of the external anal sphincter to the pressure zone in the anal canal. *Gut* 6:64–68, 1965.

Frenckner B, Ihre T: Function of the anal sphincters in patients with intussusception of the rectum. *Gut* 17:147–151, 1976.

Gowers WR: The automatic action of the sphincter ani. *Proc R Soc Med* 26:77–84, 1877.

Kerremans R: *Morphological and Physiological Aspects of Anal Continence and Defecation.*Thesis. Arscia, Uitgoven S.A., Brussels, 1969.

TABLE 5.1 MEAN VALUES (RANGE)

Degree of Continence	Number of Patients (F:M)	Resting Pressure (mmHg)	Squeeze Pressure (mmHg)	Rectal Sensory Volume (mL)	Volume for Reflex Relaxation
Complete incontinence	39 (35/4)	51 (20–100)	88 (36–200)	31 (5–120)	18 (10–50)
Partial incontinence	89 (72/17)	62 (18–144)	123 (0–420)	27 (5–33)	20 (5–50)
Seepage and soilage	42 (24/18)	62 (18–169)	178 (0–395)	40 (10–100)	21 (0–60)
Normal (controls)	**35 (19/16)**	**88 (43–164)**	**204 (62–380)**	**19 (5–60)**	**19 (10–40)**
Chronic constipation	41 (30/11)	88 (30–139)	173 (60–390)	43 (10–120)	25 (10–50)

Lane RH: Clinical application of anorectal physiology. *Proc R Soc Med* 68:28–30, 1975.

Parks AG, Porter NH, Hardcastle J: The syndrome of the descending perineum. *Proc R Soc Med* 59:477–482, 1966.

Parks AG, Porter NH, Melzak J: Experimental study of the reflex mechanism controlling the muscles of the pelvic floor. *Dis Colon Rectum* 5:407–414, 1962.

CHAPTER 6

Colon Motility and Anosphincteric Manometric Recordings by Air-Filled Balloon Technique

Marvin M. Schuster

THE BALLOON DEVICE AND TECHNIQUE

The double-balloon device that readily lends itself to recording from colon and anal sphincters consists of a hollow metal cylinder, shown in Figure 6.1A, around which double-molded latex balloons are tied, creating two compartments as shown in Figure 6.1B. One or more balloons can be inserted through the hollow core of the cylinder shown in Figures 6.2 and 6.3 for recording from the rectum and rectosigmoid and for initiating rectosphincteric reflexes. The colon balloons can be used for recording compliance and spasm.

The inner balloon of the double-balloon assembly assumes a doughnut shape when it is inflated with 7 to 10 ml of air and the outer balloon is a pear shape. Polyethylene tubing is used to communicate between compartments of the balloon and the pressure transducers. The apparatus can be inserted without proctoscopic visualization simply by distending the anus with the finger. The rectal and colonic balloons can be composed of condoms and are tied so that when filled with 50 cc of air they are fully inflated but not distended. The colonic balloon is first inserted, and the steel cylinder is then gently guided up along the rectal catheter, which acts as a guide wire. The device is inserted into the anus until only a small part of the external balloon remains visible. The internal balloon, when inflated with 10 ml of air, is surrounded by the internal anal sphincter, and the external balloon when similarly inflated is encircled by the superficial bundle of the external sphincter. The device is seated by rapidly inflating and deflating the rectal balloon with 30 to 50 ml of air. The resultant reflexes that occur (relaxation of the internal sphincter and contraction of the external sphincter) automatically

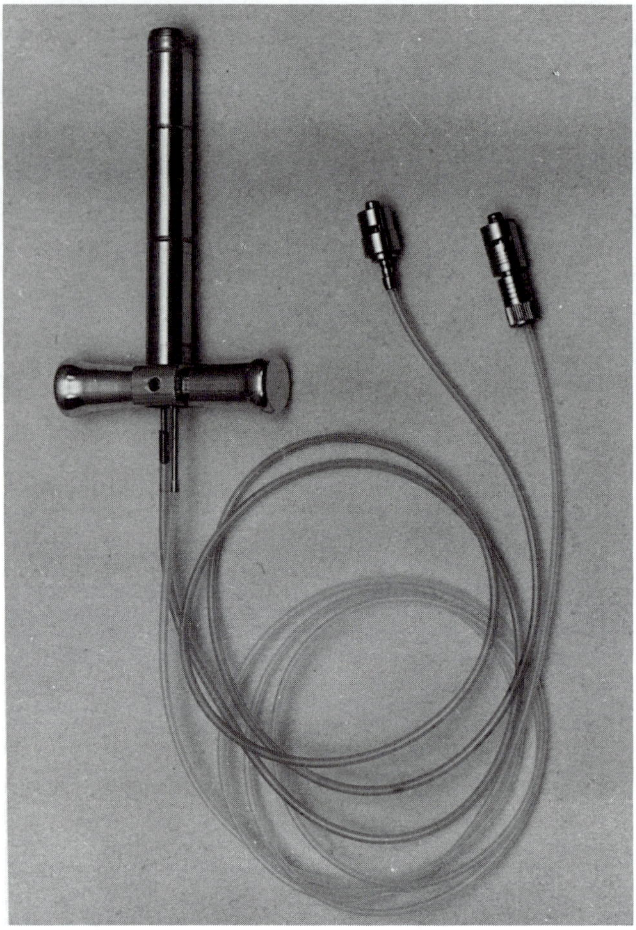

A

FIGURE 6.1 Pressure sensing device. **A:** Hollow metal cylinder with needle soldered in a core and opening to the surface.

seat the device in its appropriate location (Fig. 6.2). This hollow steel cylinder is 4 inches long and contains two 16-gauge needles soldered to the inner surface and they open into its outer surface into each balloon compartment. The balloons are tied with No. 4 silk in such a manner that each compartment can be inflated separately. There are small grooves on the steel cylinder indicating where the ties are to be placed. Balloons and cylinders are made in three sizes, infant, pediatric, and adult. The infant size is used for infants up to 1 to 2 months of age; the pediatric size up to 1 year of age; and the adult size for ages beyond those ages. The rectal catheter is composed of polyethylene tubing that is stiff enough so that it does not double over on itself.

Advantages

This apparatus can easily be inserted without the proctoscope. It seats itself uniformly in the same position in the same patient for repeated studies. Since it is

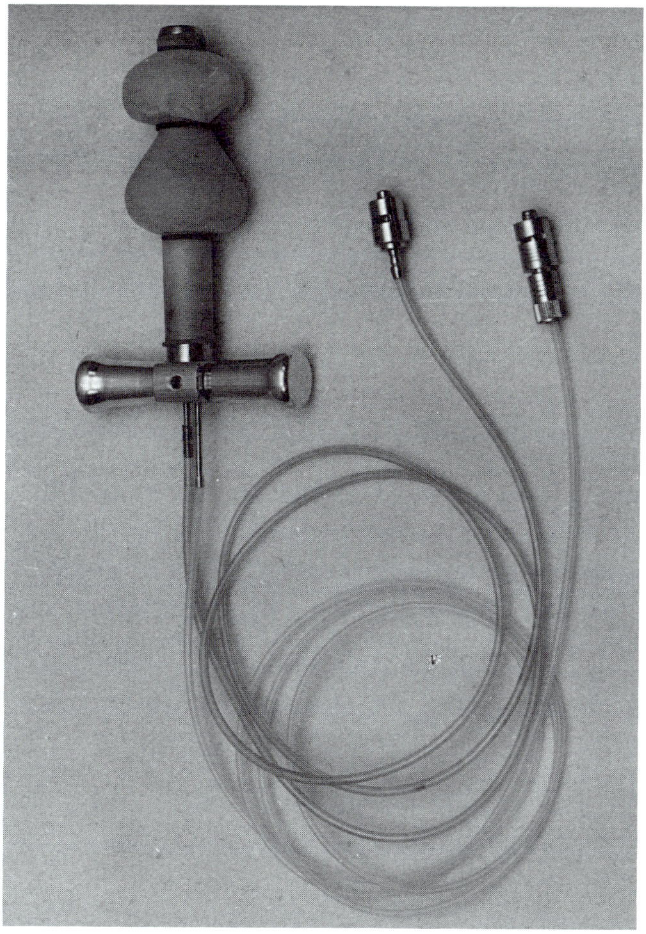

B

FIGURE 6.1 (Continued) **B:** Double balloon tied around a cylinder creating two compartments.

an air system, it does not need cleansing or drying internally, and the rubber lasts for many uses. The relatively large balloons reflect the pressures from within a large area of the sphincters. Another advantage is that the balloons stay in place readily by themselves even in infants and therefore require only one operator.

Disadvantages

The major disadvantage is that the larger the balloons, the more artifact they create; therefore, one cannot make assumptions about basal resting pressures, but rather one can record changes in pressures. These changes can be voluntary contractions and relaxations or pharmacologically, electrically, or mechanically induced changes.

Distentions may be transient (Fig. 6.2), repetitive, or prolonged (Fig. 6.3). A threshold can be established for these responses and they are different for rectum, internal sphincter, and external sphincter responses (Fig. 6.4 A and B).

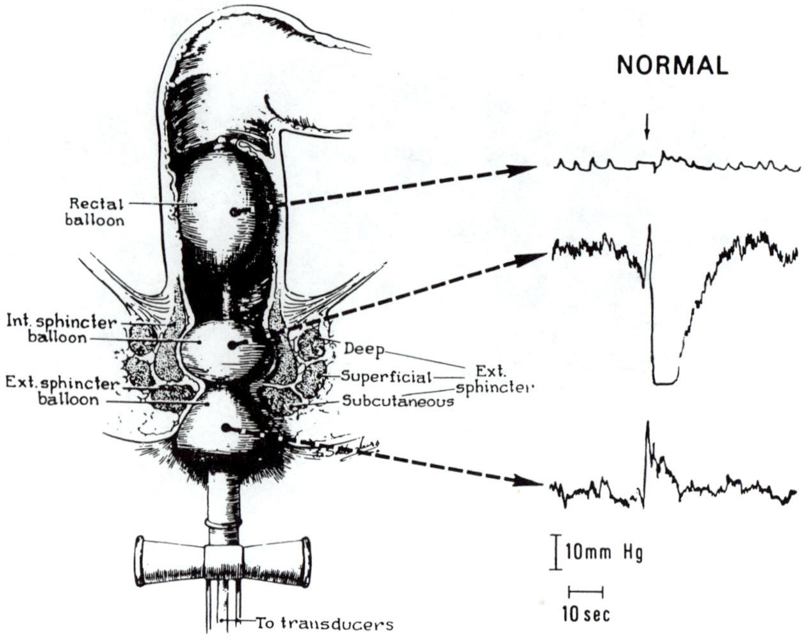

FIGURE 6.2 Schematic diagram on the *left* shows the internal sphincter balloon surrounded by internal sphincter and the external sphincter balloon surrounded by the subcutaneous bundles of the external sphincter. Rectal balloon is attached to a catheter that passes through the hollow core of the metal capsule. This balloon is kept inflated with 10 ml of air for basal recordings. All balloons connect with polyethylene catheters to pressure transducers that communicate with direct writing recorder. Tracings on the right demonstrate internal sphincter relaxation (*middle tracing*) and simultaneous external sphincter contraction (*lower tracing*) when the rectal balloon is transiently distended with air (*arrow*). (From Engel BT, Nikoomanesh P, Schuster MM: Operant conditioning of rectosphincteric responses in the treatment of fecal incontinence. *N Engl J Med* 290:646–649, 1974.)

Measurements

This apparatus readily separates out internal sphincter responses from external sphincter responses and can diagnose and differentiate disorders that selectively affect either smooth muscle or striated muscle, autonomic nervous system or somatic nervous system. For example, patients with aganglionosis (Hirschsprung's disease) fail to show internal sphincter relaxation (Fig. 6.4B).

Internal sphincter relaxation, and autonomically innervated voluntary response, occurs despite voluntary contraction (Fig. 6.5). Response of the external sphincter to perianal pinprick can also be measured.

By placing small surface electrodes on the internal sphincter balloon, one can measure myoelectric activity from the internal sphincter (Fig. 6.6). In the basal resting state a constant sinusoidal slow wave (BER, or basic electric rhythm, also called electrical control activity) can be measured from the internal sphincter (Fig.

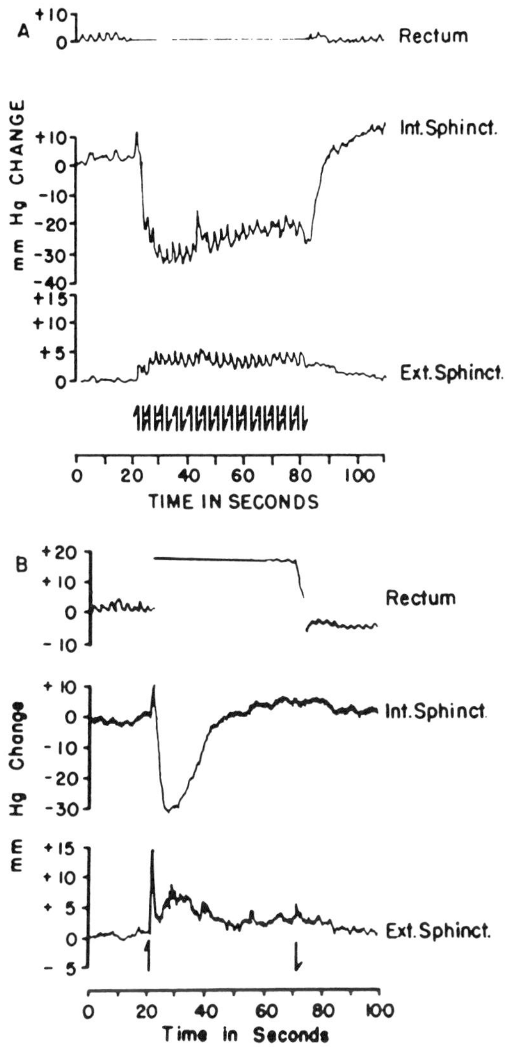

FIGURE 6.3 Comparison of the effect of intermittent transient rectal distention **(A)** with continued prolonged distention **(B).** Sphincter responses to intermittent distention persist for longer periods than with prolonged distention. (From Schuster MM, Hookman P, Hendrix TR, et al.: Simultaneous manometric recording of internal and external anal sphincteric reflexes. *Bull Johns Hopkins Hosp* 116:79–88, 1965.)

6.7). Distention of the rectum results in inhibition of the slow wave (BER, or basic electric rhythm) and consequently in relaxation of the internal sphincter (Fig. 6.8, pg. 45).

An "on the road" adaptation can be simply made, using an aneroid manometer attached to the catheter that emanates from the internal sphincter balloon. The device is inserted in the usual manner, and stopcocks are used to keep the internal and external balloons inflated. The aneroid manometer is attached to that balloon

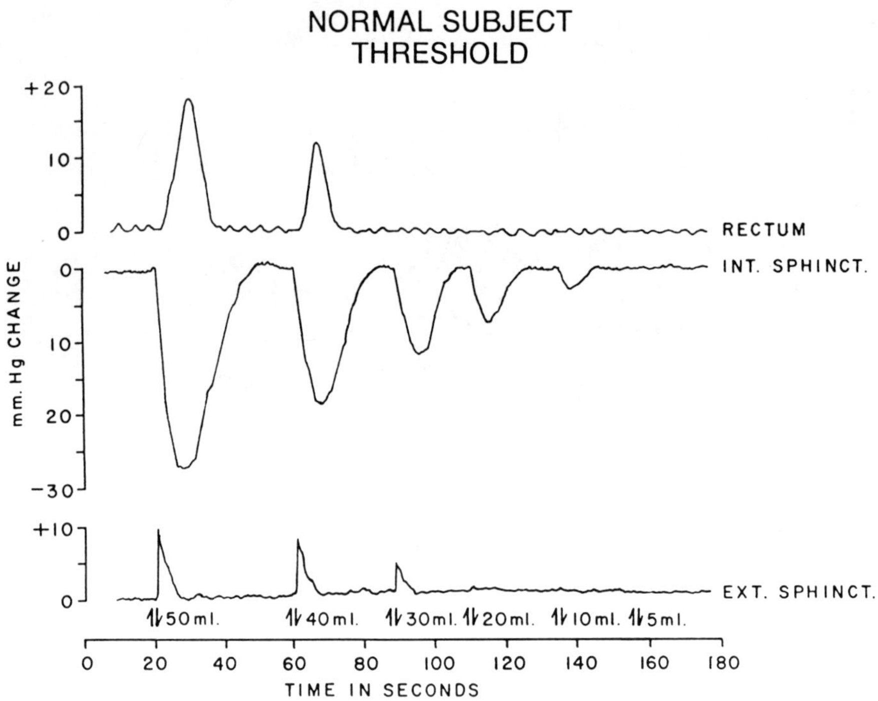
NORMAL SUBJECT
THRESHOLD
+20
10
0
RECTUM
INT. SPHINCT.
10
20
-30
mm. Hg CHANGE
+10
EXT. SPHINCT.
50 ml.
40 ml.
30 ml.
20 ml.
10 ml.
5 ml.
0 20 40 60 80 100 120 140 160 180
TIME IN SECONDS

A

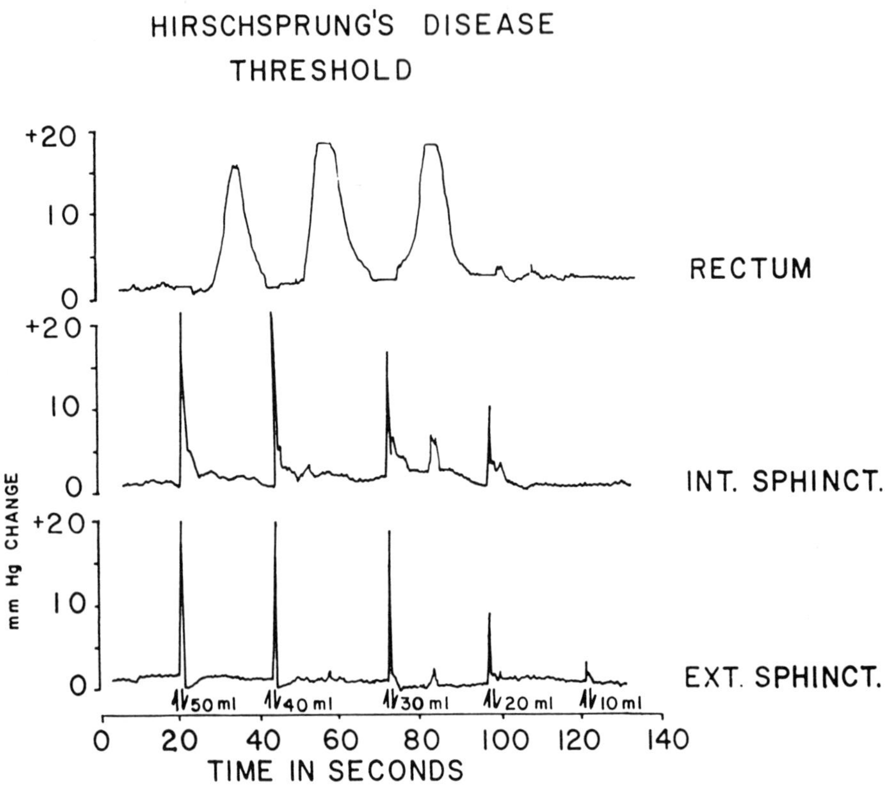
HIRSCHSPRUNG'S DISEASE
THRESHOLD
+20
10
0
RECTUM
INT. SPHINCT.
EXT. SPHINCT.
mm Hg CHANGE
50 ml
40 ml
30 ml
20 ml
10 ml
0 20 40 60 80 100 120 140
TIME IN SECONDS

B

FIGURE 6.4 Threshold for sphincteric responses in a normal subject **(A)** and a patient with Hirschsprung's disease **(B).** As decreasing volumes of air are instilled for rectal distention the amplitude and duration of the sphincteric responses decrease to the point where none can be detected. The minimal volume that elicits a detectable sphincter response is referred to as threshold. In the normal subject **(A)** the threshold for the internal sphincter response is 10 ml, that for the external sphincter 30 ml, and that for the rectal contraction 40 ml. In the patient with Hirschsprung's disease **(B),** the threshold for external sphincter contraction is 20 ml, that for external sphincter contraction 10 ml, and that for rectal contraction 30 ml.

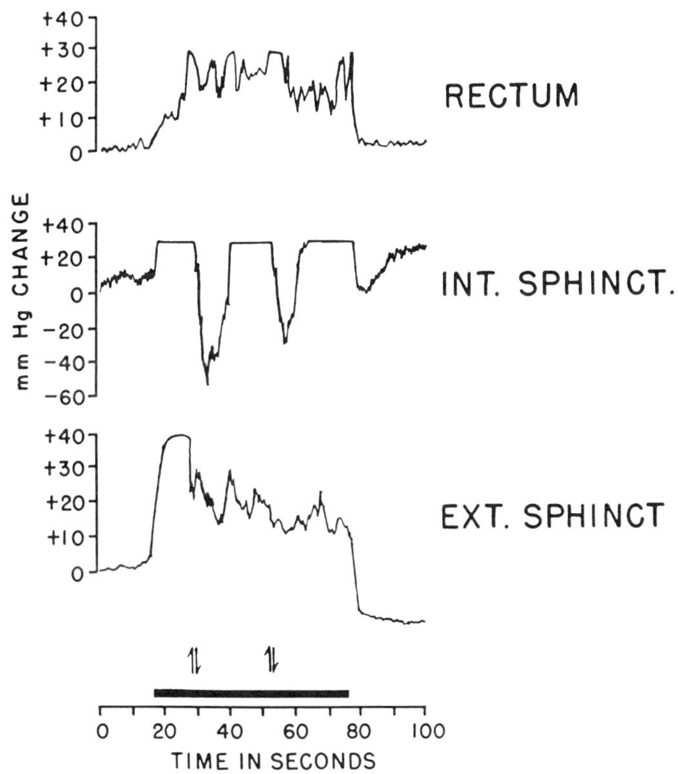

FIGURE 6.5 Distention of the rectum during voluntary contraction of anal sphincter. *Black bar* indicates duration of voluntary contraction of sphincter. *Arrows* indicate rectal balloon distention. Two transient-distentions are shown, each resulting in internal sphincter relaxation but no change in external sphincter.

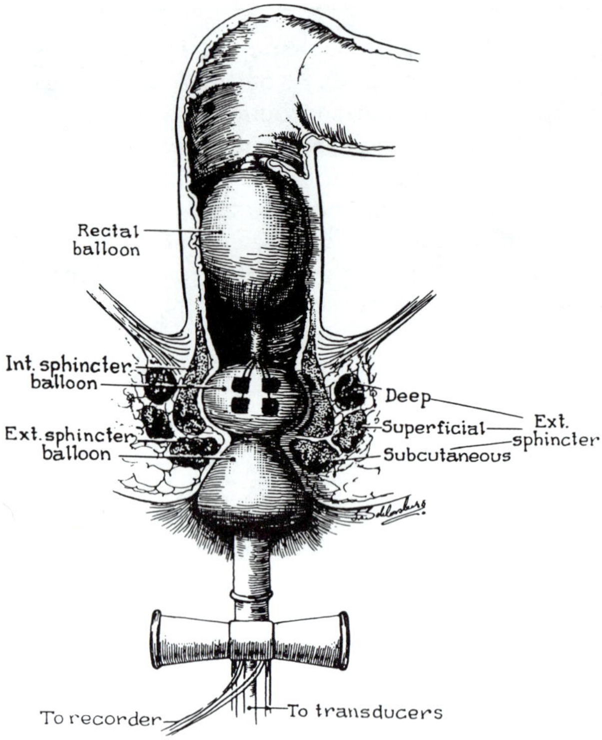

FIGURE 6.6 Schematic diagram of recording technique. The anatomical relationship of pressure-sensing device in the anal canal is shown. The flat surface electrodes used for electrical recordings are cemented onto the balloon, which is surrounded by the internal sphincter.

from which one wishes to record information, (in Hirschsprung's disease to the internal sphincter balloon) (Fig. 6.9, p. 46). The pressures that can be read from the aneroid manometer (the internal sphincter balloon) during rectal distention are shown in Figure 6.10 (pg. 46) for normal subjects and in Figure 6.11 (p. 47) for patients with Hirschsprung's disease who lack internal sphincter relaxation, but instead may have contraction.

Any number of additional colonic balloons may be added as shown in Figure 6.12. When increments of 20 ml of air are added every 2 min to one of the colonic balloons, one can establish a pressure-volume curve that reflects compliance. Normal subjects react to the immediate inflation with immediate active contraction (rectosigmoid balloon in Fig. 6.13) but tolerate large volumes of distention (160 ml of cumulative volumes shown) without spastic delayed contractions. By contrast (Fig. 6.14) patients with irritable bowel syndrome (IBS) show phasic contractions that are superimposed upon tonic pressure increases.

Use in Biofeedback

This device lends itself readily to the application of biofeedback for the treatment of disorders such as fecal incontinence. This represents the first utilization of any

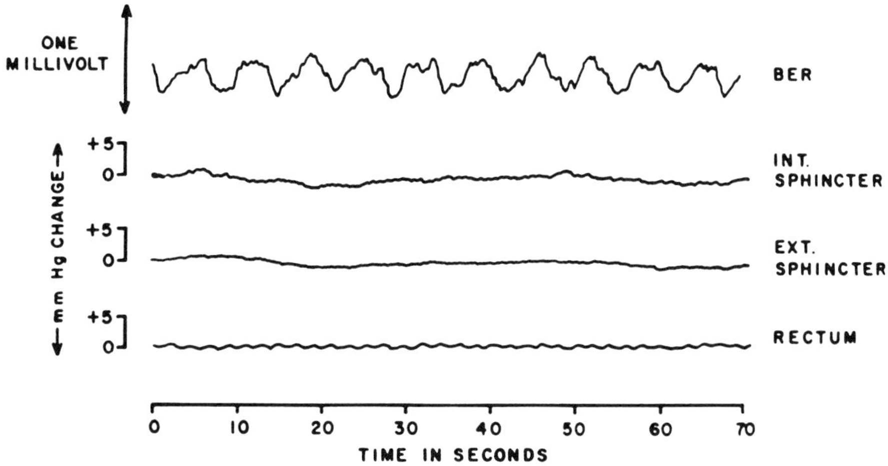

FIGURE 6.7 Constant sinusoidal BER in the resting state. A sinusoidal basic electric rhythm (BER) is recorded from the internal sphincter at a time when no pressure changes are occurring in this sphincter. The *upper tracing* is the bipolar electrical recording from the internal anal sphincter, and the *lower three tracings* are pressure recordings from the balloons placed in the designated areas. In this and subsequent figures resting pressure in each balloon is assigned a zero value on the vertical axis. Increases above this level (contraction) are designed as positive, decreases (relaxation) as negative.

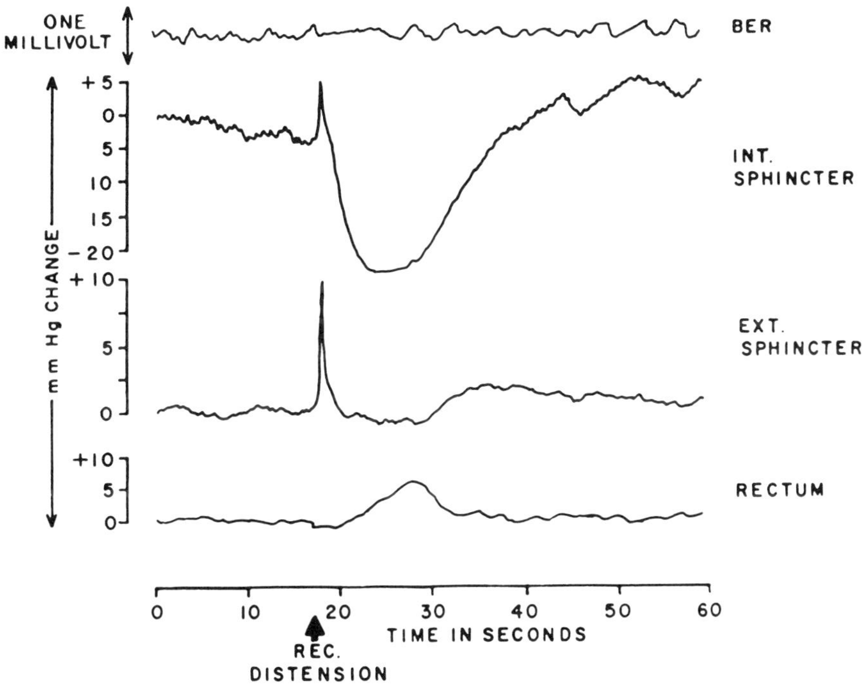

FIGURE 6.8 Inhibition of BER during internal sphincter relaxation. Inhibition of BER (*upper tracing*) accompanies the down slope of internal sphincter relaxation (*second tracing*) produced by rectal distention (*arrow*) with 50 cc of air. The BER returns at the same time that sphincter tone returns.

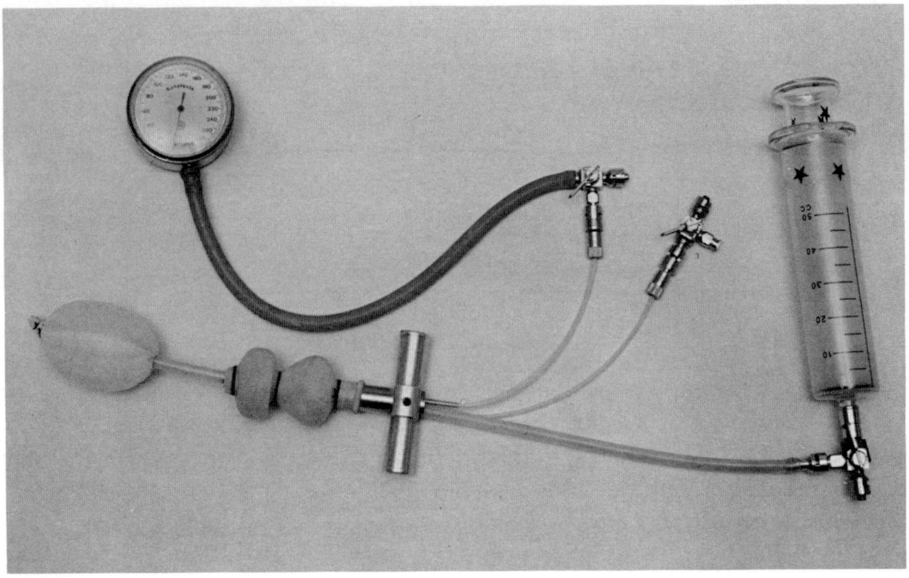

FIGURE 6.9 Device for recording internal sphincter pressure by aneroid manometer. The manometer is in communication with the internal balloon. A stopcock to the internal balloon is closed after this balloon is inflated. Rectosphincteric reflexes are initiated by transient distention of the rectal balloon via the syringe.

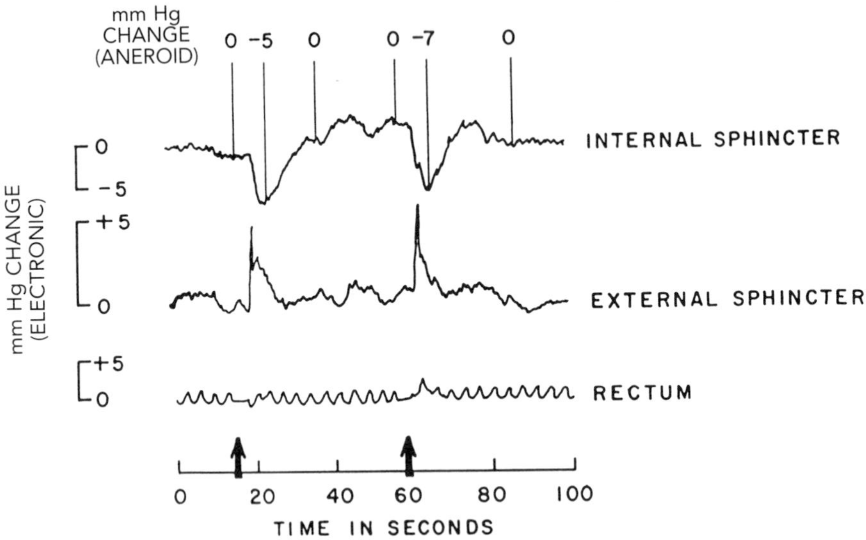

FIGURE 6.10 Normal internal sphincter response. Internal sphincter relaxation induced by transient rectal distention (at the *arrow*) is recorded on the electronic recorder as a pressure decrease in the internal balloon. Resting pressures arbitrarily assigned a zero value. Pressure increases (contraction) are designated as positive, decreases (relaxation) as negative. Pressure recordings from the aneroid manometer (*upper tracings*) correlate well with pressures recorded by the transducer in electronic recorder (*first tracing*).

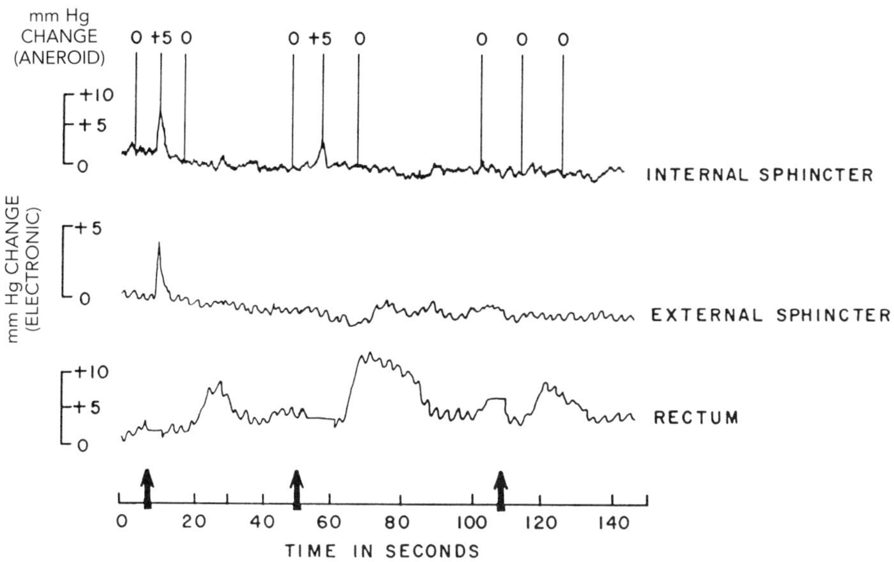

FIGURE 6.11 Abnormal internal sphincter response in Hirschsprung's disease. Rectal distention (at the *arrow*) fails to induce internal sphincter relaxation. Instead, a contraction is seen in the first two distentions. Internal sphincter contraction, when present, occurs in the absence of external sphincter contraction, as seen after the second rectal distention. In the third distention, internal sphincter failed to relax but did not contract. Pressure recordings from aneroid manometer (*upper tracings*) correlate with pressure recorded electronically (*first tracing*).

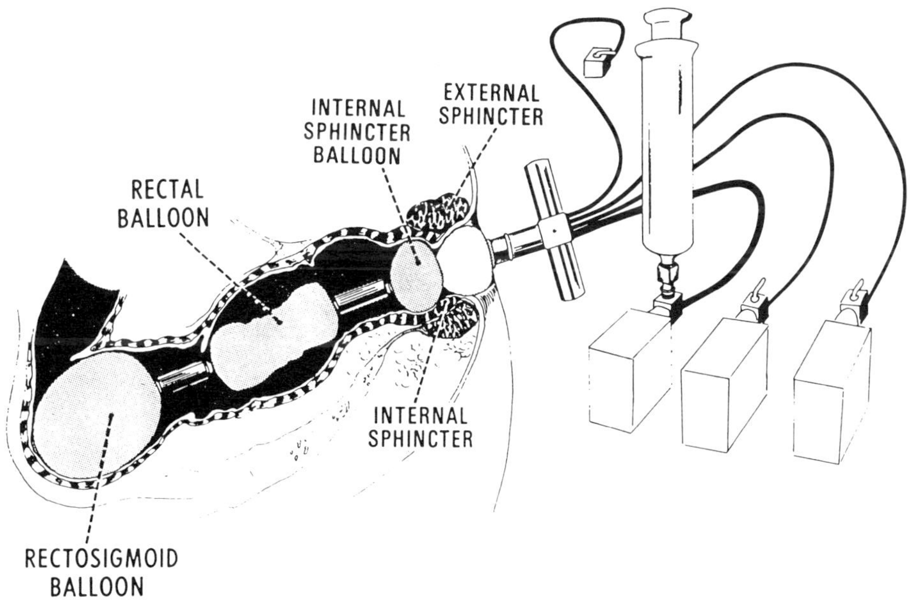

FIGURE 6.12 Balloon assembly in place for recordings from the rectosigmoid, rectum, internal sphincter, and external sphincter.

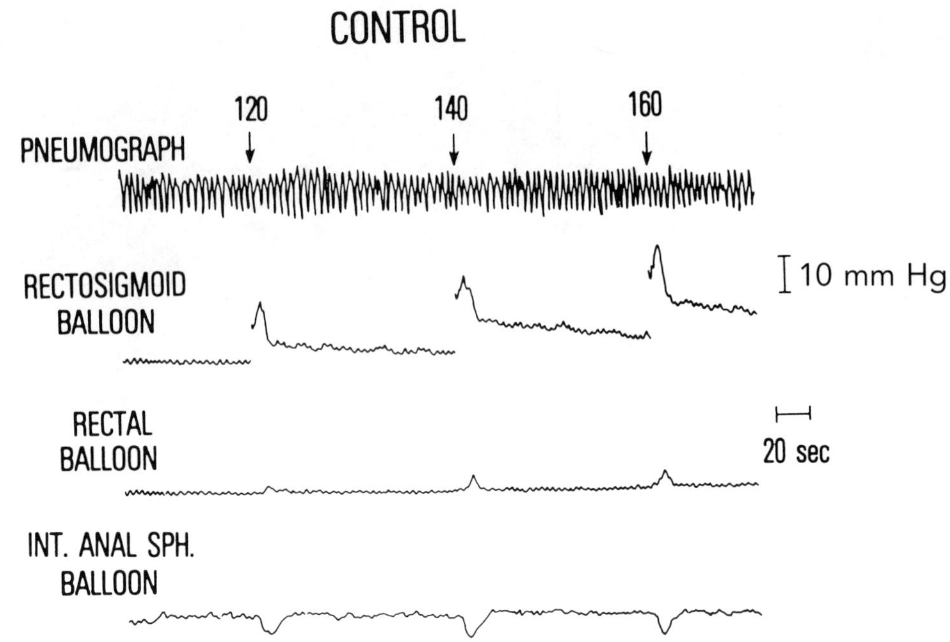

FIGURE 6.13 Manometric responses to rectosigmoid distention in normal subjects. Numbers are rectosigmoid tracing indicate cumulative volumes in the rectosigmoid distending balloon.

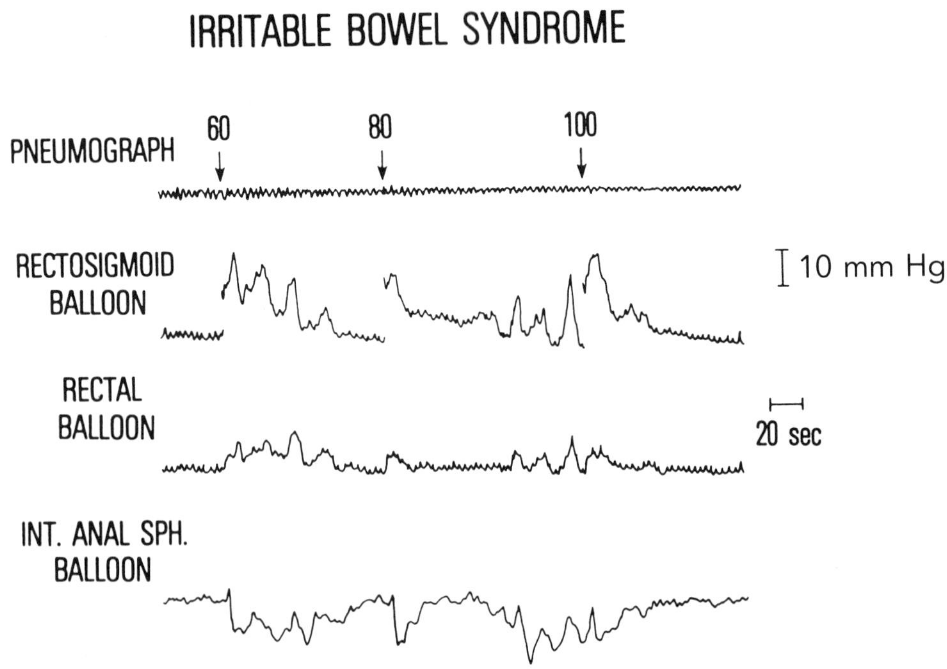

FIGURE 6.14 Phasic spastic contractions superimposed upon tonic contractions in rectosigmoid and rectum with volumes as small as 60 ml of distention in the rectosigmoid balloon in a patient with IBS.

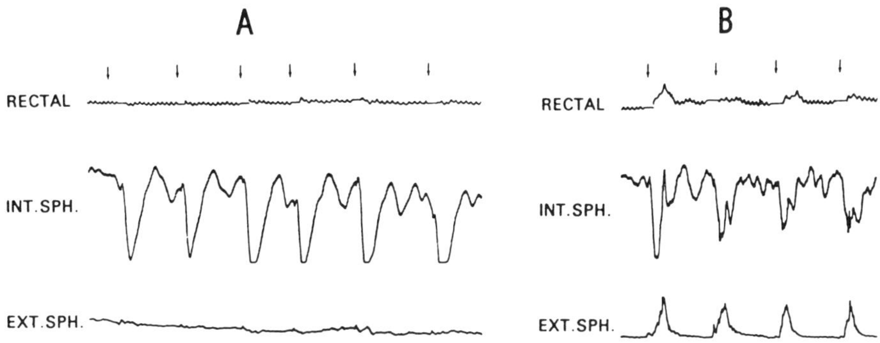

FIGURE 6.15 Rectosphincteric responses in an incontinent patient **(A)** before **(B)** after biofeedback training (From Engel BT, Nikoomanesh P, Schuster MM: Operant conditioning of rectosphincteric responses in the treatment of fecal incontinence. *N Engl J Med* 290:646–674, 1974).

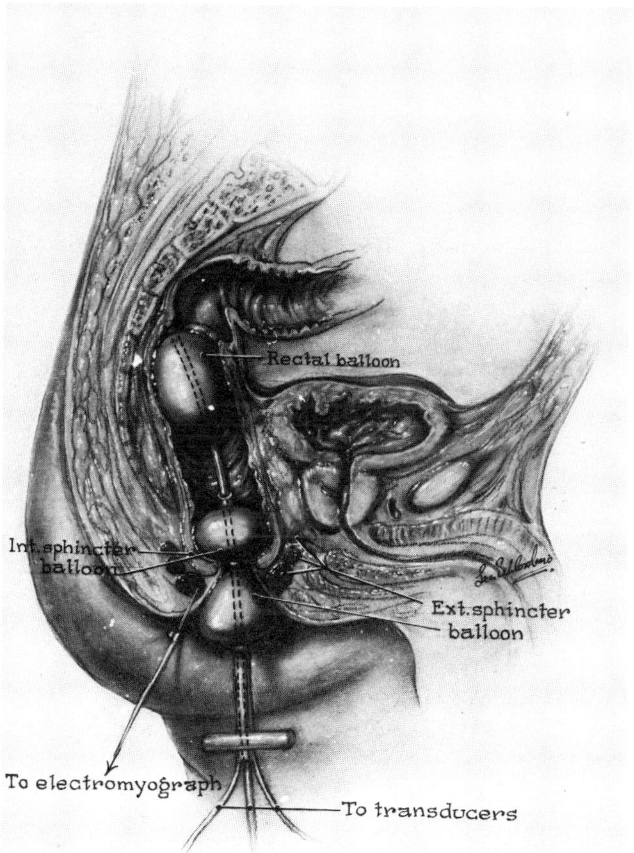

FIGURE 6.16 Diagram of recording technique. Double balloon device is shown in the anus with third distending balloon in the rectum. Electromyographic needle is inserted into the external sphincter.

motility technique for treatment as well as diagnosis. To accomplish this the table is raised so that the patient can see the recording, and the patient is instructed to contract the sphincter to make the external sphincter recording pen rise as the internal sphincter relaxes. In this matter patients who have nerve, muscle, or neuromuscular impairment of sphincter responses can be trained in one or two sessions to develop these responses (Fig. 6.15).

Modifications of the technique (Fig. 6.16) can also permit electromyographic recording by needle electrode of the external sphincter or puborectalis or by surface electrodes of the external sphincter.

SUGGESTED READINGS

Alva J, Mendeloff AI, Schuster MM: Reflex and electromyographic abnormalities associated with fecal incontinence. *Gastroenterol* 53:101–106, 1967.

Schnaufer L, Talbert JL, Haller JL, et al: Differential sphincteric studies in the diagnosis of ano-rectal disorders of childhood. *J Pediatr Surg* 2:538–543, 1967.

Schuster MM: Motor action of the rectum and anal sphincters in continence. In Code C, Prosser CL. *Handbook of Physiology,* Chapter 103. Baltimore, Williams & Wilkins 1968, pp 2121–2146.

Schuster MM: Diagnostic value of anal sphincter pressure measurements. *Hosp Pract* 8:115, 1973.

Schuster MM: Operant conditioning in gastrointestinal dysfunctions. *Hosp Pract* 9:135–143, 1974.

Schuster MM: The riddle of the sphincters. *Gastroenterol* 69:249–262, 1975.

Schuster MM: Biofeedback treatment of gastrointestinal disorders. *Med Clin North Am* 61:907–912, 1977.

Schuster MM: Anorectal disorder in irritable bowel syndrome. In Read, Nicholas W: *The Irritable Bowel Syndrome,* Chapter 17. Orlando, FL, Grune & Stratton, 1985, pp 191–200.

Schuster MM: Clinical applications of rectosphincteric manometry. *Endosc Rev* 11(2): 68–74, May/June 1985.

Schuster MM, Hookman P. Hendrix TR, et al: Simultaneous manometric recording of internal and external anal sphincteric reflexes. *Bull Johns Hopkins Hosp* 116:79–88, 1965.

Tobon F, Reid NCRW, Talbert JL, et al: Nonsurgical test for the diagnosis of Hirschsprung's disease. *N Engl J Med* 278:188–194, 1968.

Ustach TJ, Tobon F, Hambrecht T, et al: Electrophysiological aspects of human sphincter function. *J Clin Invest* 49:41–48, 1970.

Ustach TJ, Tobon F, Schuster MM: Simplified method for diagnosis of Hirschsprung's disease. *Arch Dis Child* 44:694–697, 1969.

Whitehead WE, Schuster MM: Anorectal physiology and pathophysiology. *Am J Gastroenterol* 87:487–497, 1987.

CHAPTER 7

Computerized Anal Sphincter Manometry Performance and Analysis

John A. Coller
Yash P. Sangwan

INTRODUCTION

The purpose of this chapter is to describe six basic manometric characterizations of the anorectal sphincter as performed according to specified protocols and as analyzed with a computer software program. However, before describing the specific applications, it is of value to mention the general role of manometric assessment in defecation disorders; the importance of a structured format or protocol in the performance of sphincter manometry; and the integration of a computer to the performance and analysis of manometric data.

Role of Anal Spincter Manometry in Defecation Disorders

Defecation is a complex bodily function which directly involves a number of organ systems. There is no single all-encompassing defecatory function test. If the patient perceives abnormal defecation, the initial assessment may need to be, not specialized physiologic testing with the anatomic area of perceived dysfunction, but rather with metabolic, neurologic, or psychological systems. Even if initial assessment suggests dysfunction in the pelvic region, it is unlikely that a single diagnostic study can be considered definitive. Although simplistically viewed as an obstruction to unwanted defecation, the anorectal sphincter is in fact a complex collection of structures and mechanisms closely interrelated and somewhat duplicative in function.

A quick perusal of the literature reveals abundant reports relative to manometric determinations of the anal sphincter in health and disease. It is also apparent that there is less than unanimous agreement on the relationship of manometric assessment to various disease states and consequently on the value of these studies in understanding dysfunction. Certainly, one of the principal causes of any lack of confidence in the value of manometric assessment resides in the frequent failure to appreciate that although the anal sphincter is an important element in defecation it need not be the element that is singularly responsible for dysfunction.

A close examination of the literature reveals as much variance between methodologies as there are results and would strongly suggest that one of the common denominators to this problem is the lack of uniformity of examination performance as well as definition of terms. Indeed, it is difficult to suggest uniformity and standard methodology in a field where both the understanding of the problem is incomplete and the technology of methodology is evolving. However, this lack of consensus does not give us license to disregard a precise and consistent performance technique as well as analysis and interpretive approach.

Computerized Approach to Performance and Analysis

There is nothing mystical about applying a computer to manometry. It is as reasonable to make use of a computer at the present time as it was to change from a smoked-drum to electrical recording a number of years ago. The level of enhancement that is provided by the addition of computer technology depends upon the extent and manner to which the computer is integrated into the whole system. At the lowest level of enhancement, the computer cathode-ray tube can simply serve to provide a colorful display of the conventional and rather boring X-Y plotter tracings. Although charismatic, this is an equivocal benefit.

Real enchancement does not start to take place until one uses the computer capability of digital data manipulation and storage. There are a great number of tedious error-prone manual procedures that can be relegated to the computer. In addition, there are complex mathematic algorithms that can be used that are simply not obtainable by manual means. Some of the benefits of a computerized system are listed:

1. Preliminary procedures:
   a) Automatic warm-up, alignment, and initialization of computer and manometric equipment.
   b) Automatic channel calibration and zero-baselining.
   c) Automatic identification of tracking errors.
   d) Menu selection of procedures.
   e) Indexing of performed procedures.
2. Examination performance:
   a) Automatic operation of accesory equipment, e.g., probe withdrawal motor, etc.

b) On-line prompts to produce consistent operator and patient interaction.
c) Automatic labeling of runs and annotation of comments.
d) Ability to reassign tor discard runs that deviate from protocol.
e) Ability to display in real-time or replay data on CRT or plotter.

3. Saving data:
a) Data can be stored on hard disc or on individual patient diskette.
b) Data can be archived to backup media and replayed or reanalyzed at any time.

4. Analysis:
a) Automatic reduction of raw data to a meaningful numeric characterization or sphincter function in the form of a printed report.
b) Automatic generation and printing of pressure data graphs to assist in the visualization of spincter defects.
c) Maintenance of data base logs to permit retrieval of cases for comparative study.
d) Automated analysis should not prevent the ability to perform more traditional manual assessment using conventional X-Y plotter output or CRT manipulation.

The computerized manometric system described in this chapter is the Narco Bio-Systems MMS-200.* A flat bed X-Y plotter permits conventional manual data acquisition. An IBM-compatible computer (386 or higher) with VGA monitor provides on-line color graphic display and off-line replay. A menu-driven software program is provided that assists in the automatic operations of manometric testing of the anal sphincter. Other menus are provided for esophageal manometry, pH, etc.

The Dynamic Pressure Analysis (DPA)® program is a compiled software package that is specifically designed to process the anal sphincter manometric runs that have been performed with the Narco Bio-Systems MMS-200 according to the DPA protocol. The DPA program automatically produces the numeric reports and graphic representations described in the sections that follow.

Manometric Performance According to Protocol

There is no single type of manometric performance that can completely assess anorectal sphincter function. Probes and methodologies vary considerably: recording point (1–10, or more); recording type (perfused, microballoon, microtransducer); sampling method (stationary, interrupted, continuous, pull-through); perfusion rates; etc. It is not the intent of this discussion to suggest that certain methodologies are the only or even the best methodologies. However, we will

* MMS-200: Narco Bio-Systems, 7651 Airport Boulevard, Houston, Texas 77061.

clearly describe a specific way of assessing sphincter function that may be consistently compared to similarly performed analyses. The consistent acquisition of manometric data in a standard fashion is termed PROTOCOL performance of manometry.[1]

When performing sphincter manometry according to Protocol, the responsibility for accurate assessment is placed very clearly where it should be—during *acquisition* of data. Establishment of a specific Protocol is designed to maximize the amount of useful, retrievable information from each manometric run while minimizing the likelihood of producing spurious results from real data.

If a manometric examination is performed according to a specific examination Protocol, the data generated may be processed in exactly the same way each time and the computer can automatically and reliability determine the desired parameters and result values according to a predefined algorithm. Hence, if information is entered in a prescribed fashion, the computer can do a great deal of the work that used to be done by hand. If entered in a haphazard fashion, the computer capacity is essentially limited to simply recording random data. With or without the aid of a computer, such data is still "Garbage in . . . Garbage out."

There are specific protocols that will be described for each basic type of manometric run. To the extent possible, the computer program will actively perform or assist in this regard—e.g. automatic probe withdrawal, screen prompts, etc.

However, there are general requirements, applicable to all of the manometric protocols described herein that help to provide uniformity and reliability:

1. *Preparation of patient.* It is best that the patient is at ease during the performance of manometry. Some time should be taken before actually initiating the procedure, which permits a rapport to be established between the physician and the patient. Expeditiously placing the patient on the examinining table and promptly starting the recording of data is likely to result in variability and inconsistently of at least the initial runs. It can readily be appreciated that most patients will not immediately be at ease with unfamiliar surroundings with their bare bottom exposed to strangers while a probe is going back and forth in the anal canal.

2. *Rectal preparation.* It is somewhat controversial as to whether manometry should be performed in the "as is" state or whether the rectum should be emptied of feces before performing the examination. Reliable and reproducible results require some degree of uniformity. It is quite clear that assessment of the anorectal inhibitory reflex is dependent upon a volume change in the rectum. If a rectum is already laden with stool of a varying degree, it would be very difficult to correlate responses under those conditions with that of an empty rectum. In order to maximize uniformity, it is my personal prejudice that manometry should be accomplished with the rectum emptied of fecal debris. In addition, there also exists certain mechanical impediments to the ease of accurate probe insertion if stool is residing in the rectum. The use of one or more Fleets enemas more than 2 hr prior to the examination is advised as a general preparation. If the patient presents at the time of examination still containing stool in the rectal ampulla, then a 4-ounce enema containing only tap water is advised.

3. *Patient positioning.* All manometric runs relative to the PROTOCOLS being described will be performed in the left lateral decubitus position (left side down)

with the patient's back perpendicular to the floor surface and the spinal column parallel to the floor. The hips are flexed to as near 90° as is comfortable.

Although encouraging the patient to be as relaxed as possible is often accomplished by conversation, the patient should refrain from talking during data acquisition. Talking, breath holding, coughing, and laughing all result in changes of intra-abdominal pressure that are readily transmitted to the pelvic region. Although these artifactual contributions to the record may be noted in the comments section at the end of a run, they are not automatically discerned as artifact by the analysis programs. Likewise, since the patient is usually not aware of the difference between when one is taking data and when one is simply between runs, it is advisable to clearly inform the patient that you are about to begin a run so that any little shifting in position can be accomplished beforehand.

4. *Fluid accumulation during manometry.* Multichannel perfusion probes can result in the instillation of a sizable amount of fluid into the rectal ampulla over the course of a number of manometry runs or if allowed to simply reside in the rectum between runs. This progressive accumulation of fluid can obviously have a cumulative effect on rectal distension and thus on resting anal sphincter pressure. It is best to withdraw the probe from the anal canal, if the interval between runs is expected to be appreciable. Intermittent insertion of a red rubber catheter or Foley catheter simply to allow excess fluid to be evacuated is advisable.

5. *Respiratory recording.* It is essential that simultaneous respiratory recording is performed during manometry. This record is very useful to refer to when trying to determine if a curious pressure peak in the anal sphincter was a "real" phenomenon or merely the result of a cough, deep breath, etc. Comparison with the respiratory record is essential when assessing the validity of motility slow waves.

BASIC MANOMETRIC PROTOCOLS

There are six basic manometric protocol types. Each is constructed to provide a specific characterization of the sphincter.

Before selecting a specific protocol, the computer program will assist in the automatic preliminary procedures of zero baselining, probe calibration, and system checks. Perfusion channels that are not electrically and hydrostatically intact will be identified. Menu selection of a specific protocol will automatically display the appropriate on-line viewing screen.

LONGITUDINAL RESTING PULLOUT (PO) PROFILE PROTOCOL

Purpose

The purpose of the Longitudinal Resting Pullout profile protocol is to obtain a continuous pressure profile of the entire sphincter from the proximal anal canal to the anal verge. This is accomplished by motorized withdrawal of an eight-channel

Protocol	Sphincter Characteristics
Longitudinal Resting Pullout	Length Maximum average pressure Pressure volume Cross-sectional asymmetry
Longitudinal Squeeze Pullout	Length Maximum average pressure Pressure volume Cross-sectional asymmetry
Stationary Squeeze	Voluntary augmentation Fatigue Rest vs. squeeze cross-section
Motility	Slow waves Ultraslow waves

Balloon Reflex	Rectal sensation
	  Volume of initial sensation
	  Volume of urge to defecate
	  Maximum tolerable volume
	Rectoanal inhibitory reflex (RAIR)
	Rectoanal Excitatory reflex (RAER)

Squeeze/Beardown	Rectal pressures Proximal anal canal pressures Distal anal canal pressure

radial cross-sectional probe. Simultaneous longitudinal profiles are obtained 45 degrees apart, throughout the sphincter. Consequently, as a result of the analysis program, both cross-sectional and longitudinal graphic and numeric assessments of the spincter can be obtained. The pressure characteristics of the resting internal sphincter are primarily responsible for this profile.

Equipment

PROBE. A type A probe (Fig. 7.1) with eight radially oriented channels in cross-section is used. The probe is axially oriented and fixed to a probe holder so that Channel 8, of the clockwise numbered channels, is situated in the posterior midline. Channel 1 will record from the right posterior-lateral quadrant, Channel 2 from the right lateral quadrant, and so forth. A ninth, centrally located intraluminal perfusion channel may be present.

PROBE WITHDRAWAL DEVICE. A computer-controlled probe withdrawal device is required for continuous longitudinal profile manometry. Manual removal of the probe results in erratic and unreliable data collection. The probe withdrawal

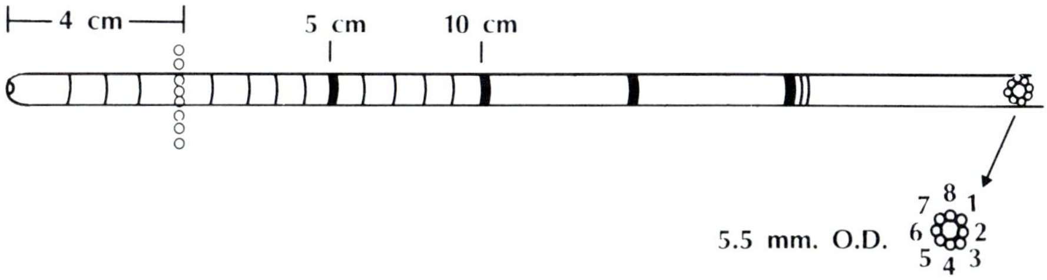

FIGURE 7.1 Anorectal motility probe. A minimally compliant flexible probe with eight radially oriented channels used for resting and squeeze Longitudinal Pull-out runs, stationary motility runs, and stationary or station pull-through runs.

device is a clamp which accepts the probed or a probe holder, in the proper radial orientation, to the device. This author uses a withdrawal rate of 1 mm/sec for a total of 100 sec resulting in a total excursion of 10 cm.

ANAL VERGE MARKER. A 2″ × 2″ gauze pad is used to mark anal verge.

Preliminary Procedure

ZERO BASELINING. Zero baselining of the probe is generally performed with the probe at the level of the anal verge. However, for the Longitudinal Pullout protocol all channels are automatically corrected to a rectal pressure of zero before analysis.

Examination Procedure

LONGITUDINAL PROFILE DISPLAY. From the Procedure Menu select the option to perform the Longitudinal Resting Pullout Profile.

PROBE INSERTION. A gentle digital examination is performed using a very well-lubricated glove. This permits the examiner to determine that an unsuspected anatomic or fecal obstruction will not interfere with probe placement. It is also well to note the direction that the rectal ampulla takes as this will facilitate probe insertion.

The well-lubricated probe is gently inserted into the anal canal, retracting the buttocks to ensure that redundant anal tags are not causing a blind fold resulting in false insertion. The probe may be disconnected from the puller device during insertion or the puller device may be advanced toward the anal orifice while insertion is undertaken. If resistance is felt, then gentle back-and-forth as well as torsional movement can be used to encourage proximal entry of the probe. On occasion, it may be necessary to reinsert the well-lubricated examining finger in order to provide a guide for the probe insertion.

The probe should be inserted so that the perfusion orifices are at least 2 cm above the proximal level of the anal sphincter, but no more than 10 cm above the level of the anal verge. There are probe markings every centimeter proximal (transducer side) of the perfusion orifices. It is best to make the final position of the probe such that the eighth or ninth cm mark is just visible at the anal verge. This way, since the withdrawal distance of the probe during longitudinal pullout will be a total of 10 cm, the pressure orifices will be between 1 and 2 cm external to the anal verge at the completion of the run. Under almost all circumstances, this will ensure that at least 2 or 3 cm of recording will have taken place within the rectal ampulla before the orifices reach the proximal portion of the anal sphincter. Once the probe has been properly positioned, it should be ensured that the probe holder is adequately placed in the puller device and that the puller device is positioned so that a full 10-cm withdrawal can be accomplished.

MARKING ANAL VERGE. Quite often, a patient's buttocks will overlap the anal verge to rest against the probe. The pressure of the buttocks pressing on the lateral orifices of the probe as it exits beyond the anal verge can result in artifactual pressure elevation in these pressure channels that could be interpreted as additional sphincter. A sharp demarcation of the anal verge can be accomplished by placing a moist 2″ × 2″ gauze pad to the level of the anal verge between the buttock and the probe on both sides of the probe. Gauze is placed at the verge for every pullout run even if it does not appear that there will be buttock artifact. A thick wedge of gauze should not be stuffed to the anal verge as this might result in deforming the most distal structure of the sphincter. When properly applied, the pressure registered in each of the channels when the anal verge is reached, will cleanly register atmospheric pressure as the gauze will readily disperse the fluid without producing occlusion of the orifices.

Alternatively, a glutelock can be used. This is a simple instrument developed in our laboratory to prevent pressure artifacts that may be created by the impingement of buttocks on the pressure ports as they exit from the anal canal. This device may be made, in varying lengths (2–5 cm) to accommodate different depths of anal clefts, from the sheath of a 3-cc syringe. Each piece is then wrapped in foam tape to provide smooth contour for patient comfort. The catheter is then threaded through the lumen of the glutelock, which is then placed at the anal verge. This maneuver prevents overhanging buttocks tissue from encroaching on the ports of the catheter.[2]

DATA ACQUISITION. It should be ensured that the patient is at ease and well relaxed. The patient should be informed that for the next approximately $1\frac{1}{2}$ min you will be collecting pressure data that will be inaccurate if there is any appreciable movement, coughing, talking, etc. It is helpful to assure the patient that there will be no surprises or uncomfortable stimuli during the recording period. Upon starting the recording, one should make a quick check to ensure that the puller motor is indeed withdrawing the probe. The pressure readings as they appear on the CRT should be examined. These should be residing either on or very close to their respective zero-baseline level. If at the onset of the run, one or more channels is appreciably (e.g., 10 mm Hg or greater) above the zero level, this is suggestive of the probe orifices being pressed against the rectal wall, possibly representing too deep an insertion. If the offending channels promptly return to a near zero level within the first few seconds, then it is best to stop the run and hit the indicated key to restart the run without the need to reposition the probe. If the pressure readings are grossly elevated, it is possible that the probe has been curled back on itself during insertion and should be repositioned.

When even the well-lubricated probe is changed from a stationary position to moving, relative to the sphincter, there may be mechanical stimulation of the sphincter which could produce a transient, erroneous pressure change even though this is not sensed by the patient. Once the probe is being smoothly and continuously withdrawn through the anal sphincter, any such mechanical artifact is not significant.

The relationship between the probe movement and the spincter should be observed throughout the course of the run to ensure that this movement continues to be steady and smooth. If the probe appears to be exiting from the sphincter in small increments rather than as smooth continuous withdrawal, it is probable that the friction between the probe and the sphincter tissue is high. Consequently, in small increments, the probe would be trying to pull the anal canal along with it, and the tissue of the anal canal would jump back in place every millimeter or so. The probe should be relubricated.

The analysis program assumes that the first 20 sec of data recording is from the rectal lumen and sphincter data reduction is based upon uniform intrarectal pressure during these first 20 sec. If the sphincter is encountered before this data segment has been obtained of if erratic readings are included in this segment, baseline reduction may be inaccurate.

At the completion of the run, the CRT screen should demonstrate that the pressure recordings have uniformly returned to the baseline. The eight radial pressure recording orifices of the probe should be external to the anal verge. Check to see that the small gauze pads used to mark the anal verge are still in place. If the lateral pressure channels on the CRT appear to have a pressure elevation extending 0.5 to 1 cm distal to the other quadrants, it is quite likely that the gauze markers for the anal verge were not in the proper position. As an extra check on run performance, it is advisable to measure the distance between the pressure orifices on the probe and the anal verge using the marker lines on the probe. This number should be included in the comment section for the run. This distance can be compared with the end of sphincter distance as displayed on the graph following analysis. This is particularly helpful when sphincter pressures are exceptionally low or when there is considerable sphincter deformity. As overall sphincter pressure decreases towards a level that approaches baseline, the reliability of mathematical data reduction decreases.

Saving the Data

Following the completion of each Longitudinal Resting Pullout run, one has to decide whether the run appears to be satisfactory from the technical standpoint;

whether it should be included as part of the mathematical and graphic assessment for the patient. Actually, you won't know if a given run is representative of the patient's sphincter until after the analysis and after there has been at least one other run for comparison. However, there are a number of simple guidelines to help you decide as to the adequacy of a run and whether to save it.

- Do all channels appear at a uniform level during the first 20 sec of intrarectal recording before reaching the proximal sphincter?
- At the end of the run, are the pressure orifices beyond the anal verge?
- Was the patient relaxed, quiet and free from voluntary squeezing during the run?

1. *Technically acceptable run.* If the run appears to be technically acceptable; was performed according to protocol; then the menu choice to save the run, as is, may be selected.
2. *Technically unacceptable run.* If the run clearly contains artifacts, e.g., coughing, that result in pressure readings that are not representative of a resting sphincter, then it should not be saved as a run that conforms to the resting sphincter protocol.
3. *Technically acceptable, but questionably representative.* Some sphincters may be severely deformed from injury or may have additional intrinsic physiologic phenomena, e.g., large ultraslow waves that produce bizarre pressure patterns. Observing the raw data on the CRT, especially on the first or second run may be confusing. Under such circumstances, you will not know these pressure patterns are representative of the individual sphincter until you have seen them in several runs. Therefore, a technically acceptable, but questionably representative run can be saved, as is. Such a run can be deleted from Analysis if it is not in keeping with other runs.
4. *Technically unacceptable, but interesting.* It may be apparent that a run does not conform to the protocol for characterizing the longitudinal profile of the sphincter and should not be included with those runs that have been performed appropriately. However, there may be some aspects of the run that you would like to examine more completely and for which you don't want to lose the data, e.g., the patient coughed and you want a record of what happened in the sphincter when the cough occurred. The run designator may be changed so that it will not be included during analysis with runs that conform to protocol.

Comment Entry

If a choice is made to save a run, the operator will be asked to type in a comment. Any information that pertains to the integrity of the run should be entered. There is no way that one will remember the uniqueness of individual runs several months later. After a Resting pullout, I like to include in the comment the distance that the pressure-recording orifices are from the anal verge, e.g., "3 cm out". This is helpful to compare with the graphic display of the distal sphincter limit after

DPA particularly in the grossly deformed low pressure sphincter. It is also a good idea to note if the gauze segments that mark the anal verge have been displaced from the proper position. If the distal lateral quadrants are prominent and the gauze was dislodged or not in place, this might account for an aberrant profile.

Number of Runs

A minimum of three Longitudinal Resting Pullout runs should be performed. There is sufficient variation in the physiologic characteristics of the anal sphincter to make reliance on one or two runs a bit cavalier. The details of sphincter characteristics will not be apparent until after the raw data has been analyzed. If gross differences of sphincter characteristics are suspected from run to run during examination performance, then it is best to perform additional runs to ensure that there are at least three runs with gross uniformity.

Analysis

The purpose of the automated Dynamic Pressure Analysis program is to take the raw data of all pressure channels and present them in a meaningful numeric and graphic manner. An example of the raw data as it appears on the CRT after a Longitudinal Resting Pullout run during data acquisition, as compared to after analysis is given below:

At the onset of Analysis, the program assumes that the first 20 sec of recording occurred before the perfusion orifices reached the sphincter. From this 20-sec data segment, the rectal pressure is corrected to an average pressure of zero by a

Raw Data Graph *Before* Analysis

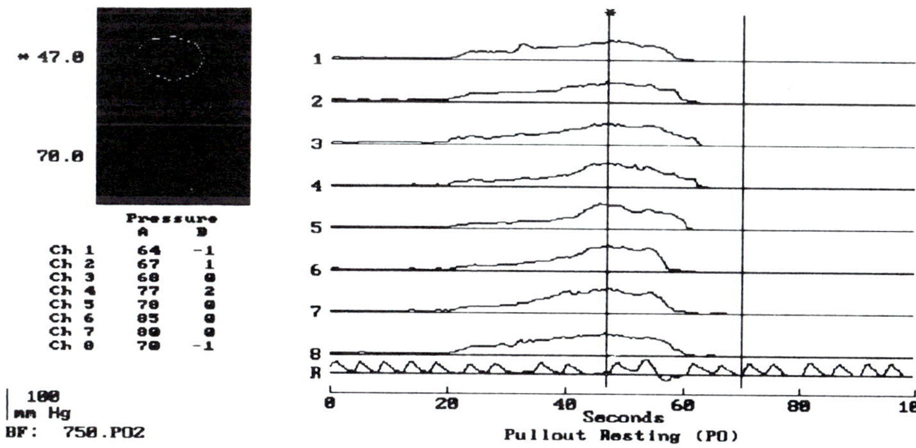

Processed Data Graph *After* Analysis

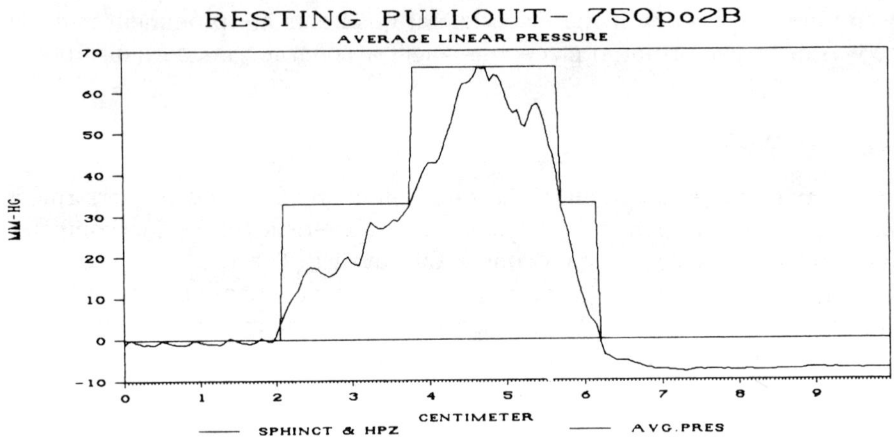

least squares regression method. This pressure correction factor is applied throughout the run. At the distal end of the sphincter, the eight-channel average pressure will fall below the zero baseline by an amount that is equal to the rectal pressure relative to atmosphere. The essentials of a longitudinal profile are displayed below.

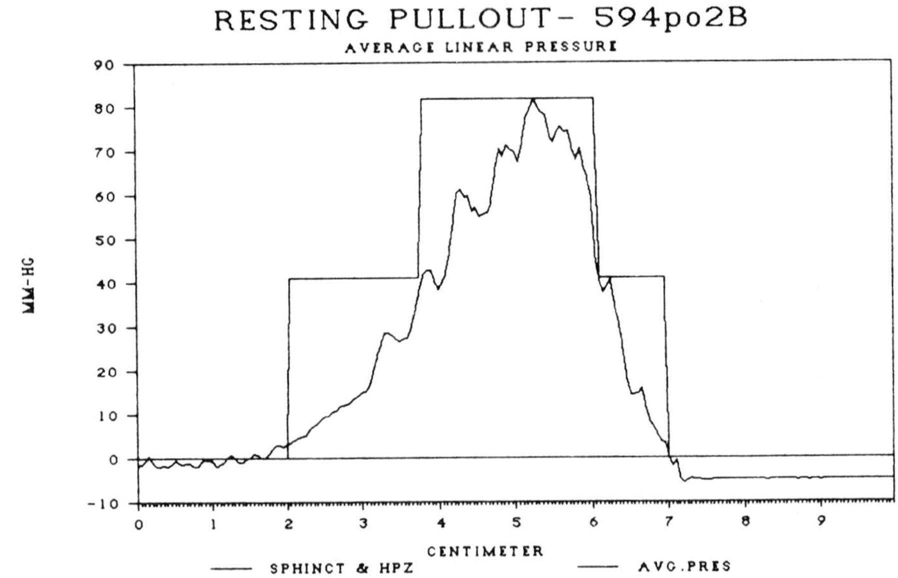

The eight-channel average pressure is displayed. The longitudinal profile is encased in a pair of rectangular outlines. The lower rectangle outlines the proximal and distal limits of the sphincter, in this case, a 49.5 mm length. Note that the proximal margin starts right at 2 cm. Had the probe been inserted less deep than it was, a less accurate reduction of rectal pressure would have been obtained. The probe could have been inserted an additional 3 cm and still have captured this rather long sphincter before the end of the run.

The upper rectangle outlines that portion of the sphincter that contains pressures that are equal to, or greater than, 50% of the Average Maximum Resting pressure which in this case is 81.7 mm Hg. The portion of total sphincter that resides within this upper rectangle is referred to as the high-pressure zone (HPZ). Please recognize that this use of the term HPZ is different from the traditional use which is to refer to the entire sphincter as the HPZ.

It should be noted that the profile is not necessarily a smooth line. As demonstrated in this profile, there are a number of regular occurring bumps. These are *not* due to mechanical stimulation from the smoothly sliding probe. They are the result of a rather substantial slow wave.

Sphincter measurements are relatively easy when dealing with an intact healthy profile as shown. However, when a sphincter has exceptionally low pressures, e.g. 10–20 mm Hg maximum pressure or has profound architectural distortion, it is very difficult to ascertain accurate parameters either by mathematical methods or by eyeball examination. In such circumstances, this program will interpret as sphincter only that portion which forms the largest continuous data segment corresponding to the criteria for sphincter inclusion. An indication of how much possible sphincter length may have been excluded from the mathematical sphincter determination is provided in the numeric report under the heading of length accuracy. In this case, length accuracy is 100%.

NUMERIC REPORT. The pertinent data segments from each resting longitudinal pullout profile run are incorporated into the appropriate section of the Numeric Report as follows:

RESTING PULL-OUT: type	FileID	AvgMax Pres	Single Max Pres	length (mm)	length accuracy	verge to max pres
PO	594PO2	81.7	90.8	49.5	100.0%	17.0
PO	594PO3	84.7	99.2	48.5	100.0%	18.5

verge to max pres	Vol^3	¦--- Asymmetry ---¦ SPHINCT	HPZ	Density	lumen pres
17.0	330894	27.1%	11.2%	6685	4.4
18.5	327052	27.1%	10.8%	6743	3.7

In addition, the data segments from each run are added to a data base on the hard disc.

Average Maximum Pressure. The maximum value for the average of the eight radial channels is provided.

Length. The sphincter length, in millimeters, is listed.

Verge to Maximum Pressure. This length in millimeters is the distance from the anal verge to the point of maximum average pressure.

Volume.[3] This is the summation of the area of each 45-degree pressure vector in mm Hg^2 for cross-sections that comprise what has been determined to be the sphincter. This pressure–volume result is a quantitation of the overall "umph" of the sphincter.

Asymmetry Sphincter. Each cross-section is assessed for asymmetry. If all eight channels in a given cross-section had identical pressures, the asymmetry for that cross-section would be 0.0%. If seven channels had identical pressures and one channel had a pressure of zero, the asymmetry would be 25%, etc. The average asymmetry of all cross-sections that comprise the sphincter is the Sphincter Asymmetry.

SUMMARY REPORT. The average value for each of the major numeric parameters for all of the resting Longitudinal Pullout profile runs is subsequently incorporated into the one-page Summary Report.

```
Longitudinal Sphincter Profile
 (continuous pullout):
 RESTING PROFILE:   # of runs            2
|-------------------------- -------------- -------------|
   Maximum Avg. Pressure             83.2 mmHg       1.5 sd
   Pressure-volume                 328973 mmHg3     1921 sd
   Sphincter length                  49.0 mm         0.5 sd
   Verge to Max Pressure             17.8 mm         0.8 sd
   Rectal lumen pressure              4.1 mmHg       0.4 sd
  Cross-sectional Asymmetry
   Sphincter                         27.1%
   HPZ                               11.0%
```

In addition, the data segment of this average value is added to a data base on the hard disc.

Graphs—Individual

Although numeric analysis is essential to the proper quantitative characterization of sphincter function, it is the graphic display that is likely to most readily convey this information to knowledgeable physicians.

A set of 14 graphs is created for each run. The most salient of these follow:

GRAPH A—LONGITUDINAL PROFILE WITH P3/A3

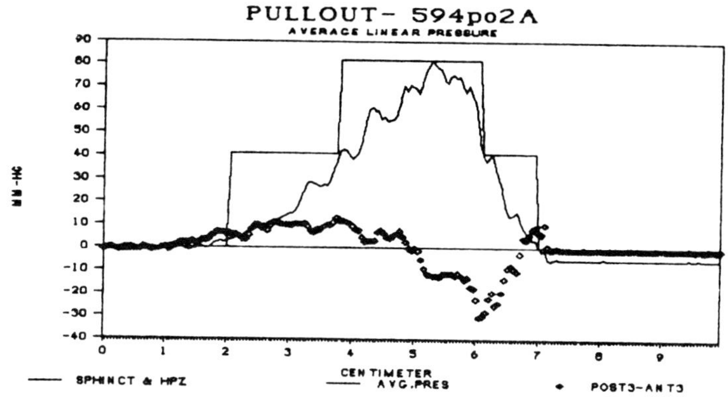

This graph is the same as described above except that an additional graph line has been added—P3/A3. This line describes the relative contribution of the posterior and anterior pressure components throughout the sphincter. The anterior pressure vectors are subtracted from the posterior vectors. When above zero, posterior predominates; when below zero, anterior predominators. The cross-over is generally in the vicinity of the maximum average pressure.

GRAPH C—RADIAL CROSS-SECTION

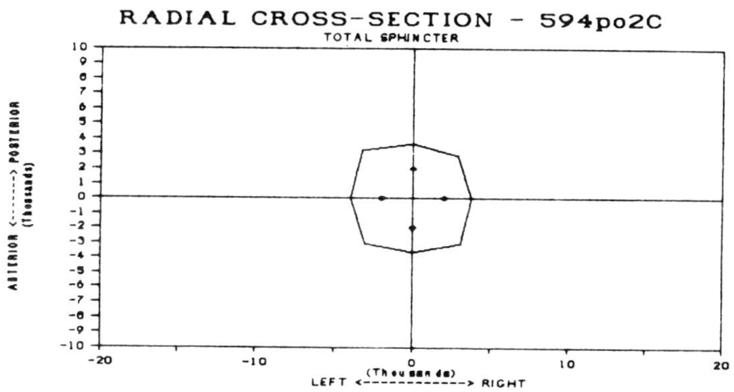

The cumulative pressure vectors for each 45 degrees of all cross-sections that compromise the sphincter are displayed. The view is as if one were looking at the sphincter, end-on, with the patient on a protoscopy table; posterior is at 12 o'clock. The units are arbitrary and have no true scale value. The tic marks on the X and Y axis have equidistant value from the center to assist in judging asymmetry should the graphs be plotted with a scale other than that for which they are designed. A more thorough view of cross-sectional asymmetry is provided in Graphs G–K.

GRAPH G—RADIAL CROSS-SECTION, PROXIMAL 20%

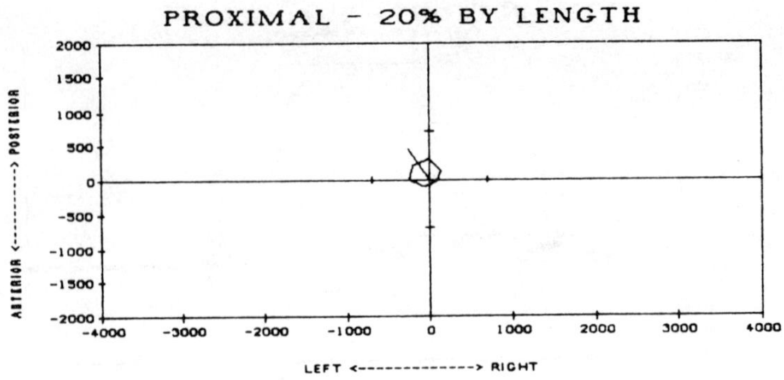

The cumulative pressure vectors for each 45 degrees of the proximal one-fifth of the sphincter, by length are displayed. The scale values are arbitrary. The X and Y axis tic marks represent equidistant values from the center. The vector line is indicative of the magnitude and direction of the net predominant pressure.

GRAPH H—RADIAL CROSS-SECTION, PROXIMAL 20–40%

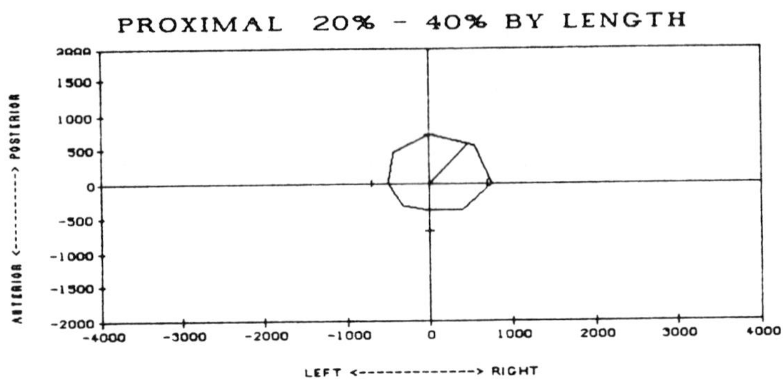

Similar to Graph G, but for the next one-fifth of sphincter, by length.

GRAPH I—RADIAL CROSS-SECTION, MIDDLE 20%

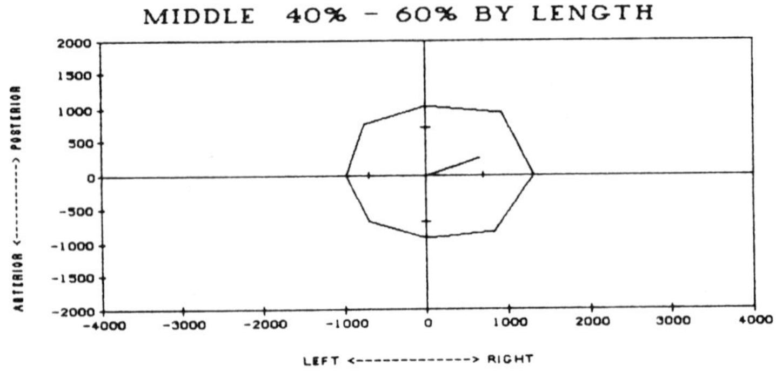

Similar to Graph G, but for the middle one-fifth of the sphincter, by length.

GRAPH J—RADIAL CROSS-SECTION, DISTAL 60–80%

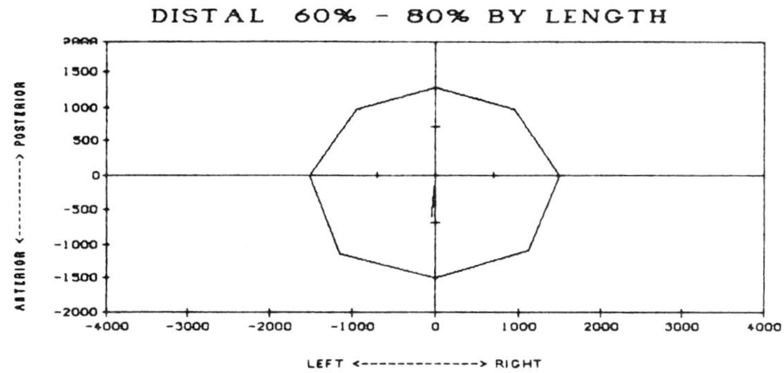

Similar to Graph G, but for the next one-fifth of the sphincter, by length.

GRAPH K—RADIAL CROSS-SECTION, DISTAL 20%

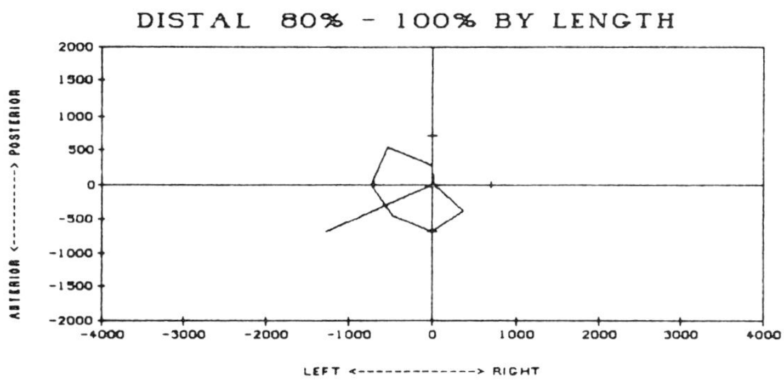

Similar to Graph G, but for the last one-fifth of the sphincter, by length.

For the most part, the above five cross-sections demonstrate a typically normal asymmetry pattern. There is a posterior predominance in the proximal sphincter; a more symmetrical appearance in the mid to mid-distal sphincter; and an anterior predominance in the most distal segment. However, in this instance, the distal 20% cross-section demonstrates a specific right lateral and right posterior quadrant deficit. Such localized segmental defects may not be readily suspected on the cumulative cross-section of the total sphincter, Graph C.

GRAPH 3-D

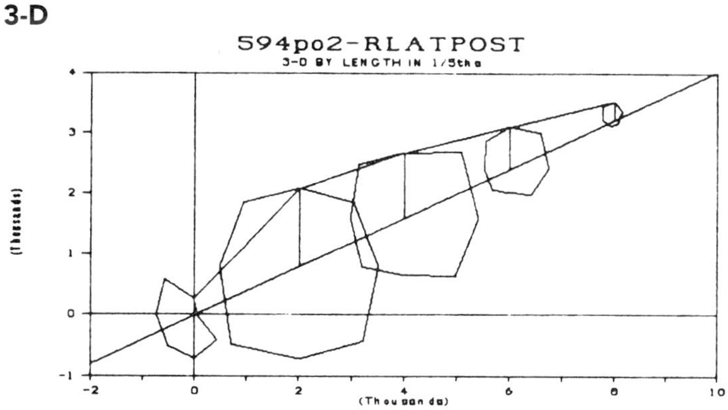

This graph is a pseudo 3-D composite of Graphs G–K. The representation is as if one were viewing the sphincter from the right posterior–lateral posterior position with the patient on the proctoscopy examination table. The rectal lumen is at the right upper corner; the anal verge is at the left lower corner.

Graphs—Summary

If a Longitudinal Squeeze Pullout profile (same protocol as Longitudinal Resting except that patient is squeezing while the probe traverses the sphincter) has also been performed, the difference between rest and squeeze will be displayed.

GRAPH DPAA—RESTING VS. SQUEEZE, MAXIMUM AVERAGE PRESSURE

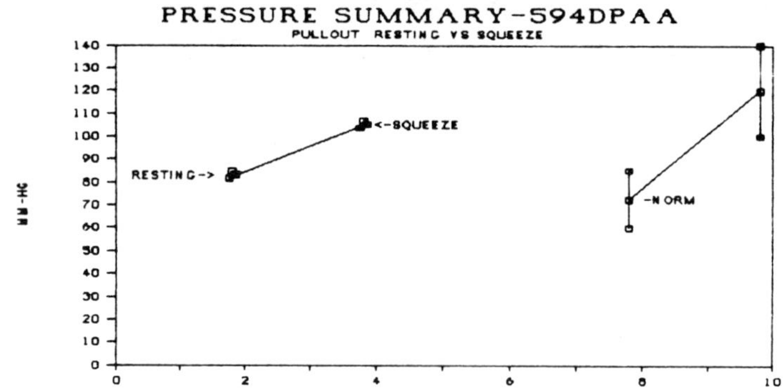

On the left side of the graph, the maximum average resting pressure for each run is plotted. If a Longitudinal Squeeze profile has been performed, the maximum average squeeze pressure for each run is plotted as the next data group. A line connects the mean of the two data groups. On the right side of the graph a "normal" resting versus squeeze is displayed. This is provided as a graphic reference comparison aid. It is not implied that results outside of the reference are necessarily abnormal. It should be borne in mind that an accurate maximum pressure during squeeze pullout will depend upon fatigability.

Examples of Abnormal Longitudinal Resting Profile

LOSS OF INTERNAL SPHINCTER

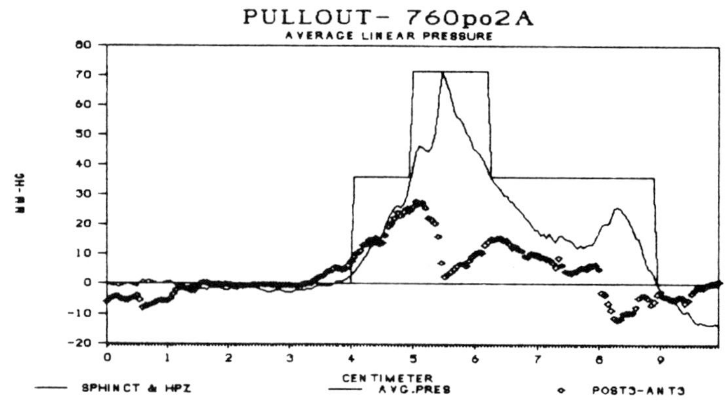

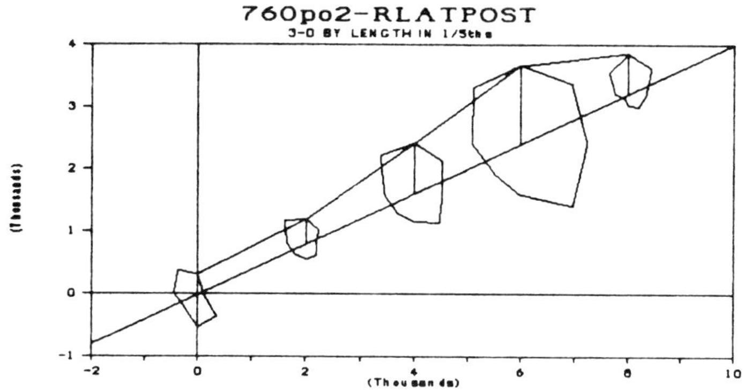

This 62-year-old male sustained injury to the anal canal resulting in morphological loss of the internal anal sphincter. His symptoms consisted of leakage and urgency without gross fecal accidents. There is marked proximal displacement of the HPZ with symmetrical loss of resting pressure in the mid and distal anal canal.

PRIMARY ANAL SPHINCTER HYPERTONIA

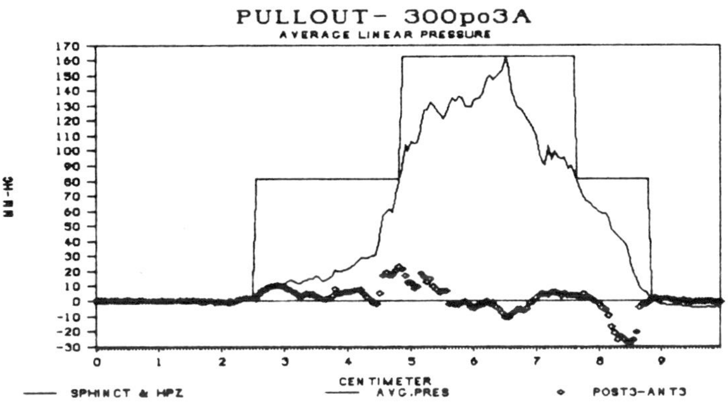

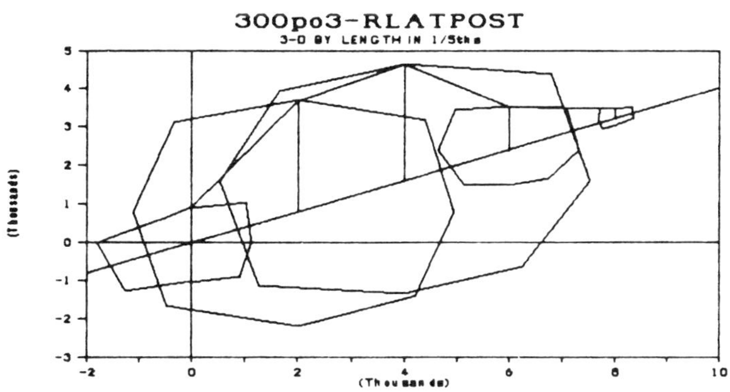

This 45-year-old male has severe pelvic discomfort and inability to initiate defecation without numerous large enemas. The overall sphincter length is excessive (6.4 cm) and the maximum average resting pressure of 162 mm Hg is exceptionally high. This is central displacement of the HPZ with nearly 3 cm of sphincter length having pressure greater than 80 mm Hg.

Longitudinal Squeeze Pullout (PS)

PURPOSE. The purpose of the Longitudinal Squeeze Pullout is to obtain a continuous pressure profile of the entire sphincter during squeeze. This is performed by motorized withdrawal of an eight-channel radial cross-sectional probe during squeeze. The protocol is conducted in a fashion similar to that which is performed during rest. Consequently, a direct comparison may be made between the resting sphincter and the augmentation that is provided by the external voluntary sphincter.

EQUIPMENT. The recording probe, probe withdrawal device, and technique of probe insertion are the same as described under Longitudinal Resting Pullout profile protocol.

DATA ACQUISITION. Before acquiring data it should be ascertained that the patient understands what is implied by squeeze because the patient's perception of squeeze may vary from simply holding the breath to bearing down; just opposite to what is desired. To avoid bringing into play unnatural forces, the examiner should use a consistent command while instructing the patient to squeeze. It is equally important for the examiner to frequently repeat the command "keep squeezing" during the recording time to prevent the patient from ceasing the voluntary effort before the run is completed.

During the recording it is essential to ensure that the instruction to squeeze is given before the recording probe reaches the anticipated beginning of the proximal sphincter. This is to avoid missing a part of the sphincter, which could occur if the patient is instructed to squeeze after the probe has already entered the proximal sphincter, thereby compromising the accuracy of the results.

SAVING THE DATA. After completing each Longitudinal Squeeze Pullout run, one needs to decide on the technical adequacy of the run. The following factors should be considered:

- Is the whole length of sphincter included in the recording; following 20 sec within the rectum?
- Was the patient squeezing in a steady fashion and not vacillating between squeeze and relaxation as shown by wide fluctuation in pressures?

TECHNICAL ACCEPTABLE RUN. If the run is technically acceptable and was performed in accordance with protocol, it may be saved by selecting Save from the menu choice. A technically adequate run will record the entire sphincter during squeeze period and this is indicated by a slow step-wise increase in sphincter pressures.

TECHNICALLY UNACCEPTABLE RUN. If the run is technically inadequate, it should not be saved. The most frequent error in performing Longitudinal Squeeze Pullout is to miss the proximal sphincter because of perineal ascent when squeeze is initiated. This is usually indicated by an abrupt pressure increase.

COMMENT. After a pullout squeeze run, it may be helpful to record the duration of squeeze effort, e.g., "sq. 20–80" and the distance the pressure recording orifices are from the anal verge, e.g. "3 cm out."

NUMBER OF RUNS. A minimum of two uniform Longitudinal Squeeze Pullout runs should be performed.

ANALYSIS. The summary report of squeeze profile is described with the same numeric parameters as Longitudinal Resting Pullout profile. Typically, during voluntary squeeze, an increase of at least 50–100% in the average maximal pressure above the average maximum resting pressure occurs.[3] Similarly, there is augmentation of pressure-volume and sphincter length during voluntary squeeze. Characteristically, the cross-sectional asymmetry in the sphincter as a whole and in the high-pressure zone within the sphincter decreases on squeeze.

CLINICAL APPLICATIONS OF LONGITUDINAL PRESSURE PROFILES. A quick glance at longitudinal profile may indicate to the investigator the likely pathology e.g., a short anal canal with globally low pressures may suggest neurogenic basis for fecal incontinence. Conversely, a localized segmental defect may indicate a traumatic sphincter injury as the possible cause of fecal incontinence. Cross-sectional analysis of longitudinal profile may precisely lateralize the sphincter defect or localize it to the proximal or distal part of the sphincter. Presence of high cross-sectional asymmetry in the entire sphincter and particularly in the high-pressure zone may indicate an unfavorable outcome after biofeedback therapy for fecal incontinence.[4] A bell-shaped pressure curve with high anal pressures is commonly seen in patients with fissure in ano.[5]

The failure of augmentation of anal canal pressures or sphincter length on pullout squeeze denotes external anal sphincter weakness. A similar conclusion may be drawn if the cross-sectional asymmetry fails to decrease on pullout squeeze.

RESTING MOTILITY WITH RADIAL (MR) PROBE PROTOCOL

Purpose

The purpose of the stationary resting motility protocol as performed with a radial probe is to identify and quantitate the presence of intrinsic cyclical activity which characterizes many anal sphincters and is attributed primarily to the internal sphincter. The intrinsic slow wave has a frequency of 10–20 cycles per minute and a relative low amplitude ranging from just above physiologic noise to 10 mm Hg. The ultra slow wave is seen on occasion and can be most dramatic. This has a slow frequency of 0.7–1.2 cycles/min with amplitudes that may exceed

100 mm Hg. Motility using the radial probe is intended to maximize the ability to identify and quantitate these waves at any one level of the sphincter.

It should be recognized from the onset that quantitation of complex, multifrequency, nonperiodic (in the mathematic sense) wave forms is an extremely complicated process. There are numerous cyclical activities (respiratory, cardiac, peristaltic, etc.) that may influence the composite sphincter wave form. This program makes no pretext of being able to distinguish the individual components with such certainty that the derived values and graphic representations can be accepted with blind faith. One must decide upon acceptance of these data by careful examination of the data, graphs, and conditions under which the procedures were performed.

Equipment

PROBE. A type A probe (Fig. 7.1) with eight radially oriented channels in cross-section is used. Axial orientation with Channel 8 at the posterior midline is maintained.

PROBE WITHDRAWAL DEVICE (OPTIONAL). Although the probe withdrawal device in not activated during motility data acquisition, it is a convenient device to use for maintaining axial orientation as well as sequential position of the probe at different points along the sphincter.

Preliminary Procedure

ZERO BASELINING. Zero baselining of the probe is performed with the probe at the level of the anal verge.

Examination Procedure

RESTING MOTILITY DISPLAY. The resting motility display is selected from the Procedure Menu.

PROBE INSERTION. The well-lubricated probe is inserted so that the radial orifices are at about the proximal level of the anal sphincters. In order to judge the level at which the probe is being inserted, pressure recording is started on the CRT. Using the manual control on the pull withdrawal device, the probe is withdrawn to the level of the sphincters from which recording is desired. If the probe is withdrawn too far, the motor can be reversed. A representative slow wave motility pattern is usually best observed at a point that is approximately half to three-quarters of the distance between the proximal end of the sphincter and the point of maximum pressure. Ultraslow waves will be best demonstrated in the vicinity of the maximum average pressure.

MARKING THE ANAL VERGE. It is generally not necessary to place a gauze to mark the level of the anal verge for motility recording. However, the depth of insertion of the radial orifice should be noted from the markings on the probe.

DATA ACQUISITION. It is important that the patient be relaxed, at rest and not move during the 100-sec recording. The patient should be reassured that there will be no surprises during the run. The CRT should be observed during the run to determine if there is indeed stability of the average pressure recording. If the run is started immediately after manipulation of the catheter, there may be an initial high pressure in all channels which promptly decreases to a steady average pressure. This indicates insufficient time for the sphincter to accommodate to the position manipulation. When this lack of steady state becomes apparent, the run should be restarted so as not to include these early artifacts. On occasion, the sphincter will exhibit large ultraslow waves in the 0.7–1.2 cycle per minute frequency. Although it may not be apparent initially that this is a pressure phenomenon rather than lack of achieving a steady average pressure state, the persistence of these waves will become evident. Under such circumstances, one will not be able to obtain a steady average state. This is really of little concern because, after all, the detection of ultraslow waves is one of the objectives of doing a resting motility in the first place.

Saving the Data

Quantitation of an anal sphincter slow wave is a delicate matter. These tend to have low amplitude (physiologic noise up to a few mm Hg) and a frequency close to that of respiration. Not infrequently, they may be overshadowed by transmitted respiratory movement obscuring the detection of any slow wave that may exist. Consequently, except for the occasional, unavoidable presence of ultraslow waves, only those runs that are technically free of artifact—e.g., unstable average pressure, cough, patient movement—should be saved as an acceptable Motility run.

Comment Entry

The depth at which the recording orifices were located relative to the anal verge should be recorded as a comment on a Motility run.

Number of Runs

The clinical usefulness of slow wave and ultraslow wave quantitation is vague at best. However, they certainly are associated with certain alterations of sphincter function. If one is going to perform a Motility run at all, it is best to perform at least two runs, at each level of the sphincter that is examined. The most rewarding level for the observation of slow waves is on the proximal side of the maximum pressure point, about halfway between the proximal end and the maximum pressure. If the recording orifices are too close to the rectum, it is likely that intrarectal pressure oscillations, primarily of respiratory origin, will be confused with true intrasphincteric slow waves. As one proceeds distally in the sphincter, there is a general degradation of the slow wave. The best location for ultraslow wave is generally in the vicinity of the maximum average pressure.

To achieve a number of runs at different levels, it is most convenient to use the puller motor with the manual switch in order to withdraw the probe 0.5 or 1.0 cm at a time.

Analysis

GENERAL CONSIDERATIONS. As stated at the beginning of this section, the identification and quantitation of an intrinsic slow wave by this program is "soft" data. The program is designed to facilitate the identification of wave forms and provide numeric results that may be accepted as reasonable representation. Neither the graphic nor numeric result should be accepted with the type of certainty that one has for an EKG tracing or serum sodium. The basic methodology used for this program is that of multiple running average reduction.

There are a number of factors that are responsible for impression in wave form analysis:

1. *Nonperiodic.* The waves under consideration are biological events of varying amplitude and frequency. They are not precisely recurring mathematical periodic signals.

2. *Multiplicity.* What we view as the slow wave is not necessarily the result of a single recurring biological event. It is certainly modulated by other factors and consequently is a composite wave itself.

3. *Amplitude.* In general, even when clearly discernible, the slow wave has an amplitude that is only a fraction of the basal sphincter pressure upon which it resides.

The highest mean amplitude that I have observed is 19 mm Hg in a sphincter with a maximum resting pressure of 64 mm Hg. This is exceptional in that the mean amplitude is usually in the 2–5 mm Hg range.

The typical low slow-wave amplitude means that it is often difficult to distinguish slow wave from biological noise or other remote influences. This is particularly true at the proximal end of the sphincter where intraluminal pressures, often associated with respiration, may have an overwhelming influence. This problem is compounded by the fact that respiratory frequency is similar to that of the slow wave.

4. *Frequency.* When attempting to discern wave forms of similar characteristics or that are marginally more prevalent than the random events of background noise, it is common to employ long recording time, e.g., 30 min to several hours. Consequently, a sampling for only 100 sec per run, during which time there may be only 12–25 full cycles of a slow wave represents a distinct limitation of precise analysis. On the other hand, the tendency to occur in burst of activity often means that a slow wave pattern will not last throughout the 100 sec. It is also readily apparent that the presence of an ultraslow wave, with a frequency of 1 cycle/minute will not be seen, if present, for two full cycles.

Despite the foregoing limitations, it is surprising how frequently, after examination of the numeric and graphic results, one can conclude that the analysis program has resulted in a reasonably appropriate quantitation. One can obtain an appreciation for the numeric and graphic representation by performing a test run, producing an artificial slow wave and ultraslow wave. After preparing the system just as you would for patient testing, raise the perfused radial probe to about 60 cm above the zero baseline level. Start a motility-radial run. Smoothly, cycle the probe tip between 60 and 70 cm above baseline every 6 sec. Repeat the run using the same 6-sec oscillation, but superimposed upon an overall probe height change that varies between 40 and 80 cm, twice during the 100-sec run. Processing these two runs by DPA will provide an appreciation of how an artificially created slow wave and ultraslow wave appear with the Analysis Program.

In accessing the validity of motility analysis, the following points should be examined:

1. *Slow-wave amplitude.* If average amplitude is less than 1 mm Hg, one should be suspicious that there is no discernible slow wave. Most likely, the transmitted respiratory wave is more predominant than any slow wave. Despite the clear appearance of the slow wave graph, it must be determined that it is not synchronous with respiration before considering it to be a valid slow wave.

2. *Slow wave frequency.* The data-values for respiration and slow wave matching should be examined. If each slow wave peak matches a respiratory peak within 0.5 sec time interval greater than 80% of the time, then one must have increased caution about accepting the slow wave as a distinct entity.

3. *Average pressure stability.* If the average pressure graph does not reflect a stable recording state throughout, the numeric result and subsequent graphs will be compromised. The program can not distinguish patient movement, cough, etc.

NUMERIC REPORT. The data segments from each motility radial run are incorporated into the designated section of the Numeric Report pages.

MOTILE2-RADIAL PROBE:			avg pres	SLOW WAVE freq	Amplitude (mm-Hg)		
type	FileId	comment	(mm-Hg)	c/min	avg	max	min
mr	594ot2	1.5 cm in	75.2	12.6	7.1	12.9	2.7

Average pressure. The average pressure throughout the entire run is provided.

Slow wave cycle/min. The derived frequency of the slow wave.

Slow-wave amplitude. The amplitude of a single cycle is taken as twice the maximum positive value of each cycle that is counted as a separate cycle. The average amplitude is the average of the individually counted cycles. The minimum amplitude is twice the lowest positive amplitude that registers as a cycle. The maximum amplitude is twice the maximum positive peak.

Respiratory rate. The rate as derived from the respiratory transducer is provided. Note: If the respiratory channel is not used, a spurious rate will be recorded from the electrical signal noise.

Respiratory/slow wave match. The last four columns provide additional data for distinguishing respiratory from slow wave. This check helps to accommodate different respiratory recording devices. The percentage of respiratory peaks that exactly match or match within 0.5 sec of a slow wave peak and the percentage of slow wave peaks that exactly match within 0.5 sec of a respiratory peak is provided. As match category approaches or exceeds 80%, one should suspect that slow wave results are actually reflecting respiration.

The data segment from each run is added to the database file on the hard disc.

SUMMARY REPORT. The slow wave frequency and amplitude values for the run that has the highest average pressure is included in the Summary Report. Although this may not be the best or most characteristic run for that patient, it is likely to be a more accurate portrayal than the average of all motility-radial runs. Automatic selection of a run with the greatest slow wave amplitude, among two similar runs, is most likely to pick the run with the greatest single artifact.

```
STA MOTILITY: RADIAL PROBE-Maximum Station:# of  runs=      1
   Avg pressure=                        75.2 mmHg
   Slow wave approximation:
       frequency=                       12.6 c/min    Min    Max
       amplitude=          Avg=          7.1 mmHg     2.7   12.9
```

Graphs—Individual

Twelve graphs are generated for each run. The three most salient graphs are demonstrated below.

GRAPH A—AVERAGE AND REDUCED AVERAGE

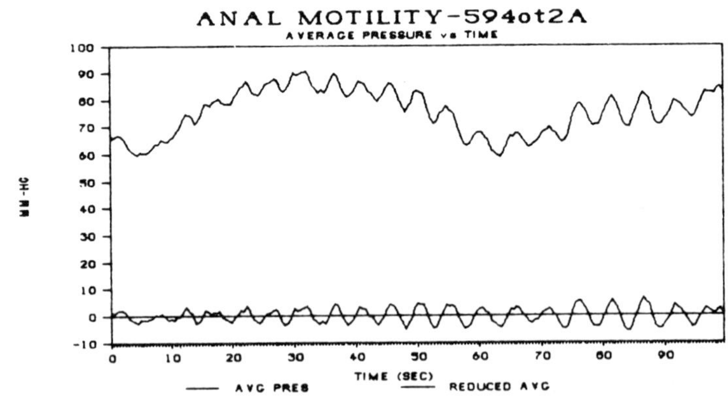

The average pressure for all channels is displayed. On the zero Y axis, the reduced average pressure is plotted.

GRAPH B—SLOW WAVE MOTILITY

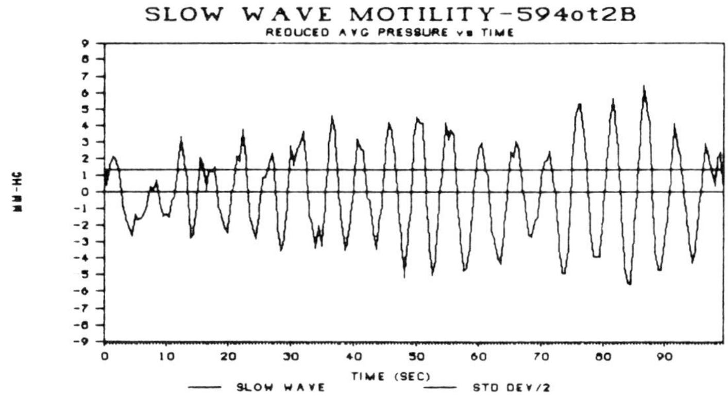

The reduced average, as displayed in Graph A, is plotted on the zero Y-axis with expanded scale. The horizontal line above the zero axis is the minimal level that must be exceeded for a positive peak to be considered for inclusion as a cycle.

GRAPH C—ULTRASLOW WAVE MOTILITY

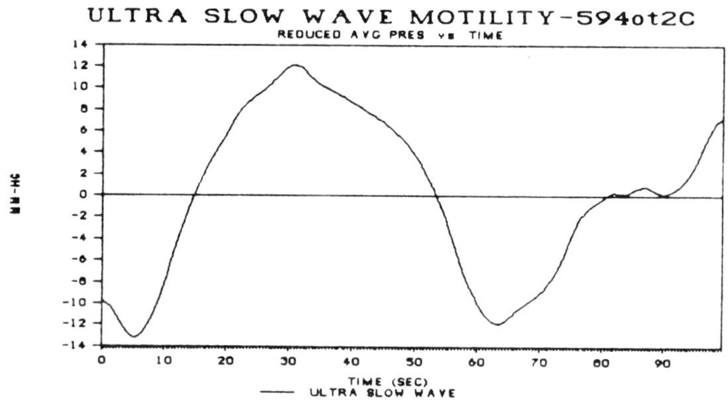

This graph represents the residual unreduced average pressure over the course of the entire run. As such, it forms a representation of the ultraslow wave activity, if present. In this instance, an ultraslow wave with an amplitude of approximately 25 mm Hg and a period of approximately 57 sec is displayed.

CLINICAL SIGNIFICANCE OF ANAL MOTILITY STUDIES. Ultraslow waves are seen more often in patients with high resting anal canal pressures, e.g., in patients with anal fissues, hemorrhoids, and primary sphincter hypertonia. The presence of prominent ultraslow anal waves and high anal pressures in patients with constipation suggests exclusion of outlet obstruction as the cause of constipation. Our recent study has demonstrated that in patients with fecal incontinence ultra-slow waves are infrequently observed.[6] While it is possible that low anal canal pressures in these patients preclude detection of large-amplitude ultraslow waves, the neurogenic basis for such findings cannot be discounted. This study has further suggested that manometric anal waves, if present, retain their normal frequency.[6] However, the diagnostic significance of manometric anal waves and their cause-and-effect relation to anal pressures remain unclear.

STATION SQUEEZE WITH RADIAL PROBE PROTOCOL (SR)

Squeeze Radial (sr)

Purpose

The purpose of the Stationary Squeeze protocol as performed with the radial probe is to obtain an assessment of voluntary sphincter capability at one or more levels in the sphincter.

The program quantitates both voluntary augmentation of sphincter tone and the fatigability of augmentation. This differs from the Resting versus Squeeze comparison provided by the longitudinal profile protocols in that only one level of the sphincter is being compared at a time. Consequently, at any point along the sphincter, this protocol may be expected to provide a more accurate picture of squeeze capabilities. Furthermore, if rapid fatigue is present, it will be apparent that squeeze assessment throughout the duration of a pullout will probably not register the maximum obtainable squeeze pressure.

Equipment

PROBE. A type-A Probe (Fig. 7.1) with eight radially oriented channels in cross-section is used. Axial orientation with Channel 8 at the posterior midline is maintained.

PROBE WITHDRAWAL DEVICE (OPTIONAL). Although the probe withdrawal device is not activated during Stationary Squeeze data acquisition, it is a convenient device to use for maintaining axial orientation as well as sequential positioning of the probe at different points along the sphincter.

Preliminary Procedure

ZERO BASELINING. Zero baselining of the probe is performed with the probe at the level of the anal verge.

Examination Procedure

STATIONARY SQUEEZE DISPLAY. The Stationary Squeeze display is obtained on the CRT.

PROBE INSERTION. Prior to probe insertion, it should be determined that the patient understands what is meant by the instruction to "squeeze." This is best appreciated with digital examination. During the instruction session, also note the degree to which the perineum moves with squeeze.

The well-lubricated probe is inserted so that the radial orifices are at about the proximal level of the anal sphincter. In order to judge the level at which the probe is being inserted, pressure recording is started on the CRT and the depth markings are noted on the probe. The probe can be positioned by hand or with the assistance of the probe withdrawal device.

Positioning with Probe Withdrawal Device. There are two advantages to using the probe withdrawal device: Radial orientation is maintained and sequential station selection is facilitated. However, it must be cautioned that the level of pelvic floor is likely to ascend during squeeze. If the probe is fixed and not allowed to move with the pelvic floor ascent, the position of the recording orifices will change during squeeze and the quantitative accuracy of the run will be compromised. Therefore, the probe external to the anal verge should not be completely taut during this type of run. If there is considerable perineal movement during squeeze, it is best to have the probe holder at an angle of about 45 degrees to the axis of the anal canal rather than straight in line as is used for the longitudinal pullout. This permits the probe to ride with the pelvic floor movement while ensuring radial orientation of the recording orifices.

Positioning by Hand. The probe may be held in place using the thumb and index finger of the left hand with the palm resting steadily on the buttock. During squeeze, the probe must be permitted to ride with pelvic floor movement. One is cautioned that maintaining axial orientation is a bit more difficult by hand.

If several stations are going to be evaluated, it is easiest to start at the proximal sphincter and work outwards, noting the depth of the probe markings with each run. If only the maximum pressure area is being assessed, the location is found while observing the CRT display.

MARKING THE ANAL VERGE. It is generally not necessary to place gauze at the level of the anal verge for Stationary Squeeze recording.

DATA ACQUISITION *Initial Resting Phase.* It is important that the patient be relaxed and at rest during the first 30 sec of recording. The patient should be reassured that there will be no surprises during the run. The CRT should be observed during the run to determine if there is indeed stability of the average pressure recording. If the run is started immediately after manipulation of the catheter, there may be an initial high pressure in all channels which promptly decreases to a steady average pressure. When this lack of a steady state becomes apparent, the run should be restarted so as not to include these early artifacts. On occasion, the sphincter will exhibit large ultraslow waves in the 0.7–1.2 cycle per minute range. Although it may not be apparent initially that this is a pressure phenomenon rather than lack of achieving a steady average pressure state, the persistence of these waves will become evident. Under such circumstances, one will not be able to obtain a steady average state.

For quantitative accuracy, it is important that the initial 30 sec is as steady a pressure level as possible.

Squeeze Phase. At 20 seconds, a prompt will appear to "squeeze." The patient should be instructed to squeeze and repeatedly reminded to keep squeezing throughout the next 40 sec. The analysis program will assess all of the pressure activity between 32 and 70 sec as belonging to squeeze. The 2-sec hiatus from 30 to 32 sec is to permit a reasonable transition from rest to squeeze.

Translating a verbal voluntary command with a consistent patient reaction is obviously as much art as it is science. The onset of squeeze should be prompt, complete, and maintained. However, the patient should not be terrified into total body tetany. Steady squeeze should be volitional rather than cycles of brief squeeze and rest. One should observe the degree of pelvic ascent and buttock contribution.

Resume Phase. At 70 sec, a "relax" prompt will appear. The patient is instructed to stop squeezing. Cessation of squeeze should not be so abrupt as to displace the probe from its position in the sphincter. The patient should not treat this phase as the end of recording. The last 20 sec of the run is used to determine if the probe is reading the pressures similar to the initial resting phase.

Saving the Data

Before saving, the CRT presentation is examined for acceptability. In order to minimize quantitative inaccuracies, runs that clearly do not comply with protocol should be either discarded or saved with an Other, "ot", designator.

The primary characteristics of a satisfactory squeeze run include stability of initial 30 sec; squeeze phase consistency; resume phase similar to initial resting phase; and absence of probe dislocation during the run.

Comment Entry

The depth at which the recording orifices were located relative to the anal verge should be the first part of any comment on a squeeze run. The entire comment will appear on the Technical Page of the report. Additional comments would include depth of probe at end of run if different from beginning; patient understanding of squeeze; pelvic floor movement; squeze with buttocks only; etc.

Number of Runs

If one is merely interested in obtaining a qualitative assessment of voluntary squeeze capability and fatigability, a single run obtained at about the level of the maximum resting pressure may suffice. This assumes that the patient clearly understood his/hor role and the run was performed with reasonable compliance to protocol. If a quantitative assessment for comparison with other patients is desired, it is certainly best practice to perform a minimum of two runs at the maximum average resting pressure level. If segmental voluntary squeeze augmentation is being evaluated, then paired runs at the level of interest should be performed. This is often the case in the distal sphincter when there has been a history of fistula surgery or delivery injury. If there is fatigue with Station Sqeeze, augmentation at various levels of the sphincter will require multiple Station Squeeze runs. However, if there is little or no fatigue, a continuous assessment of sphincter squeeze can be obtained with the Longitudinal Squeeze Pullout protocol.

Analysis

GENERAL CONSIDERATIONS. The average pressure of all eight radial channels is used to assess the station squeeze and fatigue character of the sphincter for each Station Squeeze run. A linear regression is performed on the data that is defined to be in the initial rest phase. Similarly, a linear regression is performed on the data that is defined as the squeeze interval, from32 sec and 70 sec. Finally, a linear regression is performed on the data segment between 80 sec and 100 sec onto the run. This is the pressure that the patient resumes after squeezing. It should be similar to the initial resting phase if the probe is recording at the same site.

NUMERIC REPORT. The data segment from each Station Squeeze run is incorporated into the designated section of the Numeric Report pages. This data segment is also added to the database log on the hard disc.

STA SQUEEZE-RADIAL PROB			resting		Squeeze		
		squ time	avg pres	drift	max increase		
type	FileID	(sec)	mmHg	mmHg/min	mmHg	%	delta
sr	613sr0	36	46.3	-12.8	92.9	100.7%	46.6

Squeeze				Resume	
avg increase			fatigue	avg pres	drift
mmHg	%	delta	mmHg/min	mmHg	mmHg/min
87.9	89.8%	41.6	-17.0	49.8	34.4

Average resting pressure. The average pressure of all channels during the initial resting phase is recorded.

Resting drift. The drift of the average pressure during the resting phase, as derived from the linear regression, is given in mm Hg/min. A negative value indicates an overall decreasing pressure.

Maximum squeeze increase. The maximum pressure of the linear regression line during squeeze is recorded. This is not the same as the highest recorded single pressure.

Maximum squeeze increase percent. The maximum squeeze increase is the percent increase of the maximum pressure of linear regression during squeeze relative to average resting pressure.

Maximum squeeze delta. The maximum squeeze delta is the pressure difference between average resting pressure and maximum squeeze pressure.

Average squeeze increase. The average pressure of the linear regression line during squeeze is recorded.

Average squeeze increase percent. The average squeeze increase percent is the increase of the average pressure of linear regression during squeeze relative to the average resting pressure.

Average squeeze increase delta. The average squeeze delta is the pressure difference between average resting pressure and average pressure of linear regression during squeeze.

Fatigue. The rate of pressure change in mm Hg per minute during linear regression of squeeze is indicated. A negative value indicates fatigue. A positive value indicates progressive augmentation during squeeze.

Average resume pressure. The average pressure during the last 20 sec is the average resume pressure.

Resume drift. The drift during the average resume pressure linear regression is provided.

SUMMARY REPORT. The numeric quantitation of the Station Squeeze run having the highest initial average resting pressure (the maximum station) is included in the one-page summary report. This data segment is also added to the database log on the hard disc.

```
STA SQUEEZE: RADIAL PROBE-Maximum Station: # of runs=          1
Initial resting pressure=       46.3 mmHg
Peak Squeeze=                  139.0 mmHg      92.7 delta     200.2%
Regression Max. Squeeze=        92.9 mmHg      46.6 delta     100.7%
Regression Avg. Squeeze=        87.9 mmHg      41.4 delta      89.8%
Fatigue=                       -17.9 mmHg/min       r-linear=  0.029
```

Peak squeeze. The linear regression maximum squeeze pressure value is a point on the regression line. The peak squeeze value is the single maximum average pressure value observed during the time of squeeze. It is my own impression that a momentary single unsustained peak is a less substantial characterization of effective voluntary squeeze than the linear regression derived value.

Comparison with Longitudinal Rest versus Squeeze. Theoretically, if the pressure orifices were located at the point of maximum sphincter pressure as seen on the Longitudinal Resting profile and if there was no fatigue during squeeze, the values for longitudinal pullout rest versus squeeze should be the same as the Station Squeeze run. There are a number of factors that result in a disparity between these two different assessment. On longitudinal runs, sphincter pressures are referenced to an intrarectal pressure of zero; Station Squeeze runs are referenced to atmospheric pressure. If sphincter fatigue is prominent, there will be an appreciable lessening of voluntary capability by the time the orifices reach the usual distally positioned maximum sphincter pressure during pullout. In such an instance, the Station Squeeze protocol would produce a more accurate picture of sphincter function than Longitudinal Squeeze profile.

Graphics—Individual

Twelve graphs are generated for each run. The three most salient graphs are demonstrated below:

GRAPH A—AVERAGE AND REDUCED AVERAGE

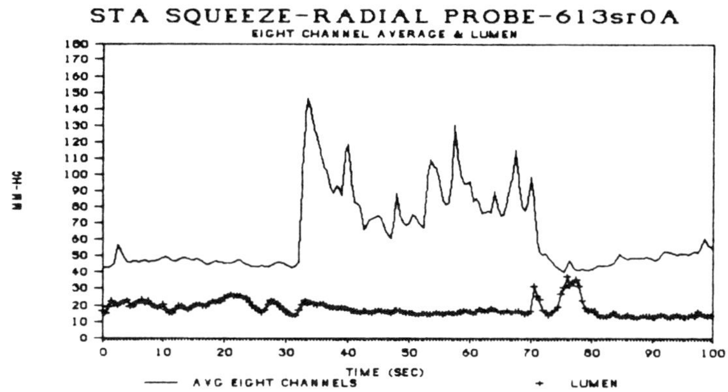

The average pressure for all channels is displayed. The reduced average pressure is plotted. Center lumen channel is plotted, if present.

GRAPH B—LINEAR REGRESSION OF REST, SQUEEZE AND RESUME

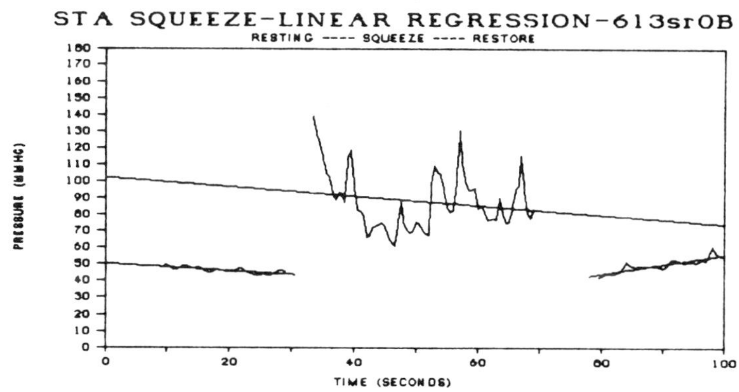

The eight-channel average pressure and the corresponding linear regression lines are displayed for the initial resting pressure phase, squeeze phase, and resume phase.

GRAPH C—RADIAL CROSS-SECTION OF STATION SQUEEZE

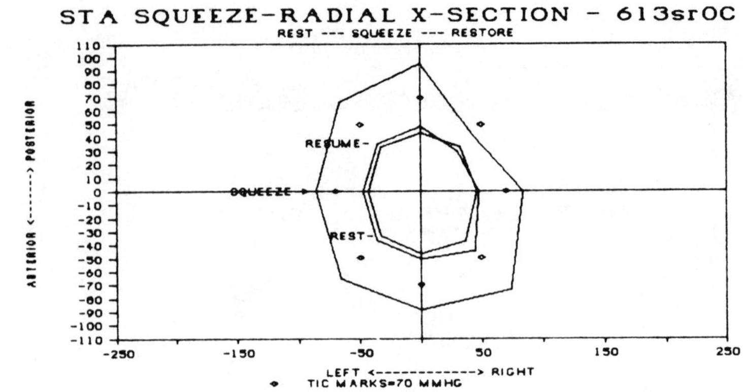

The cross-section during the initial rest, squeeze, and resume are displayed. The X and Y axis values correspond to average pressure. The unconnected tick marks are equivalant to a uniformly symmetric sphincter with average pressure of 75 mm Hg. In this case, there is a relative deficit of the right posterior lateral quadrant during squeeze.

Graphs—Summary

GRAPH DPAB

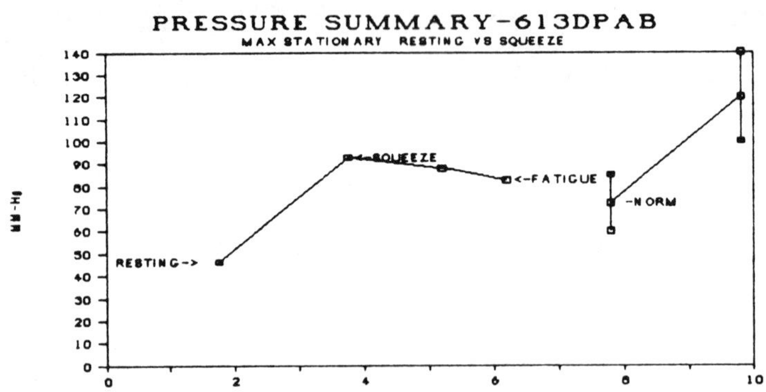

On the summary graph page, a representation of the maximum resting station graphis displayed.

BALLOON REFLEX EXCITATION/INHIBITION PROTOCOL, PROBE B-3 (bb)

Purpose

This protocol is for the quantitative assessment of the rectal anal inhibition reflex (RAIR) and the rectal anal excitation reflex (RAER). This program also provides the latency in seconds from balloon inflation to the time of maximum excitation (Le) and to the time of greatest inhibition (Li). Graphic representations display the cumulative excitatory and inhibitory components for the entire sphincter as well as for individual channels. A bar graph summarizes the prereflex resting pressure, the postinflation excitatory and inhibition response, and the final restoration pressure for each channel. A line graph displays the effect of the balloon distention on the sphincter longitudinal profile.

Standard format involves a 100-sec run. After 50 sec, the balloon is distended with 60 ml of air for 20 sec.

Equipment

1. Probe

A B-3 probe (Fig. 7.2) with eight spirally oriented channels and a balloon fixed to the top of the probe is used.

2. Balloon reflex stopcock assembly with a 140 ml Syringe
3. Anoscope

Although the B-3 probe can usually be inserted by digital guidance alone, a standard anoscope is useful for accurate positioning in some instances.

4. Narco ancillary unit for Balloon Reflex procedure

Preliminary Procedure

ZERO BASELINE. Pressures obtained during balloon reflex runs will be with respect to atmospheric pressure. Therefore, the zero baseline procedure should be performed with the probe at the level of the anal canal and with the balloon open to atmosphere.

Examination Procedure

BALLOON REFLEX DISPLAY. From the procedure menu, select the graphic display for performing balloon reflex manometry.

PROBE INSERTION. The well-lubricated evacuated balloon is guided into the anal canal with the index finger with as little mechanical stimulation as possible. Once in the ampulla, the balloon is encouraged to rest freely toward the sacral curve. The axial orientation of the probe should position the most distal perfusion orifice, Channel 8, at or within 1–2 mm of the anal verge in the posterior midline. Transient inflation of the balloon may help in positioning the balloon. Once in position, the probe should maintain its proper axial and longitudinal position without manual support.

In some circumstances, it may be easier to insert and position the probe through an anoscope.

DATA ACQUISITION. The operator should wait for about 10–20 sec after completing probe positioning before starting data calculation to permit the sphincter to settle down from any probe movement stimulation. During that interval, you should inform the patient that you will be recording information for about 2 min and that he or she should simply remain relaxed.

Before Balloon Reflex runs are performed, the integrity of rectal sensation and capacity is determined. Using a 140-ml syringe, the rectal balloon is inflated and the following are determined: minimal rectal volume perceived; volume giving rise to urge to defecate; and maximal tolerated volume. The information thus obtained may not only reveal a sensory deficit or compromised rectal capacity but is also utilized later to determine the limit of inflation that can be used safely in eliciting balloon reflex.

Prior to starting data acquisition, a syringe, filled with 20 ml of air, is affixed to the syringe port of the stopcock. During the first 50 sec of data acquisition, the pressure channels should exhibit a stable pressure level unless an ultraslow wave is prominent.

At 50 sec into the run, a prompt will appear to "Inflate" the balloon. A volume of 60 ml of air is incrusted smoothly and steadily over 3–5 secs.

During inflation, the probe position should be watched at the anal verge. Balloon distention may cause physical movement of the probe or the rectal stimulation may result in an expulsive force on the probe. Under such circumstances valuable reflex information may be obtained but the validity of quantitation may be compromised.

If the patient experiences unusual discomfort during inflation, the balloon should be deflated immediately and the position of the balloon should be checked to ensure that mechanical insult is not occurring.

At 70 sec, a prompt will appear to "deflate" the balloon. The balloon is vented to atmosphere.

The pressure reading obtained during the last 10 sec of the run will be used by the analysis program to compare with the 20-sec interval immediately preceding inflation. Comparison of these two pressure segments provides an indication of probe movement during balloon reflex. Examination of the probe at the anal verge will help to determine if probe movement has occurred. Is Channel 8 still located just at the anal verge in the posterior midline? If there is considerable difference in pressure levels for each channel for the 20 sec before inflation as compared to the level that is resumed during the last 10 sec of the run, the validity of the numeric quantitation of inhibition/excitation may be compromised. Although such a run may be numerically inaccurate, the graphic appearance of what occurs may still be informative.

The procedure is then repeated with 40, 60 and 120 ml of air as the distending volume. In patients with marked urgency or small rectal capacity, Balloon Reflex run with large volume inflation may have to be omitted or replaced with a small inflation volume to avoid patient discomfort. It is important to perform Balloon Reflex runs with different inflation volumes as outlined above because we have observed that whereas all normal subjects would reveal a reflex response at lower volumes (20 ml, 40 ml) of inflation, patients with neurogenic fecal incontinence who have blunted anorectal sensation or weak external anal sphincter may respond at high volume (60 ml, 120 ml) of inflation.[7]

Saving the Data

At the completion of the run, the decision to save or discard the data must be made. If the run has been performed according to technical protocol, then the run may be saved as is. A run that is saved as is will have a "bb" run designator indicating that this is a Balloon Reflex run performed with a B-3 probe, in accordance with the protocol. If there have been obvious breaches of protocol, e.g. patient movement, coughing, or probe movement, you may elect simply to discard the run entirely. Alternatively, if you have questions as to the validity of the run, it may be saved as an "ot" (other) run to avoid corrupting valid balloon runs. Some of the factors to examine in determining the reliability of a Balloon Reflex run are:

1. Is Channel 8 at or near zero value, indicating the distal limits of the sphincter?
2. Are the pressure readings of each channel stable during the 20 sec prior to balloon inflation?
3. Is the balloon pressure at or near zero throughout the entire time before balloon inflation?
4. Does the balloon pressure promptly increase at the point of balloon inflation?
5. Are the pressures for each channel during the last 10 sec of the run approximately equal to the pressures recorded during the 20-sec interval before balloon inflation?
6. Is the position of the probe at the anal verge at the same point at the end of the run as it was at the beginning?

Comment Entry

If the run is saved, the operator is requested to type in a comment. Any deviation from protocol or any observation that has bearing on the interpretation of the run should be included. Examples of comments that might be made include:

Sensation felt at 35 ml.
30 ml inflation.
Deflated after 6 sec.
Not valid; patient talking and/or laughing.
Probe moved outward 5 mm.
40 ml; no sensation felt, coughed at 90 sec.

Number of Runs

A minimum of four runs should be performed. The sequence of runs with progressively greater balloon volumes is best when assessing the reflex or sensation threshold.

Deviations from Protocol

An inflation time of more than or less than that which is indicated by the prompts (20 sec) can be used.

Analysis

The B-3 probe has eight spirally oriented channels that will encompass the full length of most sphincters. It is important to bear in mind that the anal sphincter is not symmetrical, either longitudinally or radially. Consequently, the spiral probe is used to obtain simultaneous longitudinal recording points recognizing that any single recording point may not be representative of the radial cross-section at that location.

During analysis by DPA, the pressure events at each location are analyzed individually and then combined to provide a composite numerical quantitation for the entire sphincter. To simplify the explanation of this analysis, an example of single channel is described. This example is in the distal portion of the sphincter (e.g., Channel 6), approximately 8 mm from the anal verge. Both excitatory and inhibitory components are present. A 60-ml balloon inflation has been used for 20 sec.

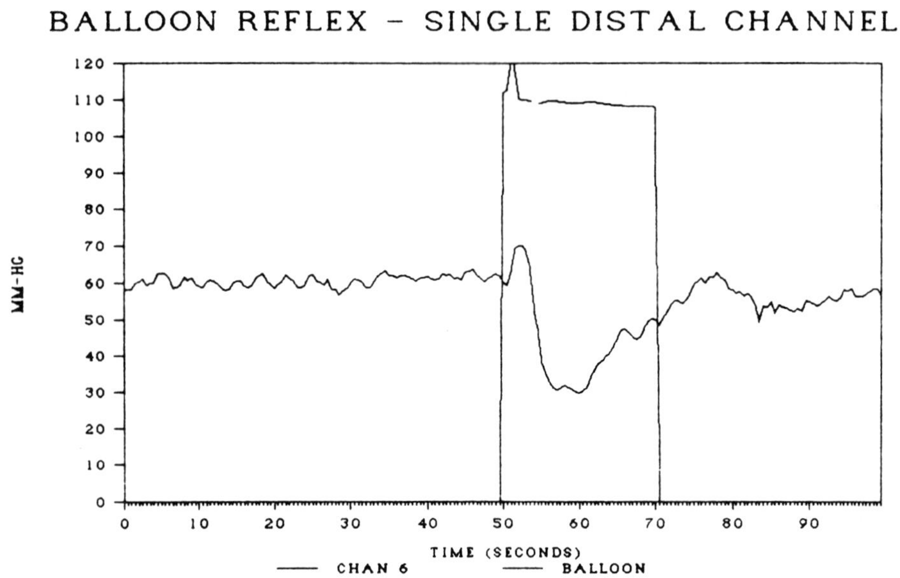

BALLOON PRESSURE DISPLAY. The balloon pressure is the somewhat rectangular plot from 50 to 71 sec. The preinflation interval is 50 sec. The balloon pressure during this interval will be displayed with a zero value. At 50 sec, during syringe inflation of the balloon, the actual balloon pressure will be displayed for pressures between zero and 100 mm Hg. Above 100 mm Hg, a balloon pressure of 100 mm Hg plus one-tenth of the balloon pressure over 100 mm Hg is displayed. At 70 sec into the run, the balloon has been evacuated and the balloon pressure returns to zero.

PREINFLATION SPHINCTER CHANNEL DISPLAY. During the 50-sec preinflation interval, the resting pressure in the sphincter channel is being recorded. The response to balloon distention will be compared to the average pressure recorded during the last 20 sec before balloon distention. In this case, a preinflation average "resting pressure" of 61.4 mm Hg is recorded during the interval between 30 and 50 sec. Only those channels that have an average resting pressure that exceeds the default "in sphincter" pressure value will be considered to reside sufficiently within the sphincter for purposes of numerical quantitation.

RESPONSE TO INFLATION.

Reflex time. DPA measures the changes that occur as a result of inflation for a predefined interval following onset of inflation. This interval is the *Reflex time,* defined as the interval after the onset of inflation during which the effects of inflation are measured. This is independent of the duration of actual balloon distention. The default Reflex time is 20 sec. Only those pressure events that occur during the first 20 sec that follow the onset of balloon distention will be considered to be a result of the reflex.

Excitation time. For each channel, excitation is considered to be present if, during the Reflex time interval, there is a pressure increase of more than 2 standard deviations (SD) above the resting pressure. The percentage increase of the maximum increase is the *percent excitation* for that channel. The time interval from the onset of balloon inflation to the maximum excitation pressure increase is the *Excitation Latency* (Le). In this case, maximum pressure of 70.2 mm Hg is reached, a 14.3% increase over the resting pressure of 61.4 mm Hg for this channel. The latency is 2.5 sec.

Inhibition Reflex. For each channel, Inhibition is considered to be present if, during the Reflex time interval, there is a pressure decrease of more than 2 SD below the resting pressure. The percentage decrease of the maximum decrease is the *percent inhibition* for that channel. The time interval from the onset of balloon inflation to the least inhibition pressure is the *Inhibition Latency* (Li). In this case, a minimum pressure of 29.8 mm Hg is reached, a 52.0% decrease from the resting pressure. The latency is 10.5 sec.

Post Inflation. The average pressure during the last 10 sec of the run is the *restoration pressure.* This is used in comparison with *resting pressure* to obtain an indication of the quality of the run especially from a probe movement standpoint. In this case, the restorative pressure is 56.4 mm Hg, an 8.1% decrease as compared to the resting pressure. Large discrepancies in the restore percent are usually the result of substantial probe movement during the run.

NUMERIC REPORT. Each individual channel, as described above, is integrated into a numeric quantitation of the entire sphincter.

The data segments from each individual Balloon Reflex run are subsequently incorporated into the appropriate section of the Numeric Report as follows. In addition, the data segment from each run is added to the database file on the hard disc.

BALLOON REFLEX-TYPE B-3 8-sphincter channels			# chan. in sphinct	Max.Avg Rest Pres.	¦---EXCITATION---------¦ # Excit Channels	% increase	Latency sec.(Le)
type	FileID	comment					
bb	5539bb3	60ml;8sec	5	54.5	2	13.5%	2.5

¦----INHIBITION------------¦ # Inhibit Channels	% decrease	Latency sec.(Li)	¦--RESUME--------¦ Avg Pres.	% change
5	64.4%	9.0	49.4	-9.3%

SUMMARY REPORT. The average value for each of the major numeric parameters for all of the balloon reflex runs is subsequently incorporated into the one-page Summary Report. In addition, the data segment of average values is added to the database log on the hard disc in the C:\DPA directory.

```
BALLOON REFLEX-cummulative approximation:   # of runs=      1
   Reference Resting Pres=       54.5 mmHg           5.0 avg # chan
   Excitation:                                       2.0 avg # chan
     linear change=              13.5% change
     latency=                     2.5 sec.
   Inhibition:                                       5.0 avg # chan
     linear change=              64.4% change
     latency=                     9.0 sec
   Restore=                      -9.3% diff from rest
```

Graphs—Individual

Eleven graphs are created for each run. Examples of four of the graphs are shown below.

GRAPH A—TOTAL EXCITATION AND INHIBITION

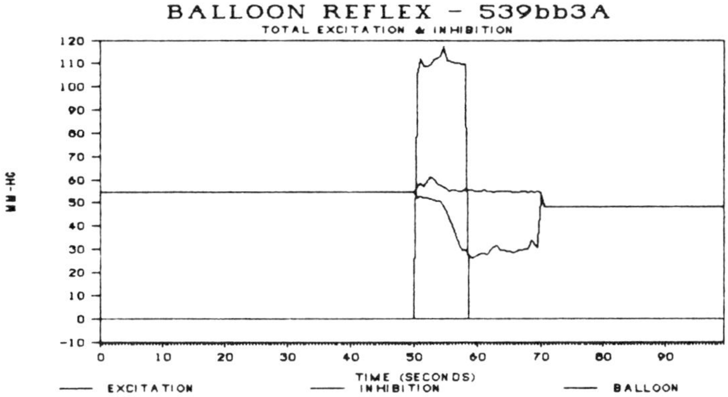

This is a composite graph designed to give an overall view of the effects of balloon inflation. The single horizontal graph line that precedes the onset of balloon inflation is the resting pressure of the channel with the maximum resting pressure, prior to balloon inflation. The summated results of channels residing in the sphincter are equated to this resting pressure. Balloon distention has been maintained for 8 sec. During the interval of reflex time that follows inflation, 20 sec in this case, the resting line splints. The upper line corresponds to the total excitatory effect of all channels as referenced to the resting pressure. The lower line corresponds to the total inhibitory effect of all channels as referenced to resting pressure. In this example, there is a total excitation of 13.5% with a latency of 2.5 sec; inhibition is 64.6% with a latency of 9.0 sec. The single horizon graph line that follows reflex time is the average restoration pressure during the last 10 sec of the run.

The difference between the horizontal resting and restoration pressure runs as a rough approximation of reliability of the run, particularly from the standpoint of probe movement during the run.

GRAPH B—INDIVIDUAL CHANNEL RESPONSE TO BALLOON DISTENTION

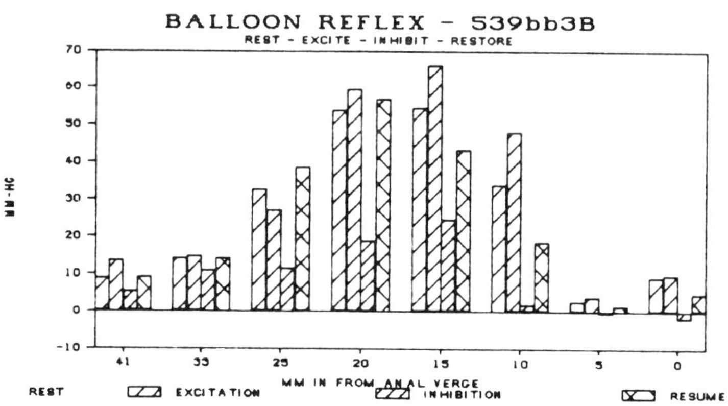

Each channel is displayed as a set of four bar graphs. The bars correspond in order to the resting pressure; the maximum excitation response; the maximum inhibition response; and the final restoration pressure for each individual channel. If Channel 8 (on the right side of the graph) is at the anal verge, the x-axis coordinate refers to the distance of the channel from the anal verge. All channels are displayed even if they are not numerically included in the sphincter.

GRAPH C—DISTENTION EFFECT ON SPHINCTER LONGITUDINAL PROFILE

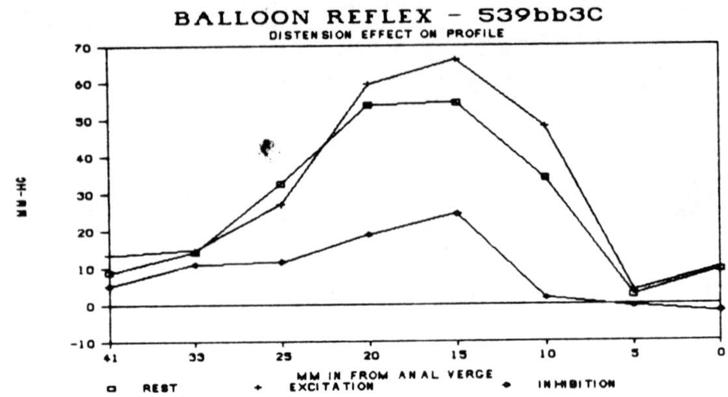

The graph line connected by the square symbols is the longitudinal profile during the resting pressure interval. The graph line connected by plus symbols is the maximum excitation profile. The graph line connected by diamond symbols is the maximum inhibition profile.

GRAPH D—PROXIMAL FOUR CHANNELS

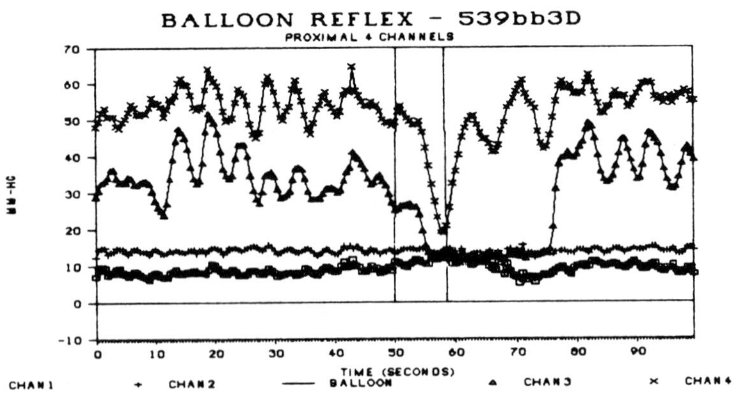

The complete recording of the pressures of the four proximal sphincter channels is graphed along with the balloon inflation marker. If Channel 8 is at the anal verge, the channels shown are proximal to the anal sphincter by the following distances: Channel 1, 41 mm; Channel 2, 33 mm; Channel 3, 25 mm; Channel 4, 20 mm.

Graphs—Summary

On the page of summary graphs, one graph is a summary of the balloon inflation results for all the balloon runs.

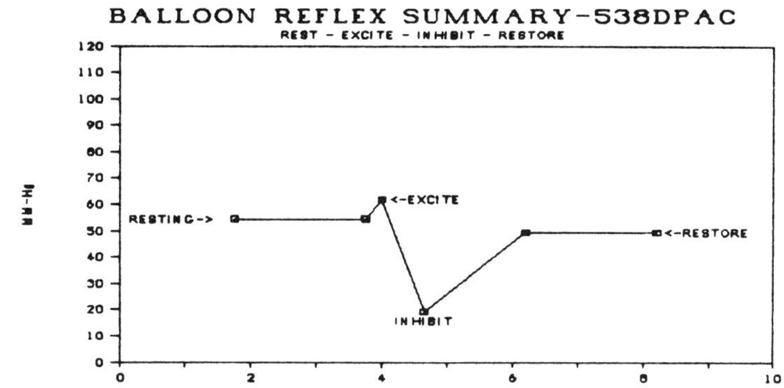

The values used to produce this graph appear on the summary report page of the report. The horizontal resting and restore graph lines correspond to the average resting and restore pressures for all of the Balloon Reflex runs that were analyzed. The space between the two graph lines represents a time interval of 20 sec, the default value for reflex time. The average maximum excitation and average maximum inhibition values are proportional to the latency in seconds of each value.

Example of Abnormal Balloon Reflex Manometry

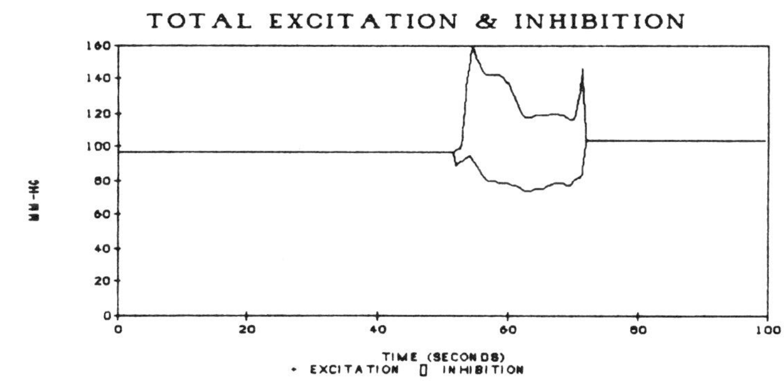

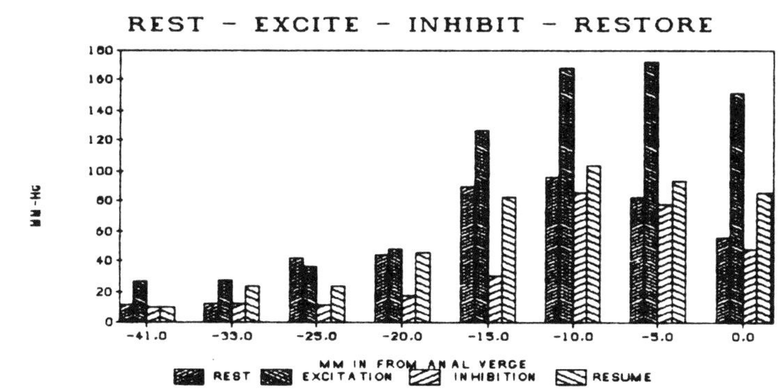

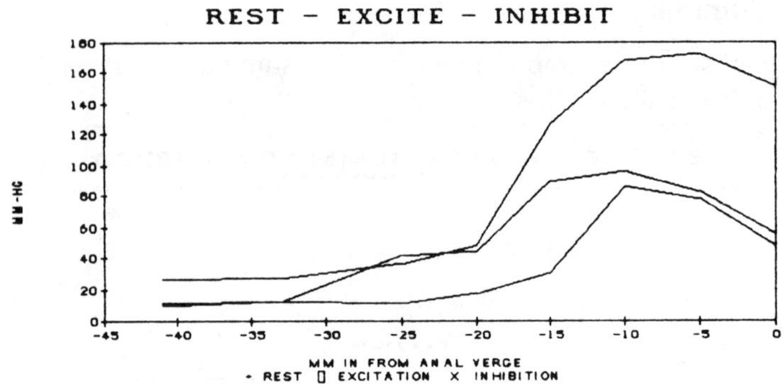

EXTERNAL SPHINCTER HYPEREXCITABILITY. This 25-year-old male has had chronic constipation since adolescence. He has a maximum average resting pressure of 125 mm Hg with proximal displacement of the HPZ and failure to silence with strain during electromyogram (EMG) testing. His transient marker study demonstrates all markers in the rectosigmoid 5 days after ingestion. The Balloon Reflex study demonstrates a marked RAER (76% increase with latency of 3.0 sec) and a diminished RAIR (27% decrease with latency of 11 sec). It is not implied that the hyperexcitability is the cause of the patient's constipation. However, this manometric pattern is frequently associated with certain constipation disorders.

CLINICAL APPLICATIONS OF BALLOON REFLEX MANOMETRY

Our recent experience has shown that different reflex patterns observed on balloon reflex manometry may reflect the pathophysiology of sphincter musculature in various pelvic floor disorders. For example, external anal sphincter denervation in neurogenic fecal incontinence may result in loss of excitatory response in distal channels.[8] Similarly, the presence of an inhibitory response in distal anal canal denotes a weak external anal sphincter unable to resist the fall in anal pressure induced by internal anal sphincter relaxation on rectal distention. However, the excitatory reflex may also be absent in extensive traumatic injury to external anal sphincter. Although similar reflex abnormalities of excitatory response may be seen in traumatic and neurogenic cases of fecal incontinence, the associated manometric findings may indicate the likely cause in a given instance. For example, simultaneous manometric distal sphincter defect with poor squeeze indicates traumatic basis for abnormal reflex response. An absence of RAIR with excitatory response in the entire anal canal[8] may indicate abnormal internal anal sphincter, although this may also be a reflection of very low anal canal pressures making it impossible to register the fall in pressure produced by inhibition. Determination of latency values of rectoanal reflexes using computerized balloon reflex manometry may also reflect the pathophysiologic basis for altered reflex response in idiopathic fecal incontinence. We have observed that in patients with neurogenic fecal incontinence, the latency of proximal excitation is usually normal as compared to the variable latency of distal excitation.[9]

The abnormalities of distal excitatory reflex on balloon reflex manometry may also be used to confirm pudendal nerve damage.[7] The distal excitatory reflex, which depends on an intact pudendal nerve for its execution, may be abnormal in patients with pudendal neuropathy. We have observed that manometrically evident reflex abnormalities, e.g., absence of distal excitation, diminutive excitation, delayed excitation or excitation at high volume of inflation only, may serve as a crude indicator of pudendal neuropathy.[7] A critical analysis of the characteristics of reflex excitation on balloon reflex manometry may serve as a suitable alternative to PNTML determination, where facilities for the latter examination do not exist.

Squeeze/Beardown Protocol

PURPOSE. The purpose of this protocol is to evaluate the effects of squeeze and beardown on rectal and anal canal pressures.

PROBE. A type B-3 probe (Fig. 7.2) with eight spirally oriented channels and a balloon fixed to the tip of the probe is used.

PROBE INSERTION. The well-lubricated, collapsed balloon is mushroomed over the tip of the catheter. It is then gently guided into the anal canal with the index finger. The catheter is aligned so that Channel 8 is located at the anal verge and situated posterior midline. The balloon reflex stopcock assembly is closed to atmosphere allowing for any change in rectal pressure to be recorded.

DATA ACQUISITION. The protocol involves invoking squeeze and bearing down response for a period of 10 sec each. Prior to and in betweeen each maneuver, there is a 10-sec recovery period.

SAVING DATA. Since these data are a variation of the balloon reflex protocol, and are to be be included with the standard balloon reflex "bb" analysis, one must save this run as a "cd" (crude) or "ot" (other) as mentioned previously.

COMMENT ENTRY. Once is it saved, the operator is requested to type in comment. It is important to be specific in this instance because it deviates from the normal Balloon Reflex Protocol. Examples of comments that may be made include the following:

cd: Squeeze 20–30 seconds, Beardown 50–60 and 70–80 seconds

NUMBER OF RUNS. Usually a single run is adequate to study the pelvic floor dynamics on squeeze and beardown maneuvers. However, if the run is compromised, the patient should be reinstructed and an additional run performed.

ANALYSIS. A graphic representation without a numeric report is generated for the Squeeze/Beardown protocol. The normal and abnormal pelvic floor mechanics for squeeze and beardown are shown in Fig. 7.2. The left half of Figure 7.2 depicts a normal squeeze-beardown response. During squeeze, the rectal lumen pressure remains virtually unchanged but the pressures in the proximal and distal anal canal increase. On bearing down, the intrarectal pressure increases significantly and this increase in pressure is transmitted to the proximal anal canal. The distal anal canal pressures decrease during bearing down.

The right half of Figure 7.2 displays an abnormal squeeze-beardown response in a patient with obstructed defecation. On squeeze, there is a pardoxical increase in intrarectal pressure which is transmitted to the proximal anal canal, but the expected increase in pressure in the distal anal canal is abnormally small. On bearing down, there is an increase in intrarectal pressure transmitted to the proximal anal canal in normal fashion, but the distal anal canal reveals a paradoxical increase in pressures (suggesting a simultaneous squeeze and beardown maneuver by the patient).

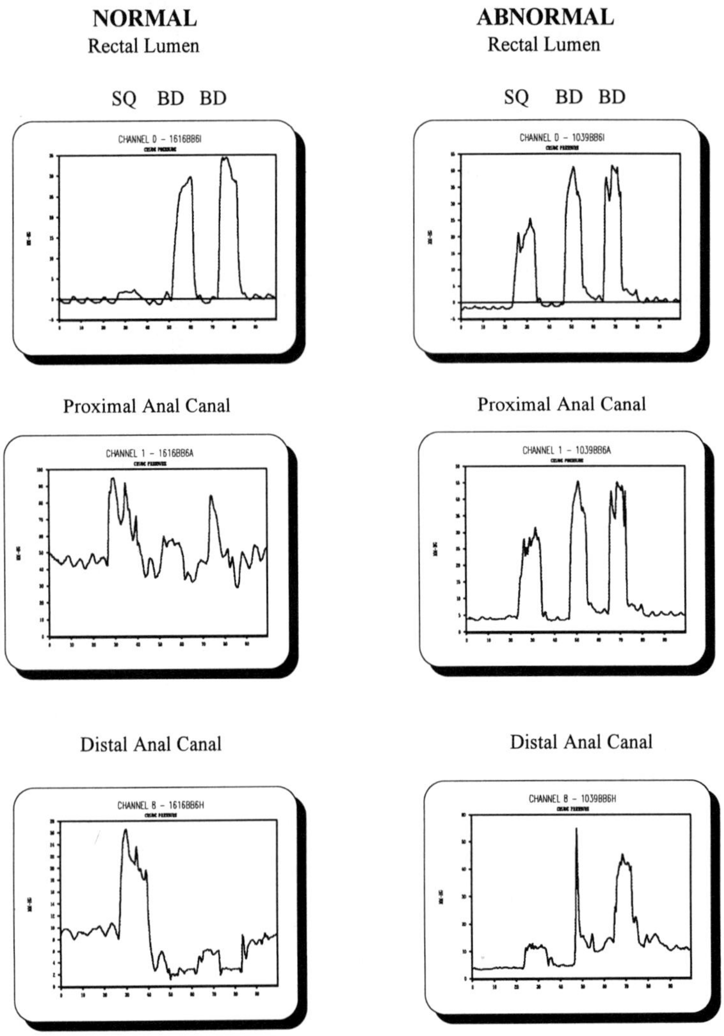

SQ = Squeeze BD = Beardown

SUMMARY REPORT OF MANOMETRY TESTING SESSION

A single page numeric report (Fig. 7.3) is automatically produced which summarizes the manometric runs that have been performed on the patient being examined. Additional numeric pages provide more detailed information on each individual run.

CLINICAL IMPACT OF COMPUTERIZED ANAL MANOMETRY

Although it is often remarked that digital examination is adequate for anal sphincter evaluation, experience with manometric validation of clinical impression repeatedly suggests that reliance on clinical examination for pressure estimation can be deceptively inaccurate. Computerized manometry performed according to a set protocol results in an accurate, reproducible physiologic assessment of anal sphincter. The information thus obtained can influence or even alter patient management. For example, low resting anal pressures in an older patient may persuade a surgeon against an ileorectal anastomosis and instead to opt for a well-constructed ileostomy after a subtotal colonic resection, particularly if the length of residual rectal stump is unduly short. Similarly, ultimate outcome after ileoanal pouch surgery is as much dependent upon technical skills as on a competent sphincter mechanism. A well-executed ileoanal pouch may be doomed to failure in the presence of a weak anal sphincter. Increasing popularity of sphincter-saving surgery in colorectal practice suggests that in selected cases preoperative manometric evaluation of anal sphincter adequacy must be performed.

Judicious use of computerized manometry may be equally helpful in treating common anorectal conditions. In the management of recurrent minor anorectal conditions such as anal fistula, hemorrhoids, and anal fissure, the information obtained from preoperative manometric anal sphincter assessment may avert major embarrassment for both the patient and physician. For example, in patients with low anal canal pressures, conservative management of hemorrhoids by rubber band ligation or phenol in almond oil injections may avoid postoperative imperfect fecal control likely to ensue after a standard three-quadrant hemorrhoidectomy. Similarly, in patients with recurrent fistulae in ano with manometric evidence of compromised squeeze pressures, staged fistulotomy with minimal sphincter division or seton use may be indicated. Manometric confirmation of low resting anal pressures in patients with recurrent fissure in ano contraindicates a vigorous anal dilatation or a conventional sphincterotomy.

The accurate quantification of resting and squeeze anal canal pressures by computerized anal sphincter manometry suggests its continued usage in preoperative assessment of sphincter adequacy in major sphincter-saving and reconstructive surgery and minor recurrent anorectal conditions alike. The precise localization of segmental pressure defects that correspond to anatomic disruption of fisceral and somatic anal sphincter make it a valuable investigative procedure in management of patients with fecal incontinence.

FIGURE 7.3 Quantitative Anorectal Sphincter Manometry Department of Colon and Rectal Surgery: Laney Clinic Medical Center

Summary Report — Date: 14-Feb-89 — DPA#:594DPA

Name: Backside, Jane — Age: 27
LC #: 1520884 — Sex: Female

CRS MD: A.B.Smartdoc, MD — Status: Dx evaluation
Ref MD: L.P.Truecut, MD — 1' Category: Urgency
Add MD: — 2' Category: Leakage

Longitudinal Sphincter Profile (continous pullout):
Resting Profile: # of runs 3 — Squeeze Profile: # runs: 2

	Resting Profile		Squeeze Profile		Rest vs. Squeeze % change	Rest vs. Squeeze delta
Maximum avg pressure	87.6 mm Hg	6.3 SD	105.2	1.5 SD	20.1%	17.6
Pressure-volume	355233 mm Hg^3	37171 SD	615929	48141 SD	73.4%	260696
Sphincter length	46.5 mm	3.6 SD	45.0	0.5 SD	-3.2%	
Verge to max pressure	18.2 mm	0.8 SD	19.5	1.5 SD	7.3%	
Rectal lumen pressure	4.2 mm Hg	0.4 SD	0.2	2.3 SD	-95.4%	
Cross-sectional asymmetry						
Sphincter	26.3%			19.0%	-27.6%	
HPZ	10.1%			9.3%	-8.0%	

```
STA Squeeze: Radial Probe-Maximum Station: # of runs =     2                    Spiral Probe-Max: # of runs=     0
   Initial resting pressure=       73.4 mm Hg     41.4 delta     56%4                      mm Hg
   Peak squeeze=                  114.8 mm Hg     37.7 delta     51%3                      mm Hg
   Regression max  squeeze=       111.1 mm Hg     18.8 delta     25%6                      mm Hg
   Regression avg  squeeze=        92.2 mm Hg   /min     r-linear= 0.889                   mm Hg
   Fatigue=                       -64.0 mm Hg                                           mm Hg/min       r=

STA motility: Radial Probe-Maximum Station: # of runs=     2                    Spiral Probe-Max: # of runs=     0
   Avg pressure=                   75.2 mm Hg                                   mm Hg
   Slow wave approximation:
       Frequency=                  12.6 c/min       Min      Max                               c/min    Min        Max
       Amplitude=          Avg=     7.1 mm Hg       2.7       12.9              mm Hg

BALLOON REFLEX-cummulative approximation:  # of runs =     2

   Reference Resting Pres=         61.8 mm Hg            6.0 avg # channels in sphincter
   Excitation:                                           1.5 avg # channels w/excitation
     Linear change =                4.3% change
     Latency=                      10.3 sec
   Inhibition:                                           6.0 avg # channels w/inhibition
     Linear change=                59.5% change
     Latency=                       9.8 sec
   Restore=                       -13.0% diff from rest
                                                                              Reviewed _____________
                                                                                J.A. Coller, MD
```

SUGGESTED READINGS

1. Coller JA, Karulf RE, Roberts PL, et al: Protocol performance in automated computer analysis of anorectal sphincter manometry. American Society of Colon and Rectal Surgeons, Toronto, Canada, 1989.
2. Barrett RC, Oster MB, Durdey P, et al: The Glutelock prevents artifactual longitudinal anal sphincter profiles. *Dis Colon Rectum* 36:9, 1993.
3. Coller JA. Clinical application of anorectal manometry. *Gastroenterol Clin North Am* 16:17–33, 1987.
4. Sangwan YP, Coller JA, Barrett R, et al: Can manometric parameters predict response to biofeedback therapy in fecal incontinence? New England Society of Colon and Rectal Surgeons, Bolton Landing, New York, October 1, 1994.
5. Keck J, Stanunis RJ, Barrett R, et al: Computer generated profiles of the anal canal in patients with anal fissure. *Dis Colon Rectum* (in press).
6. Sangwan YP, Coller JA, Schoetz D, et al: Relation between manometric anal waves and fecal incontinence. *Dis Colon Rectum* (in press).
7. Sangwan YP, Coller JA, Barrett RC, et al: Abnormal distal rectoanal excitatory reflex: A reliable index of pudendal neuropathy? New England Society of Colon and Rectal Surgeons, Bolton Landing, New York, October 1, 1994.
8. Sangwan YP, Coller JA, Schoetz D, et al: Spectrum of rectoanal reflex patterns in patients with fecal incontinence. New England Society of Colon and Rectal Surgeons, Stowe, Vermont, March 17, 1994.
9. Sangwan, YP, Coller, JA, Schoetz DJ, et al: The latency of proximal excitation and inhibitory reflex is fixed but latency of distal excitation is variable. American Society of Colon and Rectal Surgeons, Research Forum, Orlando, Florida, 1994.

CHAPTER 8

Step-By-Step Anorectal Manometry: Small Balloon Tube

Monique Hémond, Guy Bédard, Hélène Bouchard, Pierre Arhan, Alain Watier, Ghislain Devroede

USEFULNESS OF ANORECTAL MOTILITY RECORDING

The intraluminal pressure rises progressively from the rectum to the anal margin, creating a barrier to maintain continence in the resting condition (Fig. 8.1). However, in clinical practice, recording the entire pressure profile has little practical diagnostic value. Better information is obtained when resting pressures are recorded at a specific level of the anal canal and when the rectoanal reflex activity is studied.

When the normal rectum is transiently distended, a "sampling" reflex occurs in the anal canal. It depends upon the coordination of the rectoanal inhibitory reflex (in the upper anal canal, the internal sphincter relaxes) and the rectoanal contractile reflex (in the lower anal canal, the external internal sphincter contracts, see Fig. 8.2). As a result of these reflexes, the anorectum assumes the shape of a funnel. Rectal contents that trigger the reflexes descend into the cloacogenic zone (at the dentate line and just above) and their character is "sampled" (sensed). Yet, continence is preserved because of the tight closure of the external sphincter. In contrast, this does not occur in Hirschsprung's disease (Fig. 8.3).

During straining, normally the pelvic floor relaxes permitting the stool to pass. This does not occur in patients with rectosphincteric dyssynergia. To the contrary, while straining to defecate the anal canal is squeezed, behaving in a dissociated manner. Controversy exists about the terminology for this condition, but the term *anismus,* initially coined by analogy to vaginismus, is probably the most suitable one since it may be a marker of sexual abuse. This paradox can be looked for during anorectal manometry by asking the patient to strain while recording motility.

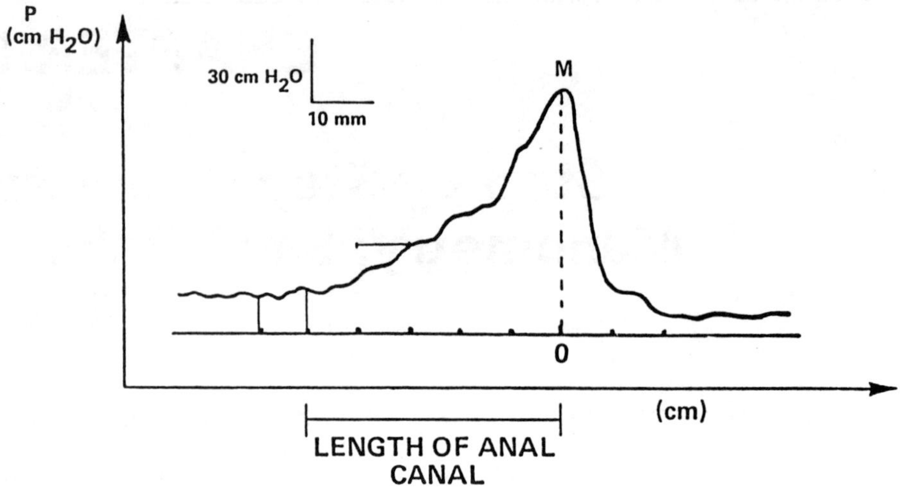

FIGURE 8.1 Normal anal canal profile. The configuration of the anal canal pressure profile changes from the rectum to the anal margin. There is a retrograde pressure gradient.

BALLOON VERSUS PERFUSED SYSTEMS

Water-perfused systems are a source of error. A "pressure" in a sphincter is not recorded as in a hollow viscus, but it is a resistance to distension. When a water-perfusion system is used, an artificial cavity is created, full of the perfused fluid and surrounded by the sphincteric muscle. As the perfusate amount increases, a full capacity is reached eventually. Then fluid leaks into the rectum and out the anal margin. More infusion increases neither the artifical cavity nor the level of the pressure. The term *yield pressure* is used to describe the situation.

When a fluid perfusion system is used, leakage of fluid is a source of technical artifact and error in the accurate measurement of pressure. The level where fluid begins to leak from the anal sphincter is reached faster if the peak perfusion rate is faster. Thus, the rate of perfusion is critical. Values below the yield pressure are meaningless because they are dependent on the rate of perfusion and only reflect the size of the artifical cavity that has been created by the perfusate. However, when leakage occurs, most people will instinctively contract their external anal sphincter (Fig. 8.4).

For the readership versed in basic science notions, it must be emphasized that the anal sphincter is essentially not a high-pressure zone. It is a zone of resistance to flow. This resistance can be indirectly evaluated by measuring the strain that results from an imposed deformity, whose value depends on the direction of the recording site.

Over the years, our preference is for systems with balloons. Balloons can be of variable size and distended with air or with water. Standardization is important and several laboratories have obtained similar measurements of anorectal pressures under standardized conditions. There is a compliance phenomenon in the

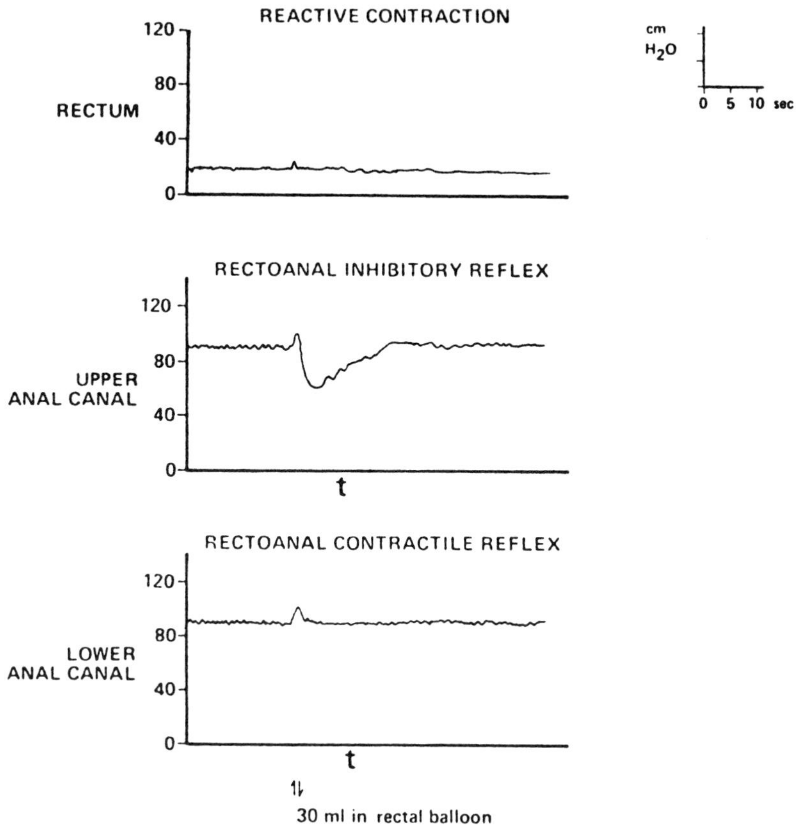

FIGURE 8.2 The result of transient rectal distension, in terms of pressure recorded in the anorectal area.

anorectal area and if it is filled by a balloon successively distended and deflated, there is a hysteresis phenomenon, i.e., both pressure–radius curves (distension/deflation) are not superimposable and the level of pressure is lower on return, for similar levels of distension. Thus, probes with larger balloons yield greater pressure in the same subject than probes with smaller balloons. Moreover, faster distension generates higher pressures (Fig. 8.5).

Air is compressible. For this reason and to facilitate duplication, we have used a system of small balloons filled with water (Fig. 8.6, top).

ANORECTAL MANOMETRY

Definition

Anorectal manometry is a diagnostic examination providing information about anorectal muscular tone and coordination between the rectal wall and the anal sphincter activity.

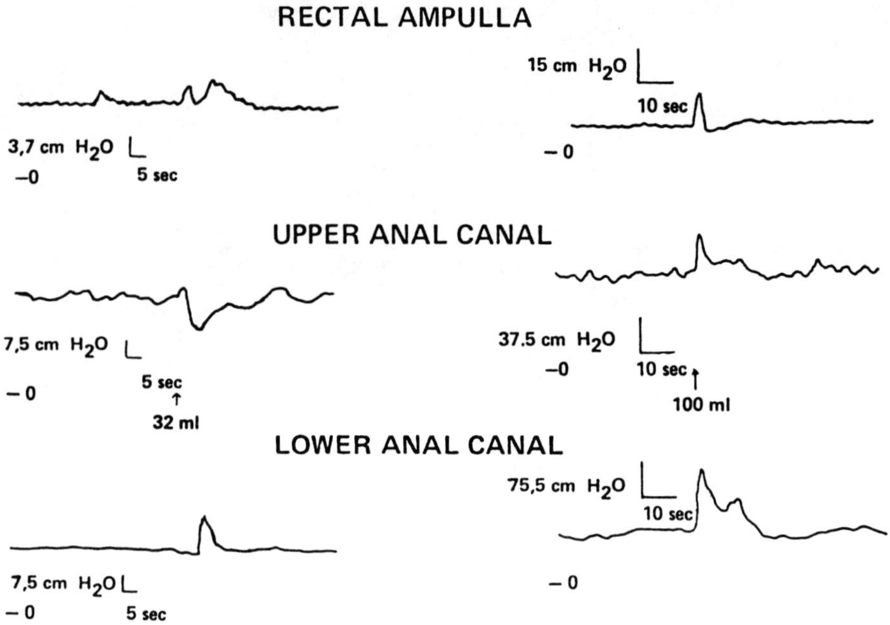

FIGURE 8.3 In contrast to the normal reflexes shown on the left, in Hirschsprung's disease shown on the right, there is no rectoanal inhibitory reflex. On the right, rectal distension has been increased to 100 ml; the patient who has this disease does not have a relaxation but may have a contraction of the internal anal sphincter, recorded in the upper anal canal.

MODIFICATION OF THE RECTOANAL INHIBITORY REFLEX DURING ANAL CANAL PERFUSION

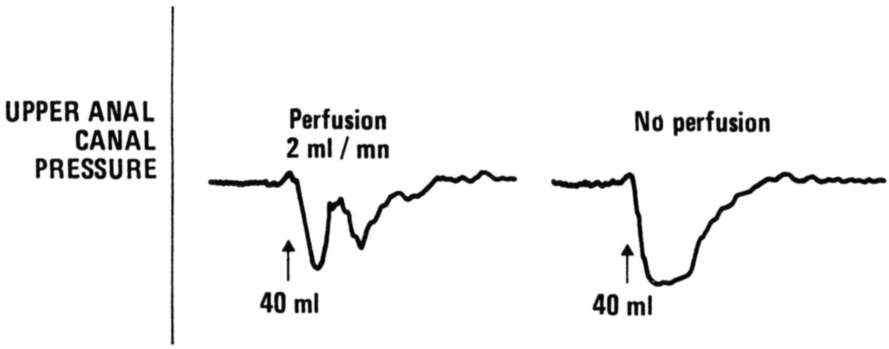

FIGURE 8.4 Rectal distension with 40 ml of air, in the same subject, with *(left)* and without *(right)* water perfusion into the open-tipped catheter, placed into the anal canal to record pressure. By increasing the rate of perfusion it is even possible to abolish the rectoanal inhibitory reflex. *When this reflex is absent, suspect a technical error, until proven otherwise, if an open-tipped perfused catheter is used, rather than a balloon system.*

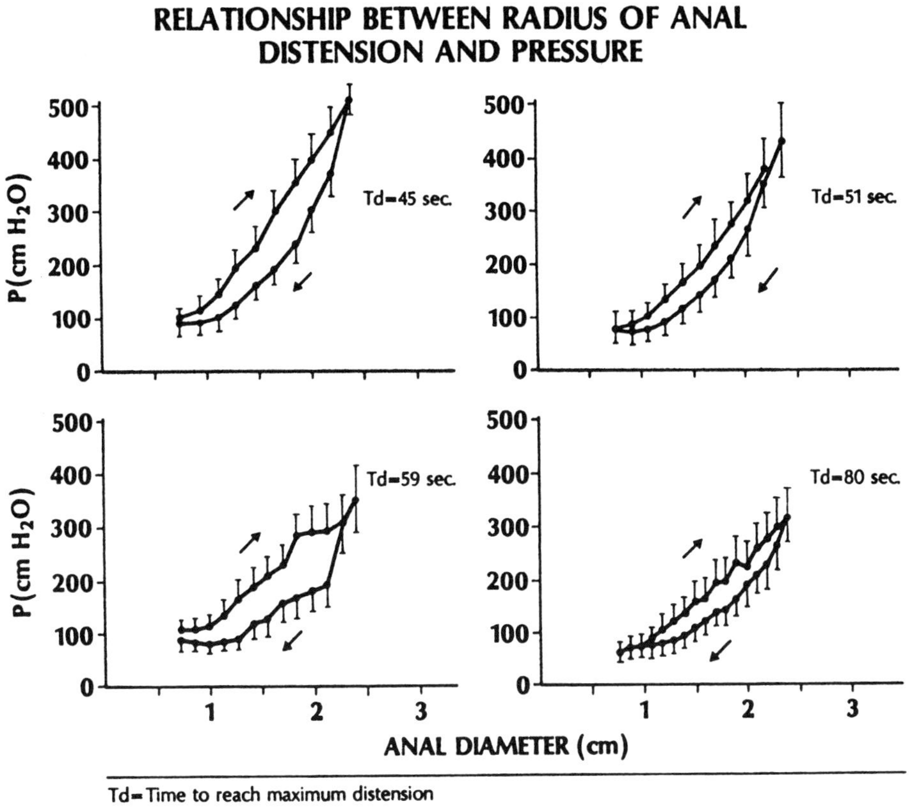

FIGURE 8.5 The anal canal has been constantly distended, while a pressure–radius curve was recorded. When returning to no distension status, the pressure is lower (hysteresis phenomenon). It should be noted that rapid distension generates higher pressures, and this is important to remember when using water-perfused systems.

Required Materials and Equipment

1. Polygraph recorder with three recording channels.
2. Pressure transducer (3) from 0 to 400 mm Hg.
3. Perfusion pump providing continuous flow at 0.6 ml/min.
4. Sphygmomanometer to calibrate the polygraph.
5. Three-way stopcocks to connect the probe and the recording equipment.
6. Filling needles of 1 mm diameter, 200 cm length, used to expand the water-filled annular balloons (for example Marquat C57) (Fig. 8.7).
7. Water-soluble lubricant.
8. Nonsterile gloves.
9. 50 ml (or more) syringes.
10. Disinfecting solution with glutaraldehyde 2%.

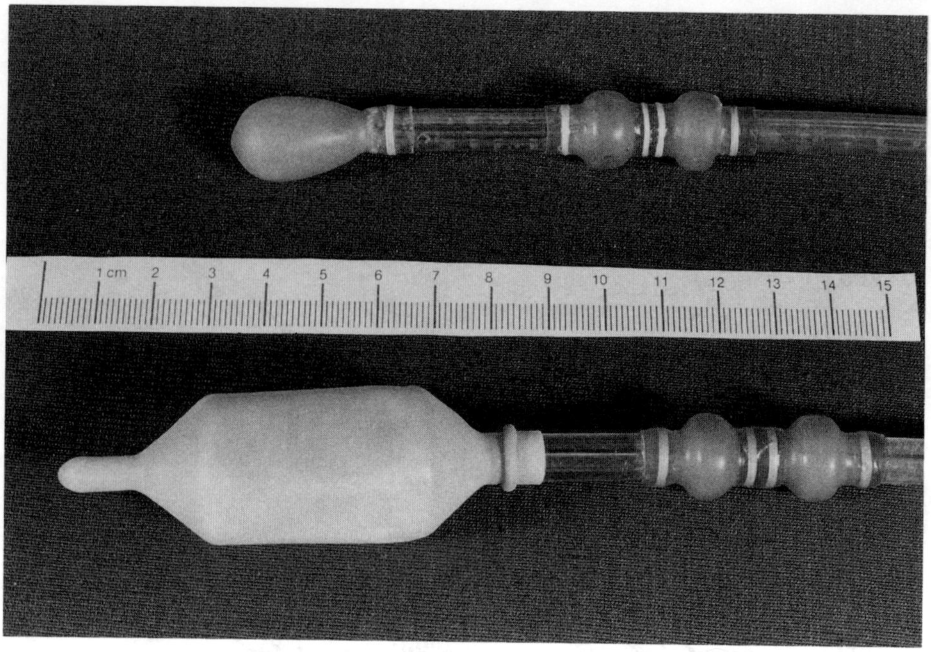

FIGURE 8.6 Small balloon tubes used to record anorectal pressures: anorectal manometry tube *(top)*; rectometrogram tube *(bottom)*.

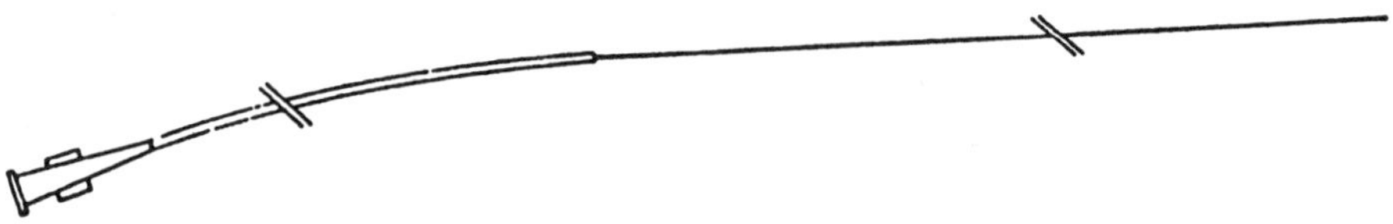

FIGURE 8.7 Needle to fill anorectal probe (Marquat C52–C53).

11. Sterile distilled water.
12. Adjustable examination table.
13. Anorectal manometric probe.

There are probes for adults, children, and infants (Fig. 8.8). Probe characteristics are summarized in Table 8.1. These probes are reusable after proper cleaning. However, balloons sometimes need to be replaced when the latex is not firm, a balloon is deformed or perforated, or there is other suspected abnormality in the balloon. When replacing a balloon, choose the appropriate sized balloon according to the type of probe and the site on the probe. Be careful not to obstruct the perfusion orifice when attaching the balloon. Balloons may be fixed with silk, but we find unwaxed dental floss to be ideal.

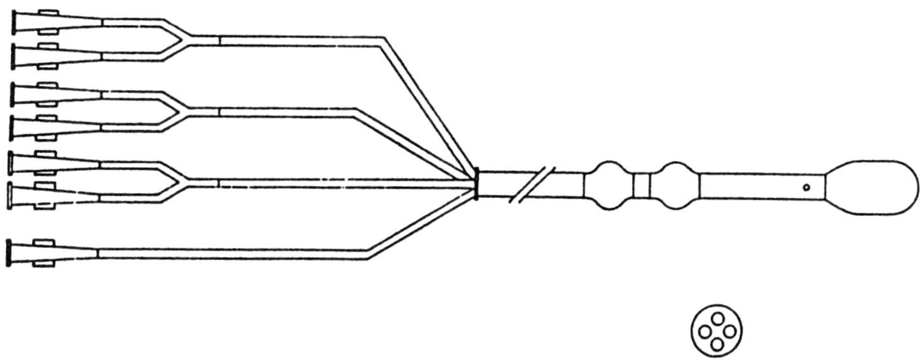

FIGURE 8.8 Technical design of the probe for anorectal manometry.

Preparation of the Patient

Preparation of the patient simply requires a saline enema (Fleet enema is an example) on the evening before the examination. If the patient is incontinent, has a fecal impaction or is suspected to have a megarectum, the preparation may be adapted to ensure and empty rectum.

Immediately before the examination the patient is asked if there is a history of anal surgery, pelvic trauma, urinary or fecal incontinence, or perineal or abdominal pain. Inquire whether the patient feels emptied after the enema. Then, ask the patient to void residual urine and feces completely.

TABLE 8.1 POLYVINYL CHLORIDE PROBES WITH 4 CHANNELS AND 3 BALLOONS USED TO RECORD ANORECTAL MOTILITY*

	(C52 A) Adult Probe	(C52 E) Child Probe	(C52 N) Infant Probe
Diameter	7 mm	7 mm	5 mm
Length	100 cm	100 cm	75 cm
First channel (rectum)	To balloon at end	To balloon at end	To balloon at end
Second channel (rectum)	To perfused opening	To perfused opening	To perfused opening
Level	10 mm from end	10 mm from end	10 mm from end
Third channel (upper anus)	To ring-shaped balloon†	To ring-shaped balloon†	To ring-shaped balloon‡
Level	50 mm from end	35 mm from end	35 mm from end
Fourth channel (distal anus)	To ring-shaped balloon†	To ring-shaped balloon†	To ring-shaped balloon‡
Level	68 mm from end	50 mm from end	50 mm from end

* Marquat Company
ZAC de la Haie Griselle
9, rue du 8 Mai 1945, B.P. 11
94471 Boissy-Saint-Léger Cedex, France
Tel: (33) 1-45-69-20-62
Telex: 210 311 F2223
Fax: (33) 1-45-69-66-68

† Diameter: 15 mm.
‡ Diameter: 12 mm.

Preparation of the Equipment

The material and equipment should be prepared in cookbook fashion as follows: (1) Calibrate the polygraph according to the instructions of the manufacturer. (2) Connect each channel to the transducers. (3) Verify the condition of the balloons of the probe. (4) Fill the tube, balloons, pressure transducers, and perfusing pump with water, making sure the system is clear of air bubbles. If there is air in the system, remove it with the filling needles. (5) Squeeze the balloons to check for leakage of water. (6) Adjust the baseline of the polygraph to 0 mm Hg. (7) Verify that the pressure transducers, the pump, the probe, and the bed are at the same level. Failure to do this is a frequent source of error in laboratories.

Positioning of the Probe

Positioning of the probe requires another series of maneuvers to be checked: (1) With the patient lying in the lateral decubitus position, introduce the lubricated probe. The distal (lower anal canal, external anal sphincter) balloon must barely disappear into the anal canal. Note if the introduction of the probe triggers abdominal pain: it is a symptom of sexual abuse. (2) Ask the patient to relax. (3) Start the perfusion pump. (4) Wait at least one minute. (5) Position the probe so that the maximal pressure is recorded at the level of the two annular balloons (resting pressure recording). The rise in pressure at the level of the lower anal canal is usually higher or equal to that of the upper anal canal. A technical error is possible if the probe is not located properly to record the external anal sphincter activity: simply reposition the probe. The patient may not understand the instruction; some contract the abdominal wall, the buttocks, or the thighs, but do not squeeze the anal canal. The patient may not be able to comply with the order (the disobedient sphincteric syndrome); this is not a conscious refusal to obey, but an unconscious mechanism of dissociation. The problem may be organic such as due to muscular damage (postpartum tears, trauma) or neurological problems (meningomyelocele, impaired innervation). (7) Inject 20–30 cc of air in the rectal distending balloon to induce the rectoanal inhibitory reflex (RAIR) (Fig. 8.2). In the rectum, a reflex contraction follows. In the upper anal canal, a reflex contraction is usually recorded and routinely followed by a reflex relaxation. A contraction in this condition is akin to anismus. In the lower canal, a reflex contraction is recorded usually, but occasionally a relaxation is recorded.

Sometimes, no rectoanal inhibitor reflex is recorded. The following may solve the problem: (1) Ask the patient not to contract the external anal sphincter during rectal distension, since this can completely mask a RAIR (Fig. 8.9), which is present, but counteracted by striated muscle activity. (2) Make sure there is no fecal impaction. (3) Increase the volume of rectal distension. In the case of megarectum, it is common to have to distend the rectum with 150 cc of air before the volume is large enough to touch the rectal wall, a prerequisite to have a RAIR. Occasionally, it has been necessary to use 400 cc. Failure to follow these steps results in an erroneous diagnosis of Hirschsprung's disease. (4) If there is anismus and no rectoanal inhibitory reflex, anorectal manometry must be repeated after pudendal block. This will not abolish puborectalis muscle activity, because it is also innervated by the sacral plexus, but it completely paralyzes the external

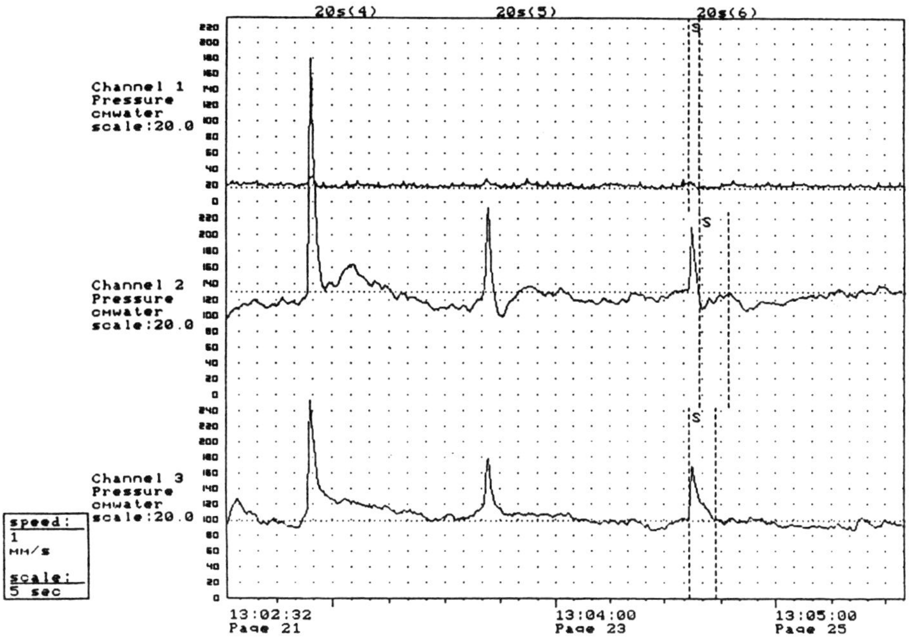

FIGURE 8.9 On the left 20 ml of air (20 s) have been suddenly injected and withdrawn into the rectal distending balloon. Note on Channel 2 that there is no rectoanal inhibitory reflex; instead, the patient has contracted the upper (Channel 2) and lower (Channel 3) anal canal. Teaching the patient not to contract the anus results in the appearance of a rectoanal inhibitory reflex as seen further right (20 s[4]) and 20 s[5]). The reflex is more clearly seen as the reflex contraction amplitude decreases. The patient still contracts on the right (20 s[6]), and this rectoanal inhibitory reflex, definitely present, is not reliable in terms of configuration.

sphincter. Thus, an apparently absent rectoanal inhibitory reflex may be found after just regional anesthesia (Fig. 8.10).

If all parameters described are not recorded, the probe must be repositioned and steps 6 and 7 must be repeated. The anatomy in Chapter 1 (Fig. 1.3) points out the muscles at the anorectum that are involved. If all systems are checked and in order, the procedure may begin.

Technical Aspects and Measurements

The mean basal resting pressure of each recording track is reproducible (Fig. 8.11, left). When beginning to record the resting pressure, the probe is positioned and a waiting period of at least 10 min is begun. The patient is asked to relax during this period. Calculate the mean basal pressure in the rectum, the upper part of the anal canal, and the lower part of the anal canal during this period before injecting air into the rectal distending balloon.

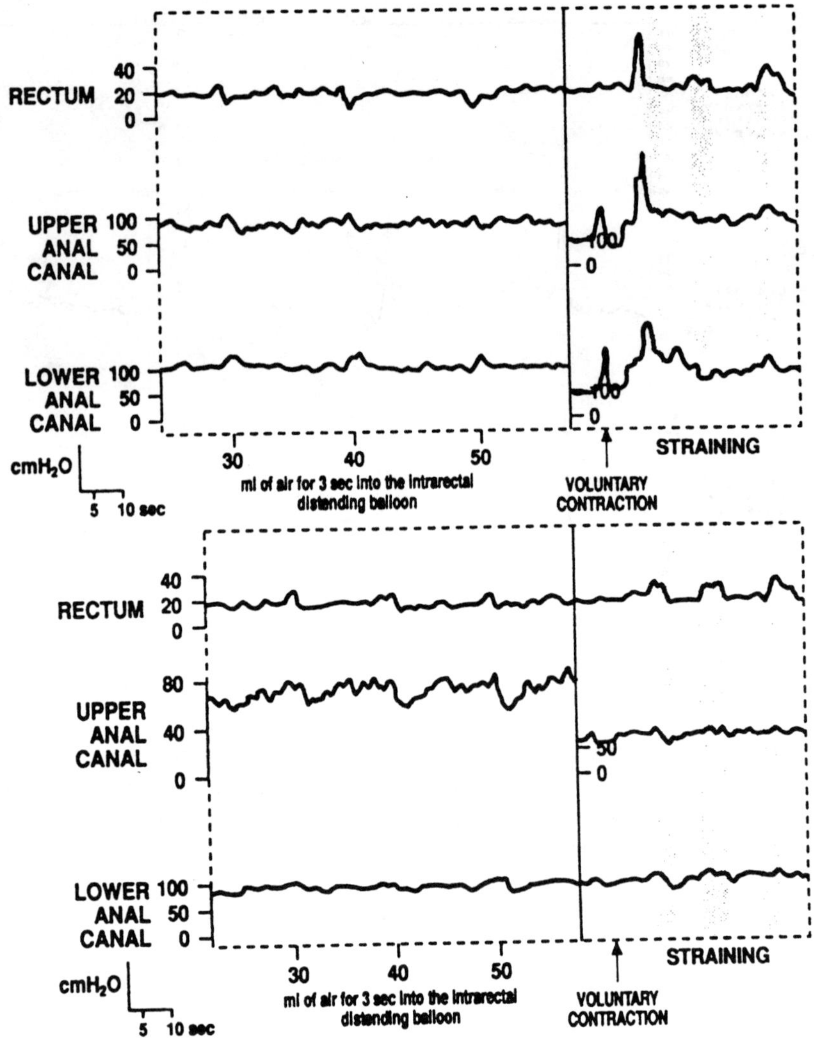

FIGURE 8.10 Anorectal manometry before *(top)* and after *(bottom)* pudendal block, in a patient consulting for severe constipation. On the left, a rectoanal inhibitory reflex is looked for. Note, on top, that there is no reflex even for a 50-ml rectal distension. On the bottom, after pudendal block, the reflex becomes evident, starting at 30 ml distension and its amplitude clearly increases, as expected, with increasing distension. The reason for the uncovering of a reflex is shown on the right of the figure, where anismus was looked for. The patient strains adequately, before and after pudendal block, as shown by the increase in rectal pressure. Before the block *(top)*, there is no relaxation in the anal canal but a contraction: this is diagnostic of anismus (rectosphincteric dyssynergia). This is abolished by the pudendal block, and a relaxation results from straining *(bottom right);* simultaneously, a rectoanal inhibitory reflex *(bottom left)* can be demonstrated.

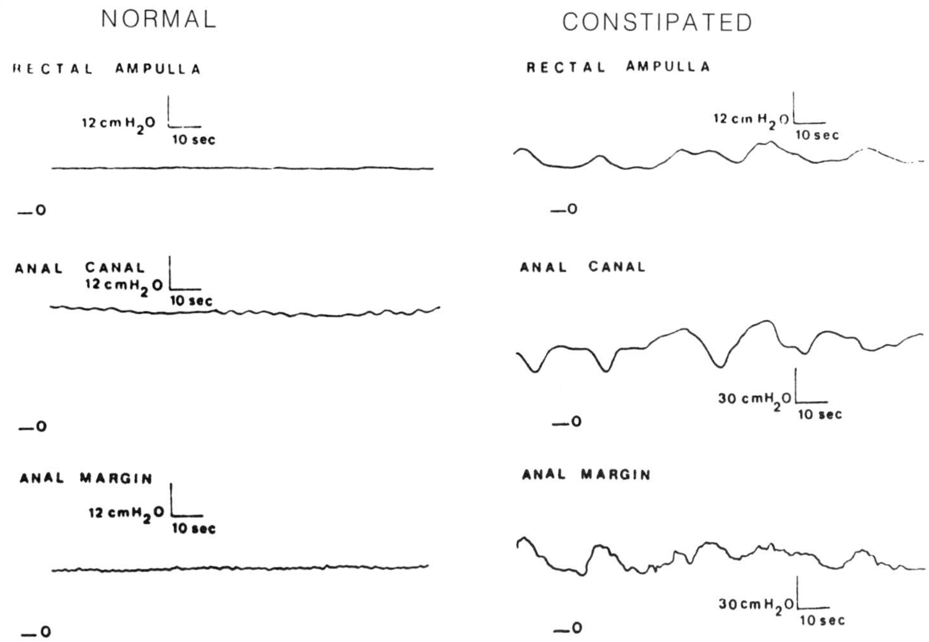

FIGURE 8.11 Resting pressures in the rectum and anal canal in a normal subject *(left)* and a constipated patient *(right).*

It can also be useful to evaluate the variations of pressure around the mean. The activity index can be calculated as 1.96 SD/mean. Unfortunately, variations are common. Changes in resting pressure in the anal canal during the waiting period may correspond to *spontaneous variations, spontaneous relaxations,* and *spontaneous contractions. Spontaneous variations* such as slow waves (Fig. 8.11, left) and ultraslow waves (Fig. 8.12) may be seen. These waves are regular and persistent variations in the resting pressure. In healthy subjects, the amplitude of variations in pressure never exceeds 20 cm H_2O in the upper anal canal and 35 cm H_2O in the lower anal canal. However, because of the prevalence of functional motor disorders in the general populations, these values should not be taken as absolute. It is possible that any change in pressure is significant. Slow waves (Fig. 8.11, left) have a frequency of 10–12 per minute and a small amplitude, while ultraslow waves have a frequency of 1–2 per minute and an amplitude that may reach over 100 cm of water; however, no study has been made to sort out these waves quantitatively. Ultraslow waves (Fig. 8.12) are only found in 10% of control subjects, and the normality of this finding is highly questionable, because these have higher resting pressures than other control subjects who have no ultraslow waves. Slow waves are present without exception in both controls and in patients with anal fissure or symptomatic hemorrhoids. Their role, because of a higher frequency in the distal part of the anal canal, is probably to promote continence, through an inward movement of anal contents; thus the absence of these slow waves is abnormal and should be noted. On the contrary, the presence of ultraslow waves is always pathological. Etiology for these waves may be a technical

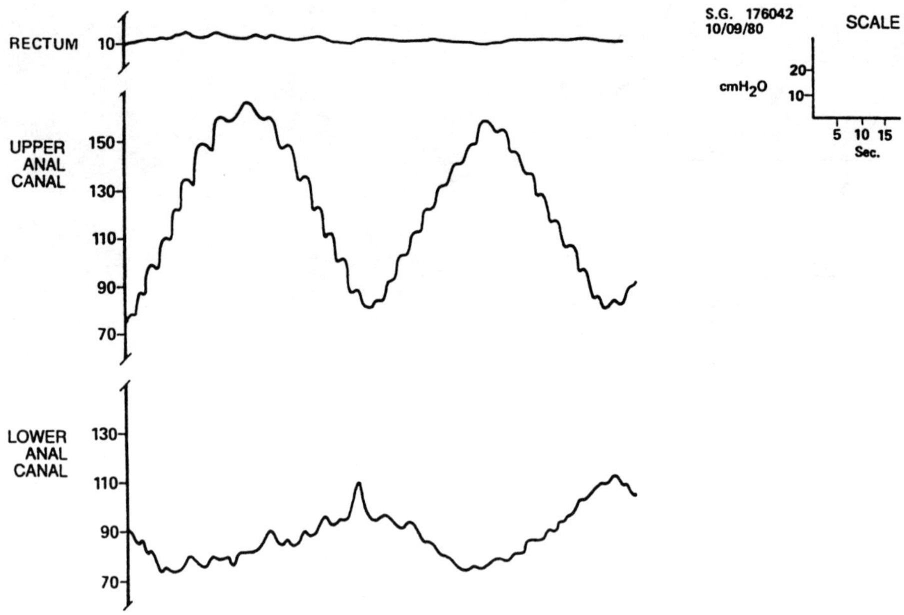

FIGURE 8.12 Ultraslow waves in the anal canal during resting conditions. Frequency is between 1 and 2 per minute; amplitude is close to 100 cm H_2O.

error, such as an enema given just prior to the examination by mistake. Pathologic conditions such as anal fissure or hemorrhoids may be associated with ultraslow waves, as well as functional problems such as constipation and the irritable bowel syndrome.

The analysis of ultraslow waves includes mean amplitude and frequency. Minimal and maximal values should be calculated from the "0" basal pressure during calibration. When ultraslow waves are present an adjustment should be made: the waiting period of relaxation before the examination should be prolonged to better calculate the variations in amplitude and frequency. Occasionally, these waves will disappear during the prolonged waiting period; this should be noted. It may be a technical artifact, or a sign of irritability.

Later in the examination ultraslow waves may interfere with recording the RAIR. It is essential to distend the rectum when the waves' curves reach a minimum value, otherwise the reflex may not be distinguished from the spontaneous changes in the pressure waves (Fig. 8.13). In analyzing this situation, it is close to impossible to quantify (amplitude, duration, surface) the reflex. Simply note that the reflex is present, but is distorted by the variations.

The second major variations is termed *spontaneous relaxation.* There are two types of spontaneous relaxations. There may be an isolated and prolonged relaxation at the beginning of the examination (Fig. 8.14). In this case the resting pressure in the upper anal canal is abnormally low, but after a while may rise and become stable at a higher level, which is the real resting pressure, present before the relaxation. This is likely due to a gaping hypotonicity of the anal canal induced by the introduction of the probe. For instance in patients operated upon for meningomyelocele, the probe is not perceived. The adjustment of the technique in

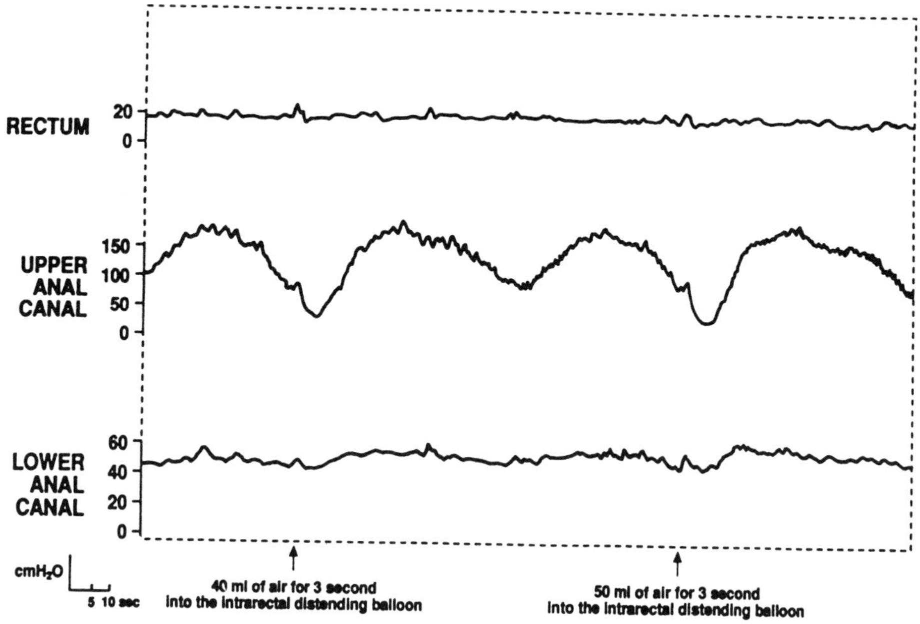

FIGURE 8.13 To determine, if there is a rectoanal inhibitory reflex, it is essential to distend the rectum toward the end of a wave, when pressure is at its lowest. Note the change in configuration triggered by the distension. In this situation, it is possible to demonstrate the presence or absence of a reflex, but quantification will be poor because of the spontaneous variations in pressure.

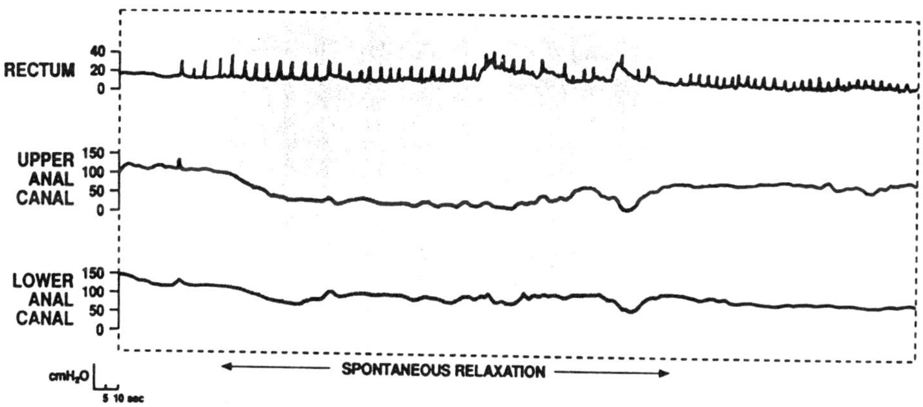

FIGURE 8.14 Spontaneous relaxation of the anal canal at the beginning of anorectal manometry. Note the initial relaxation toward the left of the figure, on the tracing obtained in the upper anal canal. It would be erroneous to attribute this phenomenon to a normal accommodation of the anal canal to the distension induced by the balloon of the probe. In fact, as one keeps waiting without any manipulation, pressure rises again and stablizes toward the right of the figure. Thus, it was a spontaneous relaxation, akin, at manometry, to gaping of the anus at rectal examination with a finger.

recording the resting pressure because of the spontaneous relaxations of this type is to ask the patient to perform a few voluntary contractions and wait for the pressure to stabilize; at analysis calculate the mean resting pressure after stabilization.

Later during the examination, there may be spontaneous isolated or repetitive relaxations of a more or less brief duration (Fig. 8.11, right). This late type spontaneous relaxation occurs at the level of the upper and sometimes in the lower anal canal, often accompanied by a rectal contraction and identified by the patient as an urge to defecate or a feeling of passing gas. This possibly represents the manometric counterpart of the sampling reflex. The etiology of this increased motor activity of the rectum may be secondary to a bowel preparation different from what is described in the protocol, or a functional motor disorder; the normality of this finding is questionable. A diagnosis of rectoanal antagonism is made when a rectal contraction coincides with an upper anal canal relaxation. This may be found in some children with chronic idiopathic constipation and in some patients operated upon for meningomyelocele.

Adjustments to the technique because of these spontaneous relaxations of the late type are made for both the recording of resting pressure and the RAIR. For the resting pressure, ask the patient to voluntarily contract the anal canal until the variation disappears. However, if the relaxation persists, check whether bowel preparation was as prescribed. If yes, advise that the preparation was insufficient to whomever ordered it. If not, reschedule the examination. After analysis calculate the mean resting pressure during the stable period. To adjust for the technique during recording of the rectoanal inhibitory reflex, wait until the resting pressure is stabilized and inject the rectal distending volumes in between spontaneous relaxations, while the recording seems stable. The analysis is as usual (see the subsequent discussion).

The third variation is termed *spontaneous contractions*. There are two types of spontaneous contractions, type I and type II. Type I spontaneous contraction of the striated muscles of the anal canal are observed at all times during the examination, neither by distension of the rectum nor by movement (Fig. 8.15). The causes of this contraction may be associated with anorectal pain or anxiety. It may also be seen in patients who have anismus, but it is not to be confused with a movement artefact.

Type II spontaneous contractions consist of one to two contractions, interrupting the rectoanal inhibitory reflex in the upper anal canal (Fig. 8.16). This is an important finding at manometry. The cause is similar in nature to that of anismus and is correctable by biofeedback with similar clinical results. As part of the analysis, note the presence or absence of such contractions in each manometry study indicating the level of rectal distension. Also, describe the configuration of these contractions.

Normally, the pressure in the upper anal canal exceeds that in the lower anal canal. However, occasionally, with a perfectly positioned probe, the pressure in the lower anal canal is higher than in the upper anal canal (Fig. 8.17). This important abnormality is referred to as an *inverted pressure profile*. This has been described in association with constipation and it indicates an excess motor activity in the striated muscles akin to the spastic pelvic floor syndrome.

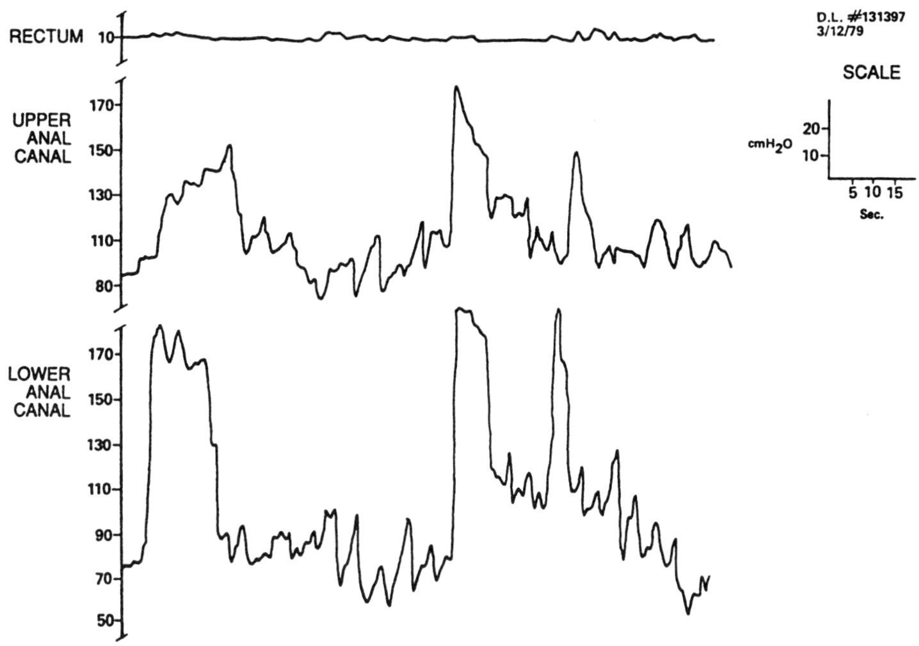

FIGURE 8.15 Spontaneous contractions type I.

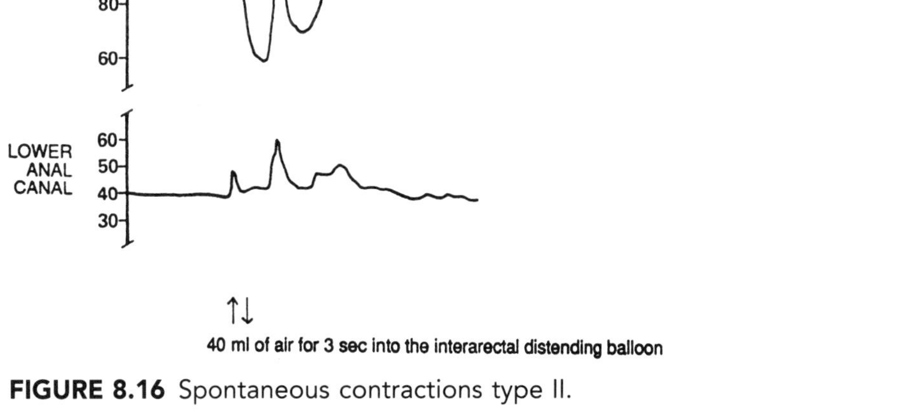

FIGURE 8.16 Spontaneous contractions type II.

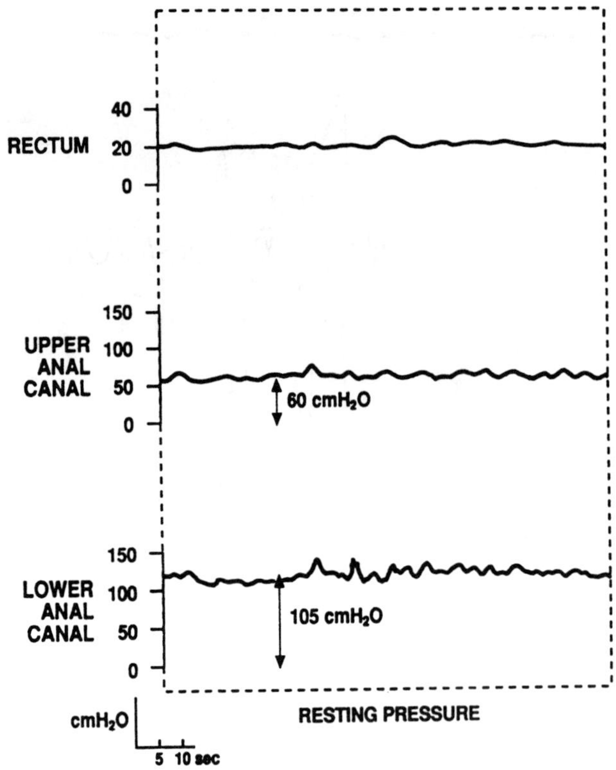

FIGURE 8.17 Pressure in the lower anal canal of this patient exceeds that of the upper anal canal, contrary to what is expected.

Voluntary Contraction

Voluntary contraction is the capacity to contract the striated muscles of the pelvic floor. The technique proceeds as follows:

1. Ask the patient for a maximal voluntary squeeze of the anal canal and then relax rapidly. The maximal amplitude is recorded (Fig. 8.18).
2. Calculate the amplitude of the first voluntary contraction of the anal canal at the three levels of recording. There should be no increase in the rectum, because it would mean the patient squeezes the abdominal wall; one may also check this by placing the hand on the abdomen.
3. Ask the patient for a second maximal voluntary squeeze of the anal canal and hold this for as long as possible (Fig. 8.18).
4. Calculate the duration and the mean amplitude of the second voluntary contraction at the three levels.
5. Observe, during voluntary contractions of the anal canal, whether the patient moves his/her legs and feet, tilts the pelvis, and/or squeezes the buttocks during the procedure. Some patients do not contract the anal canal when requested, but resort instead to such paradoxical maneuvers.

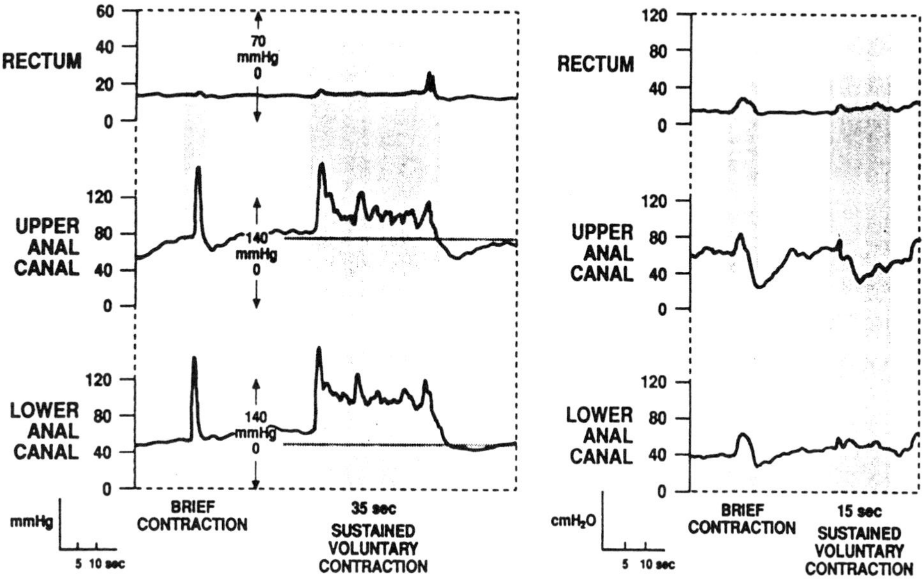

FIGURE 8.18 Voluntary contraction of the anal canal. On the left (a), the subject has an adequate contraction. In the lower anal canal, she develops 96 mm Hg of pressure above baseline level, and then succeeds to maintain 40 mm Hg for 35 sec (normally, this should exceed 20 sec), before pressure falls to zero. The best that can be done is 90 sec. On the right, (b), the patient is incontinent. She can squeeze to reach 22 mm Hg (30 cm H_2O), but this cannot be maintained at any level and pressure falls to zero within 15 sec.

Rectal Stimulation

Rectal stimulation by distending a rectal balloon elicits the RAIR. This technique entails injection of air at volumes of 5, 10, 20, 30, 40, and 50 cc into the rectal balloon to stimulate the rectum. The study is conducted in the following manner:

1. Inject the first stimulating volume and withdraw it within 3 sec. Usually after the RAIR the pressure returns to the initial baseline pressure. When the resting pressure has stabilized ask and note whether the patient felt the distension.
2. Repeat the procedure for each volume.
3. Each of the stimulations induces (Fig. 8.19) a rectal contraction (rectum), a rectoanal inhibitory reflex (upper anal canal), and a rectoanal contractile reflex (lower anal canal) which are separately recognized and analyzed.

The rectal contraction is a reflex induced by rectal distension. This contraction occurs a very short time after the stimulation. During high-speed recording, it can easily be seen that this is not contemporary to the peak of pressure triggered by the distension, but during the accommodation period of the rectum adjusting to the maintained distension. It is the result of the reflex contractile activity of the

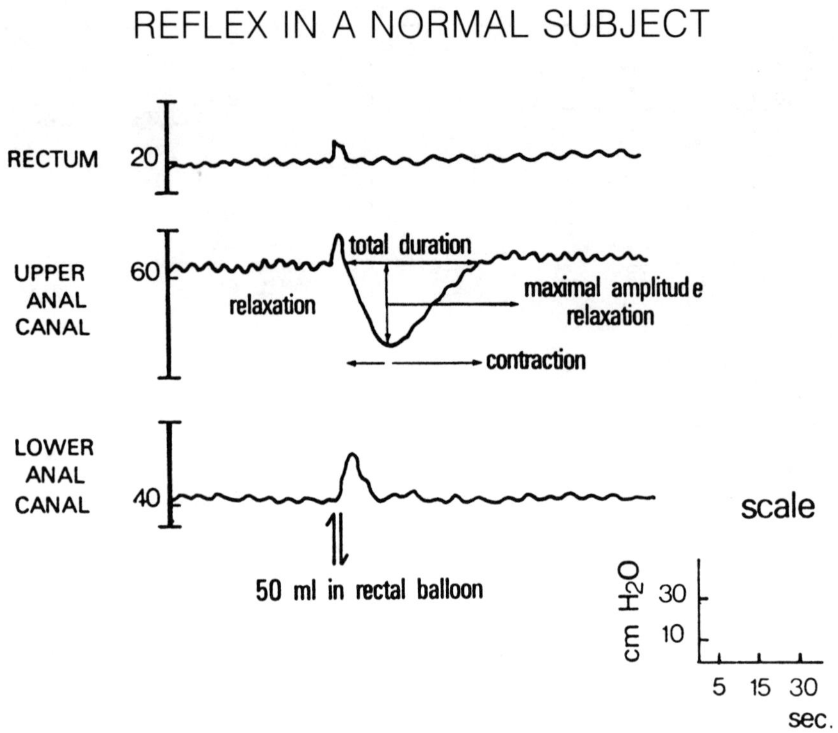

FIGURE 8.19 Reflex in a normal subject.

rectum and is abnormal in patients with functional motor disorders of the large bowel. The analysis is the recording of the amplitude of each contraction.

The rectoanal inhibitory reflex is shown as a fall in pressure recorded in the upper anal canal, secondary to the relaxation of the internal sphincter and is induced by a brief rectal distension. Of note, the rapidity and repetitiveness of the distension exerts a profound influence on the configuration of the rectoanal inhibitory reflex.

The analysis of the RAIR consists of calculation of the value of each parameter, i.e., maximal amplitude, time to maximal relaxation, time to return to baseline pressure, total duration of the reflex, and surface of the reflex obtained by planimetry. This should be done for each distension volume as follows:

1. The amplitude is the difference between the baseline pressure and the minimal value after relaxation. Usually the amplitude increases linearly with a logarithm of the distending volume (Figs. 8.20 and 8.21). If this is not the case, this should be noted as it may signify a neurological lesion such as after a trauma.
2. Time to maximal relaxation is the number of seconds between the onset and peak relaxation.
3. Time to return to baseline pressure is the number of seconds between the peak relaxation and return to baseline pressure.
4. Duration is the addition of time to maximal relaxation plus time to return to baseline pressure.

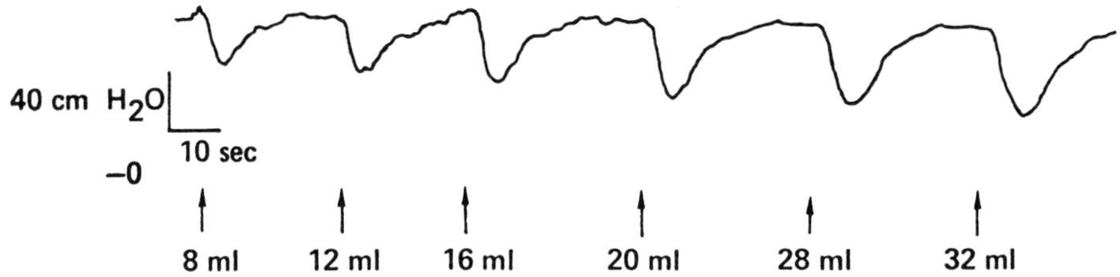

FIGURE 8.20 The amplitude of the rectoanal inhibitory reflex increases with increasing rectal distension.

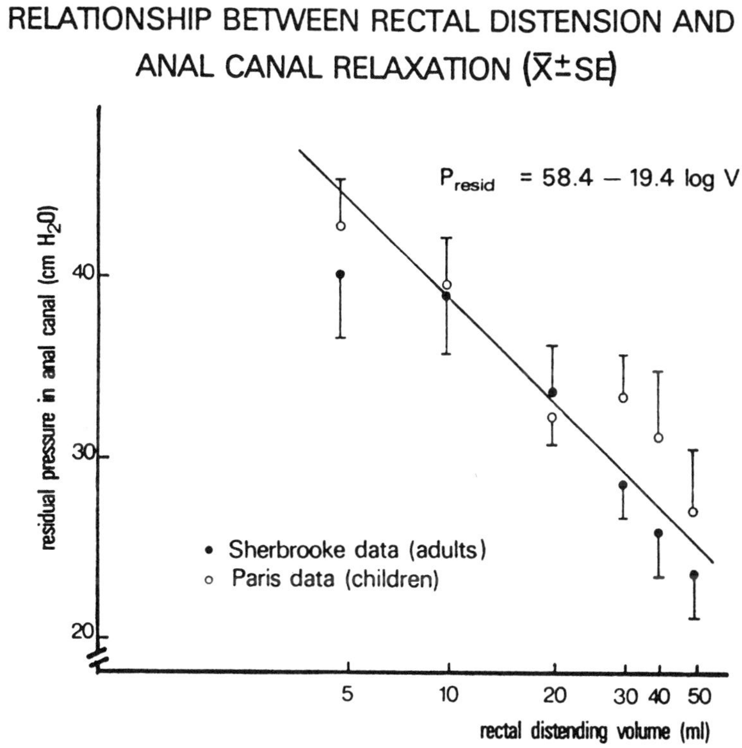

FIGURE 8.21 The amplitude of the rectoanal inhibitory reflex increases *linearly* with the logarithm of the volume of rectal distension. The figure shows the *residual* pressure after distension, thus the pressure *below* the maximal amplitude of the rectoanal inhibitory reflex (see Fig. 8.20). Note that there is no difference between adults and children.

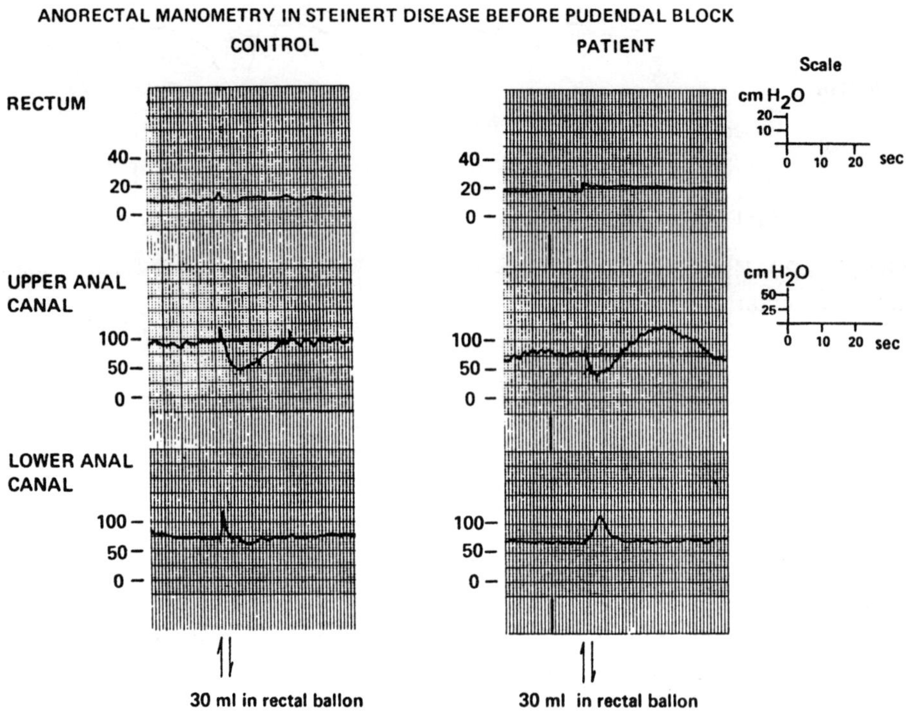

FIGURE 8.22 This patient suffers from myotonic dystrophy (Steinert's disease). Note, to the right, the overshoot of pressure after the rectoanal inhibitory reflex, well seen in the upper anal canal.

5. Planimetry is the total surface of the reflex.
6. Overshoot is defined as a return to the baseline level exceeding it temporarily by at least 20 cm H_2O (Fig. 8.22). It may coexist with spontaneous variations (Fig. 8.23), and can be found in some patients with chronic idiopathic constipation, patients with anal fissure, and patients with myotonic dystrophy. It probably is always abnormal.

The rectoanal contractile reflex is a rise in pressure recorded in the lower anal canal, secondary to a contraction of the external sphincter and the puborectalis muscles, and induced by a brief rectal distension. The respective contributions of the two muscles are not well known, but the rectoanal contractile reflex is not recorded when a pudendal block is made (Fig. 8.24).

To analyze the rectoanal contractile reflex calculate its amplitude and duration at the level of the lower anal canal. The amplitude and duration increase with increasing distending volumes of the rectum. It may be recorded in both the upper anal canal prior to the rectoanal inhibitory reflex and in the lower anal canal.

A qualitative evaluation of *rectal sensation* may be made. Rectal sensation is a subjective perception after each volume of rectal distension. A note should be made as to the minimal level that the patient perceives the balloon. This is evaluated during rectal stimulation. For a better appraisal a rectometrogram should be performed.

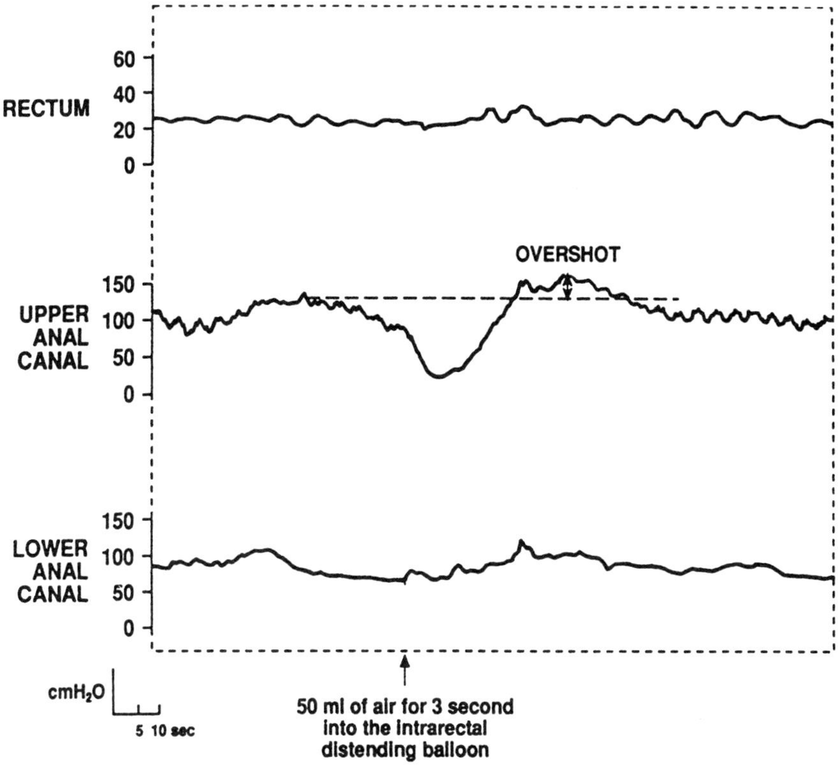

FIGURE 8.23 Overshoot of pressure after the rectoanal inhibitory reflex in a patient who suffers from chronic idiopathic constipation. Note the variations in pressure before the rectoanal inhibitory reflex is triggered. Occasionally, the amplitude of these variations is much greater and renders difficult the search for a reflex.

Another special maneuver is termed the *coughing maneuver*. This induces a rise in intraabdominal pressure and must translate into an anal canal contraction (Fig. 8.25). To achieve this, ask the patient to make a strong cough. The analysis of this cough is performed in the following fashion. First, calculate the amplitude of the reflex contraction at the three levels of recording. Then, calculate the gradient of pressure between the amplitude of the intrarectal pressure and the amplitude of the pressure in the upper and the lower anal canal. These readings should be negative, meaning the pressure remains higher in the anal canal and continence is maintained. The presence of a positive gradient is 100% specific for incontinence, but the sensitivity is only 43%, meaning that there are other factors at work to maintain continence than the anorectal structures.

Another special maneuver is termed *simulated defecation*. Simulated defecation is straining to defecate, which induces a pelvic floor relaxation permitting the passage of stool (Fig. 8.26). In some patients straining induces a contraction instead, which can include both the puborectalis muscle and the external anal sphincter muscle, or either muscle separately. It is essential to realize that this abnormality can exist in only one muscle, because biofeedback therapy should

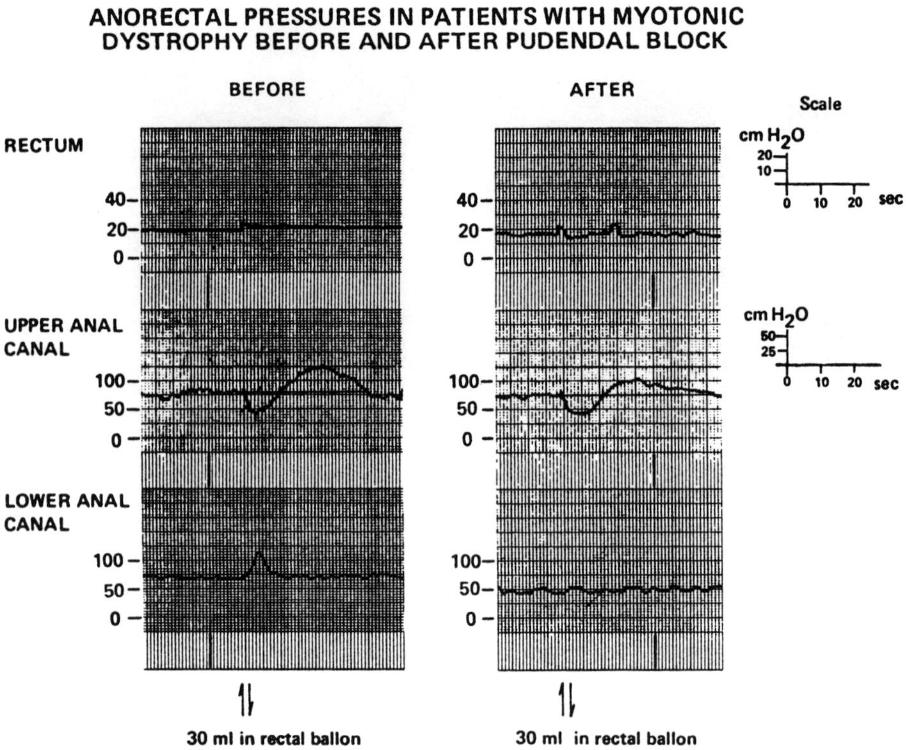

FIGURE 8.24 Pudendal block abolishes the rectoanal contractile reflex recorded in the lower anal canal. Note that the amplitude of overshoot after the rectoanal inhibitory reflex is also markedly reduced by the block, indicating it was due in part to a reflex activity of the external anal sphincter. The remaining overshoot may be due to the remaining activity of the puborectalis muscle (whose upper surface is not innervated by the pudendal nerves, but by the sacral plexus), or to internal anal sphincter activity. These tracings were obtained in a patient with myotonic dystrophy. In healthy subjects, the rectoanal contractile reflex is completely abolished by pudendal block.

encompass both for clinical efficacy. This abnormality is called anismus, but other terms are used as well. The manometric definition is for a rectosphincteric dyssynergia. This technique is performed with the patient lying down, and asked to strain to defecate. It is essential to instruct the patient not to try to withhold the probe. Ask that the straining down be performed three times. Note whether pain is experienced, and note whether the probe is expelled.

The analysis of simulated defecation is the calculation of the rise in intrarectal pressure observed during the maneuver, and the amplitude of relaxation or contraction in the upper anal and in the lower anal canal. After the straining

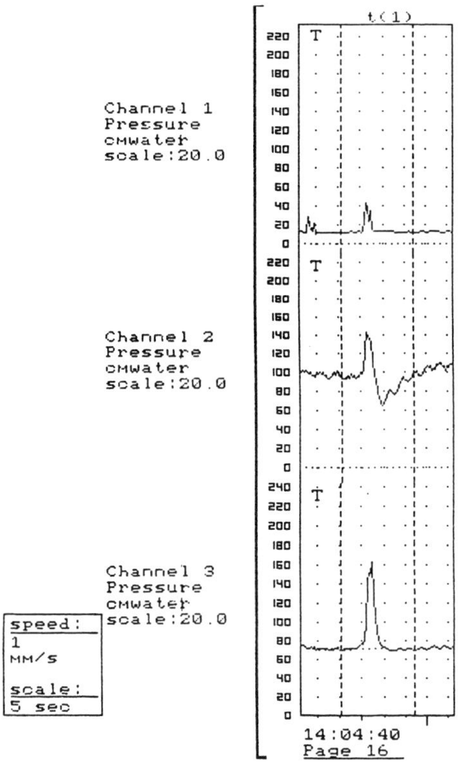

FIGURE 8.25 Cough reflex [T(1)]. Note the increase in pressure on all three channels (rectum, upper anal canal, and lower anal canal, from top to bottom). The increase in pressure in the anal canal exceeds that of the rectum, and this maintains continence.

maneuver observe the changes in pressure in the upper and lower anal canal. A post-straining contraction may follow a relaxation and vice versa (Fig. 8.27). Occasionally, repetitive contractions are recorded.

Post Manometry

The postmanometry activity is quite simple. Retrieve the probe and observe for the presence of stool. Check to see if the initial calibration is still valid. Clean and disinfect the probe adequately according to the standards of prevention of infection for use in the hospital.

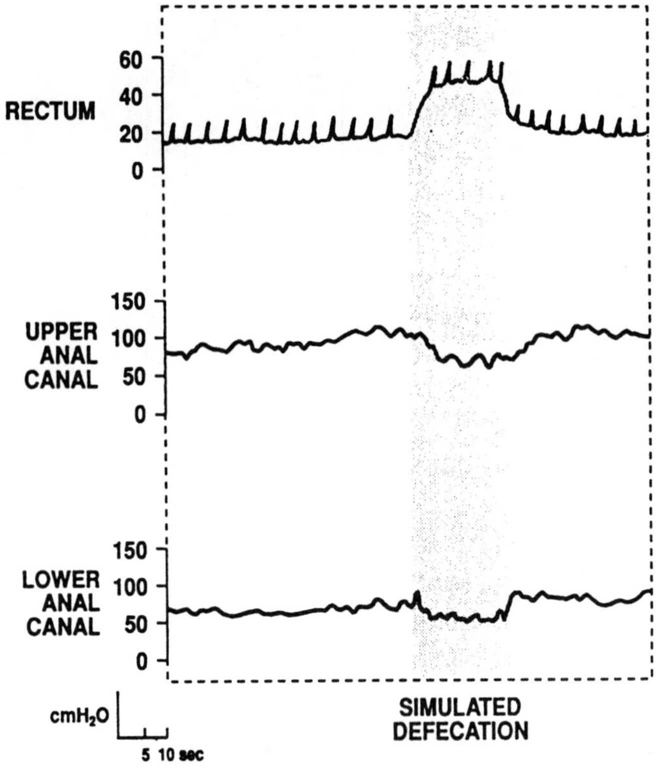

FIGURE 8.26 Straining induces a rise in rectal pressure *(top)* and relaxation in anal canal pressure *(two lower tracings)*.

RECTOMETROGRAPHIC STUDIES

The same type of probe can be used to measure the pressure within the rectal balloon, during graded distention with water. Levels of sensation and tolerance are noted.

To study the elastic properties of the rectum, pressure is recorded within the distending balloon through a separate catheter from that used for distention. This is done by inflating the rectal balloon with 10 ml of body-temperature water within 5 sec; every 30 sec another 10 ml are added. This is done until the subjects complain of lower abdominal discomfort, which always coincides with a sharp increase in the intraballoon pressure. Variations of rectal pressure (cm H_2O) with volume are recorded as a rectometrogram that is limited to the confines of the balloon. Threshold sensation volume, constant sensation volume, and maximum tolerable volume are noted. The pressure–volume curves in the balloon are first recorded in the rectum and thereafter are repeated outside of the rectum under the same body temperature and humidity conditions. Data obtained in these *in vitro* conditions are subtracted from the *in vivo* data to obtain the true rectal wall contribution to pressure changes.

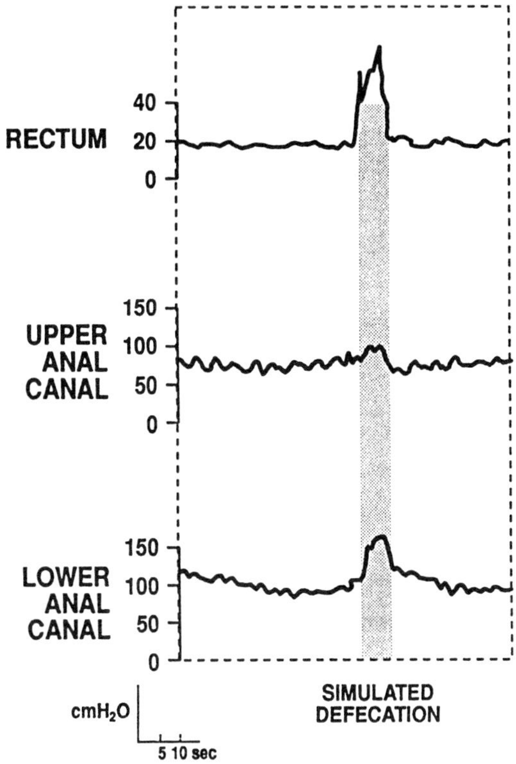

FIGURE 8.27 Anismus. See text for description.

The equipment used to obtain this rectometrogram comes from the same company.

Definition

A rectometrographic study is a diagnostic examination providing information about the rectal capacity to accommodate and its sensitivity.

Material and Equipment

1. Polygraph recorder with three recording channels.
2. Pressure transducers (3) from 0 to 400 mm Hg.
3. Sphygmomanometer to calibrate the polygraph.
4. Three-way stopcocks to connect the probe and the recording equipment.
5. Lubrifying water-soluble gel.
6. Nonsterile gloves.
7. 50 ml (or more) syringes.
8. Disinfecting solution with glutaraldehyde 2%.

TABLE 8.2 POLYVINYL CHLORIDE PROBE WITH 4 CHANNELS AND 3 BALLOONS USED TO RECORD THE RECTOMETROGRAM*

Diameter	7 mm
Length	100 cm
First channel (rectum)	To balloon at end
Second channel (rectum)	To balloon at end
Third channel (upper anus) level	To ring-shaped balloon (diameter: 15 mm) 45 mm from end
Fourth channel (distal anus) level	To ring-shaped balloon (diameter: 15 mm) 63 cm from end

* Marquat Company C53
ZAC de la Haie Griselle
9, rue du 8 Mai 1945, B.P. 11
94471 Boissy-Saint-Léger Cedex, France
Tel: (33) 1-45-69-20-62
Telex: 210 311 F2223
Fax: (33) 1-45-69-66-68

9. Sterile distilled water at 37° C.
10. Adjustable examination table (stretcher, bed).
11. Anorectal manometric probe for rectometrographic studies (Marquat Company, C53) (Table 8.2) (Fig. 8.6, bottom).

The rectal distending balloon can be made out of a finger of a surgeon's glove, 2 inches long, or commercial balloons are available (Mui Scientific, B-L4, Division of H&A Mui Enterprises Inc., 2570 Hames Road, Unit 1, Mississauga, Ontario, Canada, L4Y 4A3). The balloon must be able to contain 1,000 ml of water. This is a modification from the original equipment of Marquat, used solely for viscoelastic studies of the rectum, which necessitate only small volumes of distension of the rectum.

The importance of having two channels opening independently into the rectum is to avoid the turbulence during recording and avoid recording the pressure triggered by the force of the injecting hand.

The preparation of the patient is the same as for anorectal manometry, and so is the preparation of the material and equipment.

Positioning of the Probe

A series of maneuvers is performed:

(1) Introduce the lubricated probe while the patient lies in lateral decubitus. The most proximal (lower anal canal, external anal sphincter) balloon must barely disappear at the anal margin. If the probe cannot be introduced, a medical examination must be done. (2) Ask the patient to lie down and relax. (3) To make sure the distending balloon is adequately laid into the rectum, rather than bundled up, introduce the probe deeper, and take it out so that a peak of pressure is obtained at the level of the two annular balloons.

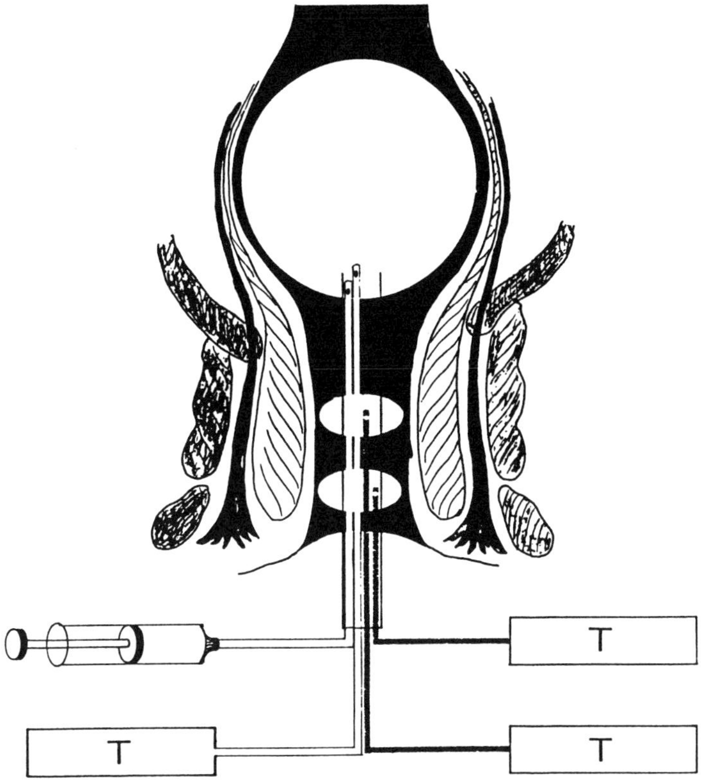

FIGURE 8.28 Technical setup for rectometrographic studies (see text for explanation).

Technical Aspects and Measurements (Fig. 8.28)

***IN VIVO* TECHNIQUE** (1) Inject into the rectal balloon 10 ml of water at body temperature, within 5 sec, every 30 sec. The *rate of distension* is absolutely key to reproducibility. Indeed, if an inflation rate of 150 ml/min is used, the tracings are not reproducible (Fig. 8.29), whereas at lesser rates, they are (Fig. 8.30). The nonreproducibility is directly related to the rate of distension (Fig. 8.31). (2) Thereafter, ask the patient to identify subjectively the following levels of sensation during the water injection:

The *threshold of sensation volume* is the perception of a short-lived sensation that will disappear before the next injection of water. This volume is not necessarily smaller than the constant sensation volume.

The *constant sensation volume* is a rectal sensation that has not disappeared before the next injection of water. This may be described as an urge to defecate, but may also be described as a rectal pain or a feeling of intraabdominal pressure.

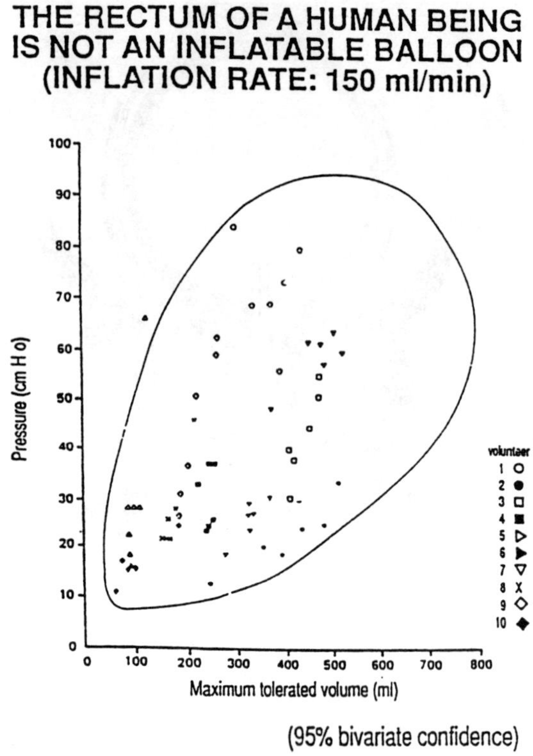

FIGURE 8.29 If the rectum is treated as an inert material, and distended regardless of the subject, wide dispersion of data is to be expected, presumably because of individual sensitivities and muscular idiosyncrasies.

Usually, on the oscillograph, a slow rise of pressure can be seen to occur between the level of constant sensation and the maximum tolerable volume (Fig. 8.32). Record this volume and take note of its description. Note that the rectoanal inhibitory reflex, recorded in the upper anal canal, does not recover at the level of constant sensation, and there is no return to baseline pressure: the upper anal canal pressure remains lowered constantly from this level of distension on.

The *maximum tolerable volume* is a perception of a sensation of fullness which corresponds to an urge of impending defecation, and, if more fluid is added, the superposition of slight pain. Some patients do not have a feeling of impending defecation before they have pain. Record this volume, and note the way the patient describes one's sensation; it may be described as a pressing urge to defecate, a pain in the pelvic floor, and a sensation of hypesthesia in the lower extremities.

Thirty seconds later, empty the rectal volume.

***IN VITRO* TECHNIQUE** *Technique:* (1) Lay the probe at the same level as the pressure transducers. (2) Repeat the procedure, as in the *in vivo* technique, to the maximum tolerable volume recorded within the rectum of the patient.

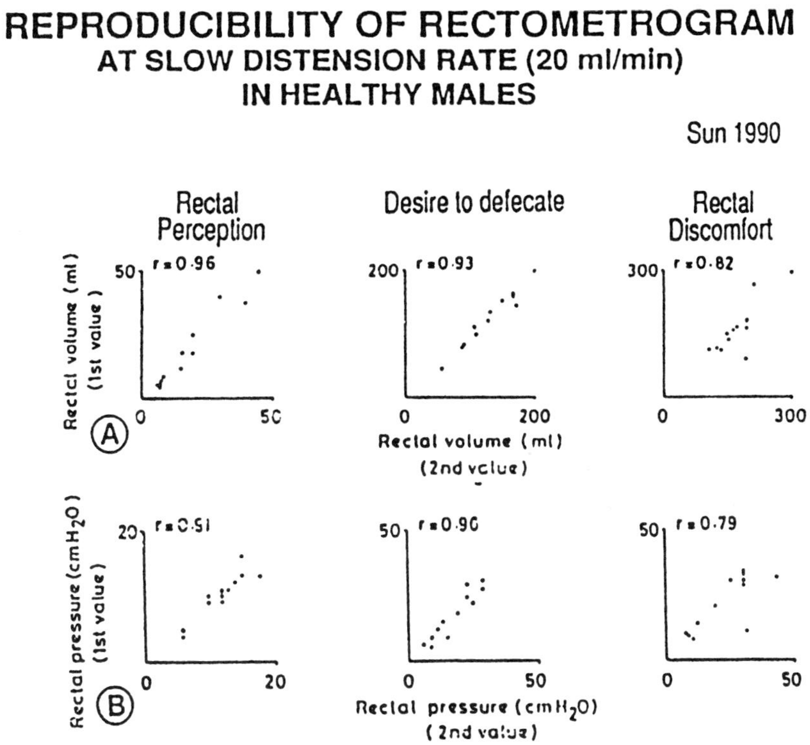

FIGURE 8.30 When properly done, rectometrographic studies are highly reproducible.

Analysis: (1) On the *in vivo* and the *in vitro* tracings, note the mean amplitude of pressure during the 3 sec preceding each volume of distension, when the accommodation of the rectum to the previous volume of distension is maximal. (2) For each volume of distension, subtract the *in vitro* pressure from the *in vivo* pressure. (3) Calculate the rectal sensitivity index:

$$\frac{\text{MTV} - \text{CSV}}{\text{MTV}}$$

where MTV = maximum tolerable volume
CSV = constant sensation volume

Diagnosis

Megarectum

Diagnosis: No control female subject has a rectal volume that exceeds 320 ml. No control male subject has one above 440. The range of normality is 140–320 ml for women and 170–440 in men. However, in stress-free controls, i.e., asymptomatic subjects who claim that stress, of any kind, does not trigger abdominal pain nor any changes toward constipation or diarrhea in bowel habits, the range of normality is much narrower, being 190–250 ml of water, and is identical in

RECTAL ACCOMMODATION IS INFLUENCED BY TECHNICAL MODALITIES OF RECTAL DISTENSION

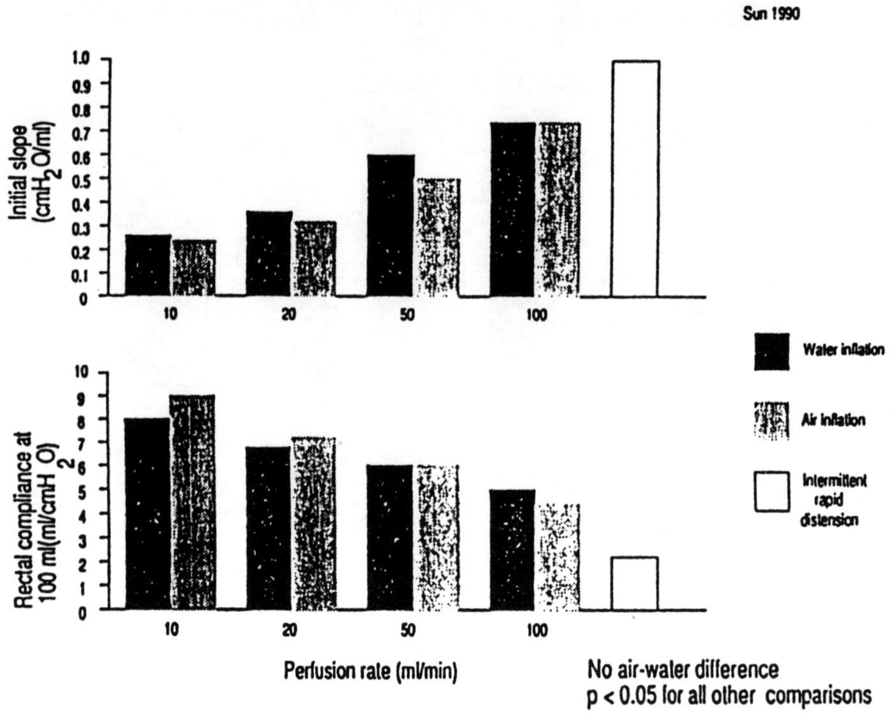

FIGURE 8.31 Rectal compliance decreases with increasing rate of rectal distension.

ELASTIC PROPERTIES OF THE HUMAN RECTUM

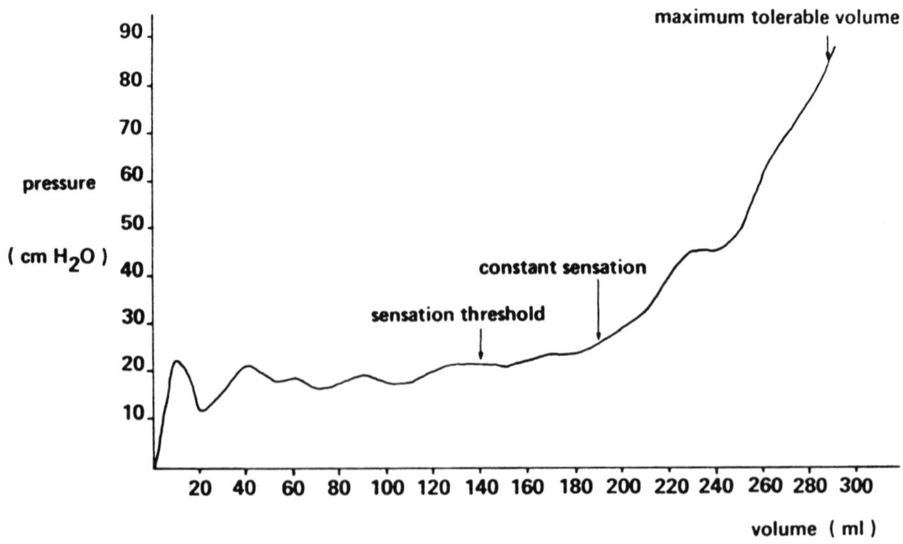

FIGURE 8.32 Pressure–volume curve during progressive rectal distension. This curve is a rectometrogram.

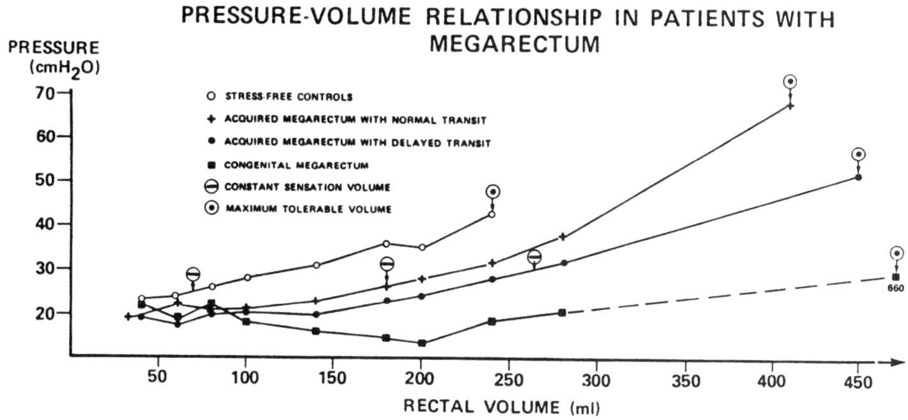

FIGURE 8.33 Mean value of pressure–volume curve in control subjects who do not react to stress with abdominal pain nor with change in their bowel habits, and in constipated patients with megarectum.

women and men (n = 11). A safe diagnosis of megarectum can be made if the maximum tolerable volume exceeds 440 ml (Fig. 8.33).

It must be clearly understood that if patients do not *feel* any rectal sensation, this does not mean that they have a problem with sensitive innervation. Indeed, Figure 8.33 shows clearly that the same sensation level in three groups of patients is reached when more fluid has been injected: it means they have elastic properties of the rectal wall differences that account for the differences in sensation. It is a *motor* disorder, rather than a *sensitivity disorder*.

Rectal Hypoesthesia: Hypoesthesia of the rectum does exist but to make such a diagnosis, the musculature contribution has to be taken into account, hence the use of the rectal sensitivity index described above. In patients with megarectum, known to have a motor problem, the lowest value of rectal sensitivity index is 0.35. Thus, no diagnosis of hypoesthesia can safely be done above that level, for fear of mixing motor and sensory components of the problem.

Microrectum

Diagnosis: A diagnosis of microrectum is made when the maximum tolerable volume is below 140 ml in women and 170 ml in men. It must be remembered that the 140–190 ml is a gray zone in terms of diagnosis, as discussed above for values found in stress-free controls.

This may be found in chronic rectal ischemia (Fig. 8.34), chronic idiopathic constipation, and irritable bowel syndrome.

The technical aspects after the procedure are the same as after anorectal manometry.

PRESSURE-VOLUME RELATIONSHIP IN THE RECTUM OF PATIENTS WITH CHRONIC RECTAL ISCHEMIA

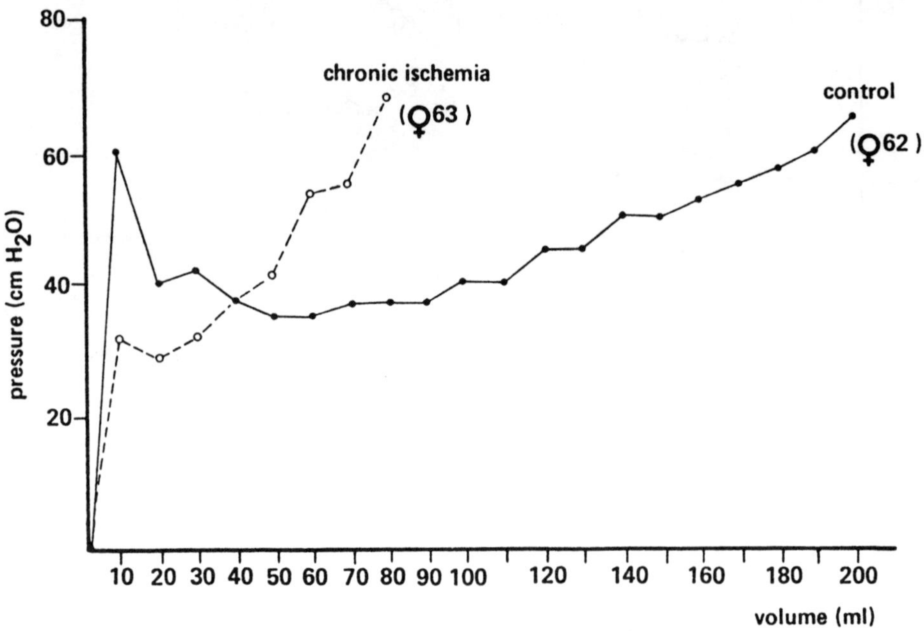

FIGURE 8.34 Chronic rectal ischemia. An example contrasting a patient and a healthy subject of the same age. Contrary to common belief, the rectal capacity does *not* decrease with age. In this case, it is a sign of underlying pathology, ischemia, commonly found with age. There is no correlation of volume and age in asymptomatic controls.

MANOMETRIC FINDINGS RELATED TO SOME CLINICAL FEATURES

This section is an attempt to sort out abnormalities, starting not from anorectal motility findings, as exemplified above, but from clinical diagnosis. For each diagnosis, one or more abnormalities may be recorded.

Aging

There is a decrease in resting pressure and in maximal squeeze pressure, which is more marked in women. A decrease in voluntary contraction and a decrease of rectal compliance have been described. Of note, these data are subject to debate because the selection of healthy, asymptomatic, stress-free controls is key. The literature on this subject is very conflictual. For instance, not all studies show a decrease in compliance, because some control subjects selected in some studies, in fact, suffered from chronic rectal ischemia known to decrease the rectal capacities to accommodate.

Anal Fissures

There are ultraslow waves in the anal canal. Resting pressure is elevated but squeeze pressure is usually normal. When eliciting the RAIR a large overshoot, a rebound contraction, occurs immediately after normal internal anal sphincter (IAS) relaxation. There is also impaired mucosal sensitivity.

Anal Surgery

Basal pressure in the upper and lower anal canal may be decreased. There is an absence of the RAIR especially after full thickness sphincterotomy. There is a decrease in amplitude of the RAIR and its surface, as measured by planimetry.

Anesthesia of the Anal Mucosa

It leads to a decrease in amplitude and duration of the voluntary squeeze pressure.

Anismus

This is defined as a paradoxical contraction of the external anal sphincter (EAS) and/or the puborectalis muscle, as the patient strains to defecate. This is recorded as a rising pressure not only in the rectum—which is evidence that the patient strains—but also in the upper and/or the lower part of the anal canal. It is essential to know that anismus may be recorded in only one of the two muscles because otherwise biofeedback may lead to failure because one of the muscle has not recovered. In addition, one can record the presence of spontaneous contractions interrupting the RAIR. There may be a decrease in amplitude with or without a decrease in surface, as measured by planimetry, of the RAIR. There may be an inverted pressure profile of the anorectum. The threshold of the rectal volume recorded to induce a desire to defecate is usually abnormally high. The threshold required to induce other sensations, on the contrary is often normal. Finally, in normal subjects anismus may be caused by the embarrassment of defecating while being watched, but this needs to be interpreted.

Brain Lesion

They may be accompanied by a decrease in resting pressure of the anal canal, secondary to a dysfunction of the IAS and EAS.

Brain Stem Lesion

There may be an absence of the RAIR in anterior lesions of the brain stem, but it may be present in posterior lesions.

Chronic Paraplegia

Resting anal pressures are usually normal in this situation.

Chronic Radiation Injury

They are accompanied by a reduced sensory threshold.

Chronic Rectal Ischemia

It may be accompanied by an absence of the RAIR or a decrease in amplitude and of surface as measured by planimetry. There may be an increase of duration of the RAIR. During rectometrographic studies, there may be a microrectum.

Chronic Respiratory Failure

The RAIR may be absent.

Complete Rectal Prolapse

Resting pressure in this situation is normal if the patient is continent, but decreased if the patient is incontinent. There is an activation of the RAIR from the advancing prolapse segment. Anorectal sensation is disturbed. Maximal voluntary contraction of the anal canal is decreased. The anal pressure does not increase above rectal pressure during increases in intraabdominal pressure.

Complete Supraconal Spinal Cord Lesions

Basal pressure in the anal canal is normal. There is absence of voluntary contraction of the EAS. There is a decrease in response of the EAS activity to increases in intraabdominal pressure, for instance, with cough. The higher the lesion, the lower the intraabdominal pressure generated, and the lower the EAS response. There is no inhibition of the EAS activity during straining. Distension with relatively minimal volumes in the rectum generates giant rectal contractions, with an amplitude of more than 40 cm H_2O for 10 sec, associated with deep anal relaxation, a markedly exaggerated normal response. There is an absence of receptive relaxation of rectal tone during rampdistension of the rectum. No specific rectal sensation occurs during rectal distension but 50% of the patients will experience a dull pelvic sensation at maximum distension. Of note, the RAIR is present in all spinal patients, but there is no correlation between volume of rectal distension and both amplitude and duration of the RAIR. On deflating the rectal balloon, anal pressures often exceed the values observed immediately before inflation (a rebound response). This response is absent in patients with high spinal cord lesions.

Diabetes

In diabetic patients, large rectal waves of more than 20 cm H_2O for more than 5 sec can be recorded. There is a decrease in rectal sensitivity and spontaneous transient IAS relaxations.

Frontal Lobe Lesion

Spontaneous rectal contractions have been described, and there is an increase in perception of threshold of rectal distension. There is no RAIR. There is a decrease in amplitude and duration of voluntary contractions of the anal canal. The anal canal is hypotonic.

Functional Colopathy/Irritable Bowel Syndrome

Findings should be noted in patients with the irritable bowel syndrome. There may be an increase in amplitude with or without increase in surface of the RAIR, as measured by planimetry, and it may be followed by an overshoot in pressure. The basal rectal pressure may be elevated or unstable. There is also an increase in basal pressure in the anal canal secondary to activity of the IAS and EAS. Spontaneous relaxation and ultraslow waves can be recorded in the anal canal. There may be an inverted profile in pressure in the anal canal. There is an increase in rectal sensitivity, a decrease in rectal compliance, and an increase in rectal contractility and anal relaxation and response to rectal distension. The rectum is hypertonic. There is an inappropriate rectoanal inhibition at lower rectal volumes and it is sustained for long periods.

Hemorrhoids

Patients with hemorrhoids have ultraslow waves and a higher than normal resting anal canal pressure. There is also an increase in threshold of sensitivity of the mucosa. The distal part of the anal canal fails to relax during rectal distension.

Hereditary Internal Anal Sphincter Myopathy

In hereditary IAS myopathy, the IAS is hypertrophied and hypertonic. It relaxes but often incompletely and after high degree of rectal distension. There is an increase of maximal anal canal pressure and marked ultraslow waves activity.

Hirschsprung's Disease

In Hirschsprung's disease the main finding is the absence of RAIR, but there are other abnormalities that can be recorded at anorectal manometry. There is an increase in rectal pressure with more frequent waves. There is an increase in slow-wave oscillation of high amplitude in the upper part of the anal canal. There is an increase in frequency (47%) of the rectoanal contractile reflex. In the upper part of the anal canal, there are more frequent spontaneous variations of pressure of lower frequency and greater amplitude than normal. There is an absence of inhibition of rhythmical activity of the IAS after rectal distension. Finally, there is a low pain threshold for rectal distension.

Incomplete Supraconal Lesions

Voluntary contraction of the sphincters is possible, but there is a weak squeeze pressure. Rectal sensation is blunted. External anal sphincter response to rectal distension and increased intraabdominal pressure is often enhanced. Rectal compliance is abnormally low. Anal relaxation and rectal phasic contractile response to rectal distension are exaggerated.

Incontinence

In patients with fecal incontinence, several findings may be abnormal. Usually, there is a decrease in maximum resting and squeeze pressure, but this pressure may be completely normal. There may be an increase of spontaneous relaxations in resting anal canal pressures, which are longer lasting and more frequent than normal. Rectal volume necessary to induce sphincter relaxation is reduced. There is a decrease in maximum tolerable rectal volume. Large rectal waves have been described. Reflex contraction of the external anal sphincter is delayed, when attempting to prevent release of feces. There is an impaired IAS tone. There is a positive gradient with a cough reflex. EAS response to rectal distension and increases in intraabdominal pressures are impaired.

Irritable Rectum

Some patients have what has been labeled *irritable rectum,* which is similar to the irritable bowel syndrome. There is an increase in rectal sensitivity and an abnormally low rectal compliance. Sustained relaxation of the IAS can be recorded and repetitive rectal contractions induced at abnormally low rectal volumes.

Low Anterior Resection

After low anterior resection, there is a decrease in rectal compliance but it may recover with time.

Low Rectal Transection

When there has been a low rectal transection, the RAIR may completely disappear at least temporarily.

Low Spinal Lesion and Cauda Equina Lesions

Patients with low spinal lesions and cauda equina lesions may exhibit several abnormalities. There may be impaired rectal sensation, reduced rectal tone, an absence of external anal sphincter response to rectal distension, and increase in intraabdominal pressure. The conscious contractions of the EAS may be impaired or absent. There may be a decrease in basal anal canal pressure due to problems with the internal and the external anal sphincter. There may be spontaneous relaxations in the anal canal and absence of a rectoanal contractile reflex. Finally, there may be no correlation between rectal distending volume and amplitude and duration of the RAIR.

Megarectum

In this situation, there is an increase in rectal compliance and maximum tolerable volume. There is reduced rectal sensation but this is not due to a problem of sensation but to a problem of viscoelastic properties of the wall, a higher volume being necessitated to produce enough stretch of the rectal muscle to obtain sensation. Secondary to the hypotonicity of the rectal wall, there may be no RAIR, or there may be a decrease in amplitude and surface, as measured by planimetry, of the RAIR. There may be a decreased duration of RAIR and their may be occasionally a decrease in basal rectal pressure.

Meningomyelocele

In patients with meningomyelocele, anorectal manometry may be entirely normal. There may be however a decrease in resting anal canal pressure due to problems with both the IAS and EAS. There may be rectoanal antagonisms, i.e., spontaneous intermittent relaxations of the upper anal canal with simultaneous rectal contractions. Anal canal pressure may be very unstable in its upper part, resembling ultraslow waves. Finally, the RAIR may be absent.

Multiple Sclerosis

In multiple sclerosis, the anal canal may be hypertonic. The RAIR may have a decrease in amplitude. There may be spontaneous rectal contractions and an abnormal threshold of perception of the rectal distension which is increased.

Obstetrical Trauma

After obstetrical trauma, there may be a weak basal pressure in the anal canal secondary to distortion of both the EAS and IAS. There may be absence of maximal voluntary contractions of the EAS.

Perfusion of Rectum by Saline and Bile Acid

Perfusion of the rectum by saline and bile acids produces an increase in rectal contractile activity and an increase in depth of anal relaxation. This may cause leakage at a much earlier stage. Presumably, this situation applies to patients who malabsorb bile salts and present for fecal incontinence. History will obtain a problem of chronic watery diarrhea but occasionally a severe burning abdominal pain only. This occurs in patients with small bowel disease such as Crohn's disease and it may also occur after small bowel resection involving the last 100 cm of small bowel. Of note, a significant number of these patients are found to have idiopathic bile salt malabsorption, presumably on the basis of dysmotility of the small bowel, perhaps of psychophysiological nature.

Physical and/or Sexual Abuse

These produce distortion in anal rectal motility. There may be a decrease in maximal voluntary contraction of the anal sphincter and little rise in anal pressure upon straining. Thus these patients squeeze little the pelvic floor and strain little. There may be a decrease in rectal sensation. Finally, anismus and other manifestations of abdominopelvic dyssynergia are frequently present.

Post Hysterectomy

After hysterectomy, one may find a decrease in rectal sensation, a decrease in sigmoid motor activity, but in some patients an increased rectal sensitivity has been described.

Pruritus Ani

In pruritus ani, resting anal pressure is usually normal but the RAIR may be exaggerated.

Pudendal Neuropathy

This is probably the long-term result of straining against a tight anus and is part of the descending perineum syndrome. There is a decrease in basal pressure of the anal canal secondary to a problem with both the IAS and EAS. There are weak conscious contractions of the EAS. There is a decrease in squeeze pressure and in duration of maximal voluntary contraction. The rectoanal contractile reflex may be decreased in frequency and amplitude, and even be absent. There is a decrease in rectal sensation and impairment of the RAIR.

Rectal Surgery

Rectal surgery may produce a decrease in amplitude with or without a decrease in surface as measured planimetry of the RAIR.

Sacral Resection

It may produce a decrease in resting anal pressure. Discrimination of anorectal contents is disturbed if nerves are sacrificed bilaterally, but it is normal if they are sacrificed unilaterally.

Scleroderma

There may be a decrease in amplitude and sometimes surface, as measured by planimetry, of the RAIR which may be completely absent. There may also be a decrease in basal pressure of the anal canal secondary to a dysfunction of the IAS and EAS.

Short Segment Hirschsprung's Disease

It is an entity which must be recognized. There is no RAIR. In this situation, radiology is useless, and in ultrashort segments Hirschsprung's disease, anorectal manometry is the sole way of making a diagnosis. In this situation, a differential diagnosis is to be done on the absence of RAIR for fear of making an erroneous diagnosis of Hirschsprung's disease on this basis. There may be a high resting anal canal pressure due to IAS and EAS activity.

Sipple Syndrome Type IIb

There may be an absence of RAIR.

Solitary Rectal Ulcer

A rectal prolapse must obligatorily be searched for. There may be a decrease in basal and squeeze pressure of the anus. The IAS activity may be perturbed and no tone be present. There is an increase in rectal sensitivity, as well as an abnormally low rectal compliance. Sustained relaxation of the IAS and repetitive rectal contractions are induced at abnormally low rectal volumes.

Spinal Anesthesia

After spinal anesthesia, there is a decrease in resting and pressure. This type of anesthesia does not abolish the relaxation of the IAS in response to rectal distension and the RAIR is still recorded.

Spinal Shock

After spinal shock, there is a decrease in resting upper anal canal pressure. There is also absence of maximal voluntary contraction of the external anal sphincter.

Steinert's Disease

In myotonic dystrophy (Steinert's disease) the RAIR is followed by an overshoot of pressure.

Ulcerative Colitis

In ulcerative colitis, there is increased rectal sensitivity and abnormally low rectal compliance. A sustained relaxation of the IAS and repetitive rectal contractions are induced at abnormally low rectal volumes.

Uninhibited Anal Sphincter Relaxation Syndrome

The EAS does not contract either reflexively or voluntarily on rectal distension.

SUGGESTED READINGS

Akervall S, Fasth S, Nordgren S, et al: Manovolumetry: a new method for investigation of anorectal function. *Gut* 29:614–623, 1988.

Arhan P: Données expérimentales sur la physiologie de l'appareil recto-anal chez l'animal et chez l'enfant. Thèse, Université de Tours, France, 1972.

Arhan P, Devroede G, Persoz B, et al: Response of the anal canal to repeated distension of the rectum. *Clin Invest Med* 2:83–88, 1979.

Arhan P, Faverdin C, Devroede G, et al: Anorectal motility after surgery for spina bifida. *Dis Colon Rectum* 27:159–63, 1984.

Barnes PR, Lennard-Jones JE: Function of the striated anal sphincter during straining in control subjects and constipated patients with a radiologically normal rectum or idiopathic megacolon. *Int J Colorectal Dis* 3:207–209, 1988.

Beuret-Blanquart F, Weber J, Gouverneur JP, et al: Colonic transit time and anorectal manometric anomalies in 19 patients with complete transaction of the spinal cord. *J Auton Nerv Syst* 1–9, 1990.

Devroede G, Arhan P, Duguay C, et al: Traumatic constipation. *Gastroenterology* 77:1258–1267, 1979.

Devroede G, Vobecky S, Massé S, et al: Ischemic faecal incontinence and rectal pain. *Gastroenterology* 83(5):970–980, 1982.

Devroede G: Constipation. In: Sleisenger MH, Fordtran JS, eds: *Gastrointestinal Disease: Pathophysiology, Diagnosis, Management.* ed 5. 1993, pp 837–887.

Edwards CA, Brown S, Baxter AJ, et al: Effect of bile acid on anorectal function in man. *Gut* 30:383–386, 1989.

Faverdin C, Dornic C, Arhan P, et al: Quantitative analysis of anorectal pressures in Hirschsprung's disease. *Dis Colon Rectum* 24(6):422–427, 1981.

Frenckner B: Function of the anal sphincters in spinal man. *Gut* 16:638–644, 1975.

Glick ME, Meshkinpour H, Haldeman S, et al: Colonic dysfunction in patients with thoracic spinal cord injury. *Gastroenterology* 86:287–294, 1984.

Gunterberg B, Kewenter J, Petersen I, et al: Anorectal function after major resection of the sacrum with bilateral or unilateral sacrifice of sacral nerves. *Br J Surg* 63:546–554, 1976.

Hamel-Roy J, Devroede G, Arhan P, et al: Functional abnormalities of the anal sphincters in patients with myotonic dystrophy. *Gastroenterology* 86(6):1469–1474, 1984.

Hamel-Roy J, Devroede G, Arhan P, et al: Comparative esophageal and anorectal motility in scleroderma. *Gastroenterology* 88:1–7, 1985.

Hancock BD: Measurement of anal presssure and motility. *Gut* 17:645–651, 1976.

Hancock BD: Internal sphincter and the nature of hemorrhoids. *Gut* 18:651–656, 1977.

Hancock BD: The internal sphincter and anal fissure. *Br J Surg* 64:92–95, 1977.

Hancock BD: Lord's procedure for haemorrhoids: a prospective anal pressure study. *Br J Surg* 68:729–730, 1981.

Kerremans R: *Morphological and Physiological Aspect of Anal Continence and Defecation.* Brussels, Editions Arscia S.A., Presses Académiques Européennes, 1969.

Kumar D, Waldron DL, Williams NS: Home assessment of anorectal motility and external sphincter EMG in idiopathic faecal incontinence. *Br J Surg* 76:635–636, 1989.

Lawson JON, Nixon HH: Anal canal pressure in the diagnosis of Hirschsprung's disease. *J Pediatr Surg* 2:544–552, 1967.

Lebel ML, Grand'Maison F: Étude électromyographique dynamique du plancher pelvien dans la constipation: importance de l'EMG à l'aiguille. *Can J Neurolog Sci* 15:212, 1988.

Leroi AM, Bernier C, Watier A, et al: Sexual abuse and functional disorders of the lower gastrointestinal tract. *Int J Colorectal Dis* (accepted for publication).

Leroi AM, Berkelmans I, Denis PH, et al: Anismus as a marker of sexual abuse: consequences of abuse on anorectal motility. *Dig Dis Sci* (in press).

Martelli H, Devroede G, Arhan P, et al: Some parameters of large bowel motility in normal man. *Gastroenterology* 75:612–618, 1978.

Meagher AP, Lubowski DZ, King DW: The cough response of the anal sphincter. *J Colorectal Dis* 8:217–219, 1993.

Nothman BJ, Schuster MM: Internal anal sphincter derangement with anal fissures. *Gastroenterology* 67:216–220, 1974.

Parks AG, Porter NH, Melzack J: Experimental study of the reflex mechanism controlling the muscles of the pelvic floor. *Dis Colon Rectum* 5:407–414, 1962.

Preston DM, Lennard-Jones JE: Anismus in chronic constipation. *Dig Dis Sci* 30:413–318, 1985.

Prior A, Stanley K, Smith ARB, et al: The effect of simple hysterectomy on anorectal and urethrovesical symptoms. *Gut* 33:264–267, 1992.

Rao SSC, Holdsworth CO, Read NW: Anorectal sensitivity and reactivity in patients with ulcerative colitis. *Gastroenterology* 83:1270–1275, 1987.

Read MG, Read NW, Haynes WG, et al: A prospective study of the effect of haemorrhoidectomy on sphincter function and faecal continence. *Br J Surg* 69:396–398, 1982.

Schouten WR, Blankensteijn JD: Ultra slow waves pressure variations in the anal canal before and after lateral internal sphincterotomy. *Int J Colorectal Dis* 7:115–118, 1992.

Sun WM, Read NW, Prior A, et al: Sensory and motor responses to rectal distension vary according to rate and pattern of balloon inflation. *Gastroenterology* 99:1008–1015, 1990.

Tobon F, Nigel CR, Reid W, et al: Nonsurgical test for the diagnosis of Hirschsprung's disease. *N Engl J Med* 278(4):188–194, 1968.

Varma JS, Smith AN: Abnormalities of colorectal function in intractable constipation following hysterectomy. *Gut* 26:581–582, 1985.

VerDuron A, Devroede G, Bouchoucha M, et al: Mégarectum. *Dig Dis Sci* 33(9):1164–1174, 1988.

Wald A. Chandra R, Chiponis D, et al: Anorectal function and continence mechanisms in childhood encopresis. *J Pediatr Gastroenterol Nutr* 5:346–351, 1986.

Watier A, Feldman P, Martelli H, et al: Hirschsprung's disease. In Haurbrick WS, Schaffner F, eds: *Bockus Gastroenterology,* ed 5, J. E. Berk, consulting editor: W. J. Snape, section editor.

Weber J, Denis P, Mihout B, et al: Effect of brain stem lesion on colonic and anorectal motility. *Dig Dis Sci* 30(5):419–425, 1985.

Weber J, Grise P, Roquebert M, et al: Radiopaque markers transit and anorectal manometry in 16 patients with multiple sclerosis and urinary bladder dysfunction. *Dis Col Rectum* 30:95–100, 1987.

Weber J, Delangre T, Hannequin D, et al: Anorectal manometry anomalies in seven patients with frontal brain damage. *Dig Dis Sci* 35(2):225–230, 1990.

Whitehead WE, Engel BT, Schuster MM: Irritable bowel syndrome. *Dig Dis Sci* 25:404–413, 1980.

CHAPTER 9

Defecography

Leonard M. Glassman

OVERVIEW

Defecography is the functional fluoroscopic evaluation of rectal emptying. While the semipublic act of defecation might be expected to inhibit patients from adequately cooperating during the examination, this has not been our experience when the procedure is explained and the number of observers in the room is held to a minimum.

Many radiology departments have been hesitant to offer defecography, worrying first that patients will not come after the chair is constructed or purchased and second that they will. In addition, there is much uncertainty in the interpretation of the results based on the radiologist's unfamiliarity with the abnormalities of defecation and the integration of those findings with the clinical complaint and results of other testing. Often abnormalities are found on the defecogram which have no correlate with the clinical problem and therefore should be disregarded. We must remember to treat the patient not the test.

We do both a scintigraphic and a fluoroscopic study in almost all patients. The scintigraphic study is done first because it is the more physiologic of the two tests and its results are therefore more indicative of normal or abnormal emptying. The scinitgraphic study also acts as a check on the completeness of evacuation when the fluoroscopic study shows poor emptying and uncertainty exists as to whether it is caused by disease or patient inhibition.

INDICATIONS

The most common reasons for referral for defecography are: the assessment of constipation or fecal incontinence; the assessment of a vaginal mass; the suspicion of anorectal prolapse or the finding of a solitary rectal ulcer.

Less frequent indications are: the assessment of the feeling of incomplete evacuation; the evaluation of local anal disease such as perianal pain, fissures, or hemorrhoids; the assessment of frequent small stools; the postoperative evaluation of repairs of previously documented pathology or postcolectomy pouch procedures.

CONTRAINDICATIONS

The presence of anorectal surgery within the past 2 weeks or a known colon perforation or anastamotic leak are the major contraindications. The exam also should not be done during pregnancy; the average dose of radiation is approximately that of a barium enema.

THE SCINTIGRAPHIC STUDY

Equipment

1. 25 gm Veegum powder.
2. 300 cc warm distilled water.
3. 2 mCi technetium-99m (^{99m}Tc)
4. Three 60-cc irrigation syringes.
5. Standard scintigraphic camera.

Procedure

The Tc sulfur colloid is mixed into the distilled water. The Veegum powder is added to the water one scoop at a time while mixing, stirring until the mixture is the consistency of toothpaste. Spoon the mixture into the three irrigation syringes and administer mixture to the patient rectally until the patient experiences fullness or the entire amount has been given.

Image using a standard scintigraphic camera in the left lateral sitting position immediately for 5 min. Then have the patient go to a private toilet and evacuate as completely as possible. Image again for 5 min in the left lateral sitting position.

Results

Use computer analysis:

64 × 64 byte static acquisition.

Draw ROI over rectum of both pre- and postevacuation images.

Compare the counts of each ROI and calculate percent emptying using the following formula:

$$\frac{\text{Initial counts} - \text{Final counts}}{\text{Initial counts}} \times 100\% = \%\ \text{emptying}$$

The study can also be done in the dynamic mode during evacuation but this duplicates much of the information obtained in the fluoroscopic study and loses the physiologic nature of defecation in private as the dynamic study must be done in the scanning room next to the scintillation camera.

THE FLUOROSCOPIC STUDY

Equipment

1. Standard television fluoroscopic table capable of supine and erect operation and filming, preferably using large films although 90 mm photofluorogram spot films are acceptable.
2. Videocassette recorder.
3. Hemorrhoid cushion filled with air or water; a water-filled cushion gives better pictures whereas an air-filled one gives only adequate images but a lower radiation dose.
4. High-density, high-viscosity barium paste such as Anatrast (55% wt/wt barium sulfate USP) or Evacupaste. These are premixed barium pastes that come already loaded in a caulking tube with a connecting tube which can function as an enema tip.
5. Standard caulking gun.
6. 50-cc irrigation syringe filled with 30 cc of liquid barium (58% wt/wt barium sulfate suspension) normally used for double-contrast enemas.
7. 240 cc of oral barium mixture as for small bowel study (40% wt/wt barium sulfate suspension) if enterocele is suspected.
8. Water-soluble lubricant for enema tip.
9. Defecography chair or bedpan on footboard of fluoroscopic table.
10. Bedpan if frontal study is necessary.

Procedure

No patient preparation is necessary.

If an enterocele is suspected, the patient should be given 240 cc liquid barium by mouth 1 hr before the examination. We do this routinely as many enteroceles are asymptomatic or thought to be rectoceles on physical examination. Occasionally special circumstances such as a patient's morbid fear of impaction prevents taking the oral barium.

The videocassette recorder is connected to the video output of the fluoroscopic system to record the procedure. The barium cartridge is placed in the caulking gun. All supplies are arranged on a table in easy reach of the fluoroscopic table (Fig. 9.1).

The patient is brought into the fluoroscopic room and the painless nature of the exam is stressed after appropriate history is obtained.

The patient is placed in the left lateral position on the horizontal fluoroscopic table and the lubricated connecting tubing is inserted gently. Using the irrigation

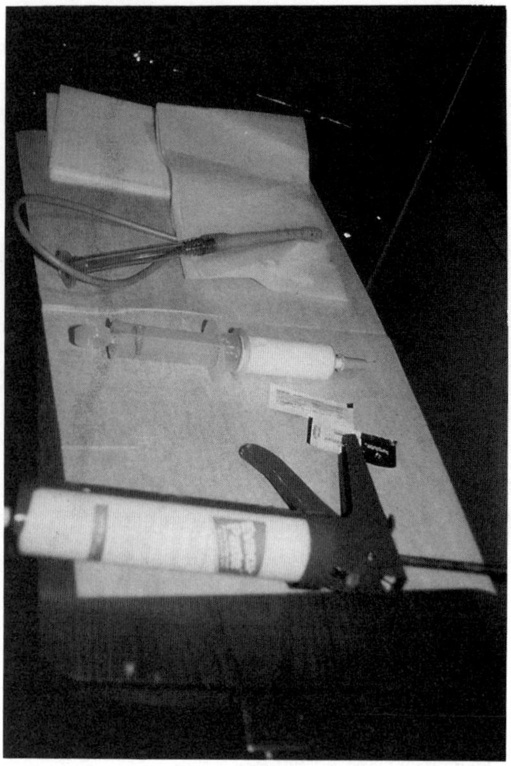

FIGURE 9.1 Table setup for fluoroscopic study includes connecting tubing here with the optional enema tip, radiopaque patient number marker, lubricant, towels, liquid barium in syringe, caulking gun loaded with barium paste.

syringe, 20–30 cc of liquid barium is injected into the tubing. This coats the mucosa of the rectum.

The tip of the caulking cartridge is then attached to the tubing and the barium paste is injected until the patient feels full or the cartridge is almost empty.

Injection is continued as the tip is removed to coat the anal canal with barium.

The patient is asked to stand while the table is put in the erect position. The chair is moved into position next to the erect table (Fig. 9.2) or, if a chair is not available, the footboard is attached at chair height and a bed pan placed on the footboard facing out to the side (Fig. 9.3). A hemorrhoid cushion is put on top of the bed pan or chair seat (cushion valve pointing posterior and down).

Fluoroscopy is performed in the lateral position.

The video recording and fluoroscopy is begun. The patient's identification number is taped to the fluoroscope in a position to be visible on the TV monitor during recording.

After a baseline fluoroscopic spot film is obtained (preferably a large film capable of visualizing both the sacrum and pubis), the patient is asked to squeeze the anal sphincter muscles to elevate the pelvic floor and another film is exposed. The patient is then asked to strain, but not empty. Then the patient is asked to empty the rectum with forceful straining. At the end of this effort, a fifth film is exposed during maximum straining.

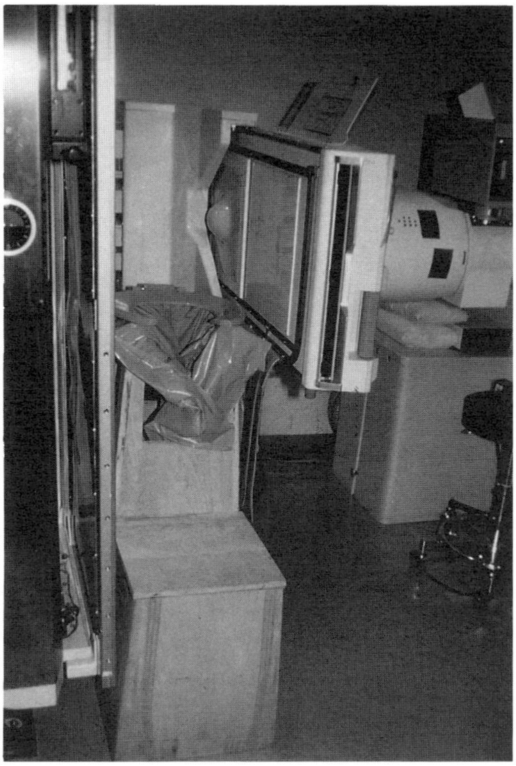

FIGURE 9.2 Defecography chair with plastic bag for collecting barium. Hemorrhoid cushion sits atop the commode seat during the examination.

The video recording is then stopped.

He or she is reminded to drink large amounts of fluids over the next 24 to 48 hrs and take laxatives as necessary to empty the small bowel barium so that impaction does not occur.

If there is suspicion of a lateral abnormality that would not be appreciated in the lateral view filming of the standard study, a frontal (anteroposterior) study can be performed. After the standard study, the rectum is refilled with paste barium only and the patient is seated semi-erect on a bedpan under the fluoroscopic tower with the table horizontal. The same maneuvers are performed with spot filming and videotaping.

Results

The data sheet (Table 9-1) is filled out using the films and video recording. It is especially helpful if a video printer is available to print representative frames of the videotape. If not, measurements can be made off of the monitor screen during freeze frame. The videotape is necessary because events happen quickly during defecation and both the examiner and the patient want to do the exam only once. The tape can be reviewed over and over again until the radiologist is sure the information has been obtained.

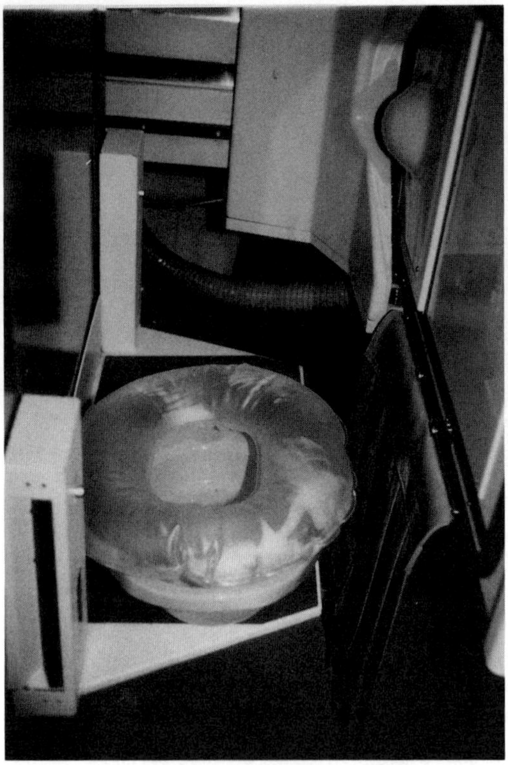

FIGURE 9.3 Bedpan and hemorrhoid cushion on the footboard of fluoroscopic table as an alternative to the defogram chair.

The anorectal angle is measured using the axis of the anal canal and the posterior wall of the rectum as the two limbs of the angle (do not use the axis of the middle of the full rectum). If the posterior wall of the rectum is curved rather than straight or if a posterior bulge (perineal hernia) is present, it may be difficult to draw that limb of the anorectal angle. In that instance, review of the videotaped exam allows the analysis of puborectalis relaxation.

Descent is measured referable to the pubococcygeal line as seen on the films (the video image does not usually cover enough area to make this measurement from the tape) or any fixed landmark on the video image.

The anal canal width and length are measured during maximal evacuation.

Rectocele and perineal hernia sizes are the maximum sizes seen during the exam.

An enterocele is diagnosed when the barium-filled small bowel is seen to indent the superior rectal surface or herniate into the rectovaginal space anterior to the rectum. It is often seen only on the straining film after evacuation because the filled rectum blocks the small bowel descent.

Prolapse is diagnosed from the films and videotape and is characterized as high, mid, or low in the level of origin and as anterior, posterior, or both anterior and posterior in site of origin.

TABLE 9.1 DEFECOGRAPHY DATA SHEET

Date:____________________ Patient ID#____________________

Patient Name:____________________ Physician:____________________

Chief Complaint:____

MEASUREMENTS

	REST	SQ	VALS	DEF
Anorectal Angle (degrees)				
Perineal Movement (cm)				

Anal Canal Length (cm) ____________________

Anal Canal Width (cm) ____________________ (minimum diameter while maximum evacuating)

Evacuation efficiency (%) ____________________ (scintigraphic technique)

MORPHOLOGY

General (capacity, contours, etc.)______________________________

____

Puborectalis Relaxation—Y/N
Megarectum—Y/N
Rectocele—Y/N Length × height (cm)____________________
Perineal Hernia—Y/N Length × height (cm)____________________
Intussusception—Y/N
Anterior Posterior Both
Low Mid High Obstructing Outlet
Enterocele—Y/N

COMMENTS

Continent/Dribbled During Vals/Dribbled at Rest/Incontinent

____

____

____________________M.D.

BAO 9/8/89

LMG 2/9/94

THE NORMAL EXAMINATION

There is a wide range of normal values depending on the technique used, landmarks identified for measurement, and the quality of the images obtained. The changes in these values during an individual exam are most helpful as the patient becomes his or her own control. In patients with multiple exams over time without intervening treatment, it is surprising how reproducible the findings are, giving credence to the usefulness of the exam in depicting normal and abnormal anatomy and physiology.

The anorectal angle should decrease during squeezing and significantly increase during effective straining and defecation. This increase in the angle during defecation reflects the relaxation of the puborectalis muscle. The concept of the anorectal angle is an old one and in my opinion outmoded now that videotaping of the exam has become standard. The relaxation of the muscle is obvious, if it occurs, on review of the tape and often the measurement of the angle is arbitrary or confusing if the posterior wall of the rectum is curved or a perineal hernia is present.

Perineal movement should be up during squeezing and down during straining and defecation but not more than 4 cm of movement in either direction. Classically, perineal movement is measured referable to the pubococcygeal line but many modern fluoroscopic machines are not capable of taking large films, therefore this line is not constructible. In that instance, measurement against any fixed point *within the patient* is acceptable.

Evacuation should be relatively complete. Normal evacuation should be at least 90% in the intact rectum and 60% in a ileo-anal pouch as measured on the scintigraphic study or estimated from the fluoroscopic examination.

A small rectocele (<3 cm) is very common and clinically insignificant. Small folds in the rectum at the end of defecation are also normal.

The upper rectum should remain in apposition with the sacrum during the entire procedure. The rectum may be relatively horizontal or vertical without being abnormal. The contraction wave forms a funnel shape during defecation.

The anal canal should remain closed except during defecation.

The frontal exam, if performed, is viewed only for lateral bulges and abnormal collections of small bowel but no measurements need be taken as they were done in the standard study.

THE ABNORMAL EXAMINATION

Scintigraphic emptying of less than 90% is abnormal. Occasionally the fluoroscopic emptying is normal in the face of an abnormal scintigraphic result. In the absence of size criteria for megarectum (9 cm in the anterior-posterior diameter), the normal fluoroscopic result is reported as correct. Lower numbers can be indicative of incomplete emptying secondary to megarectum, spastic puborectalis muscle, or retention of stool in a rectocele.

If the nuclear study is normal or near normal and the fluoroscopic study shows little emptying, rely on the nuclear study and assume that the poor emptying during fluoroscopy is related to the semipublic nature of the test.

The fluoroscopic study is analyzed using the data sheet (Table 9.1). The measurements of the anorectal angle, if performed, reflect the relaxation or nonrelaxation of the puborectalis muscle. Fixation of the muscle or paradoxical contraction during defecation is abnormal suggesting spastic pelvic floor syndrome.

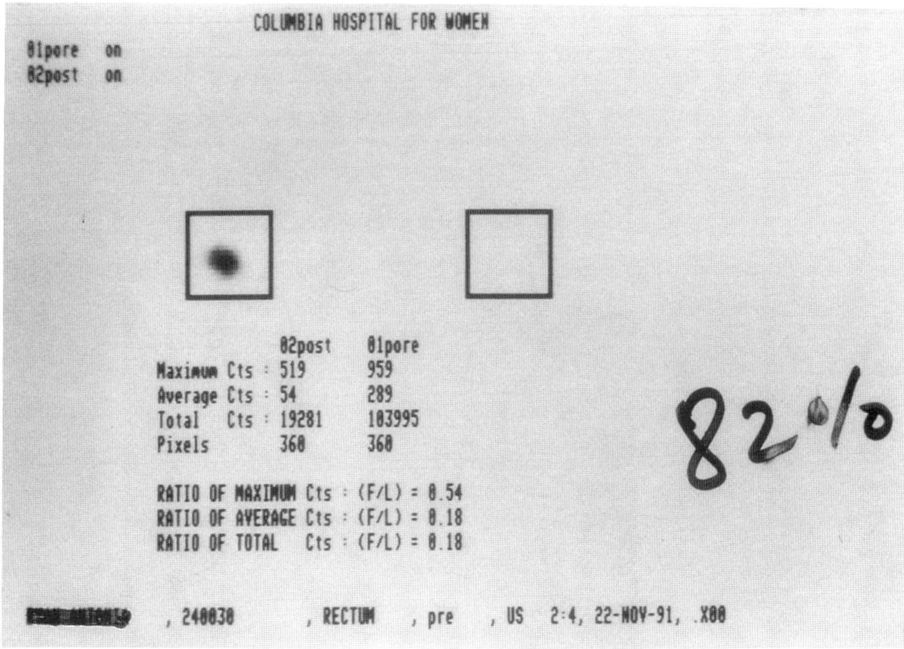

FIGURE 9.4 Scintigraphic study showing below normal emptying of 82%.

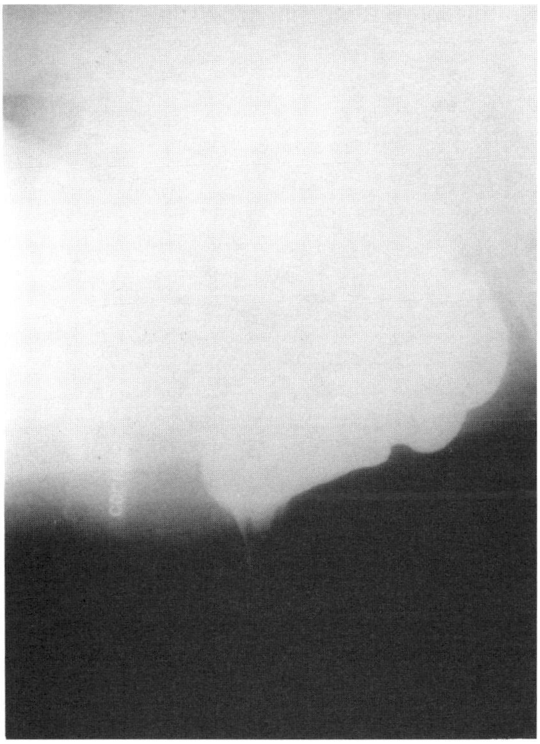

FIGURE 9.5 Normal resting view (anterior is on the left) showing a normal small anterior bulge and moderate posterior impression of the puborectalis muscle.

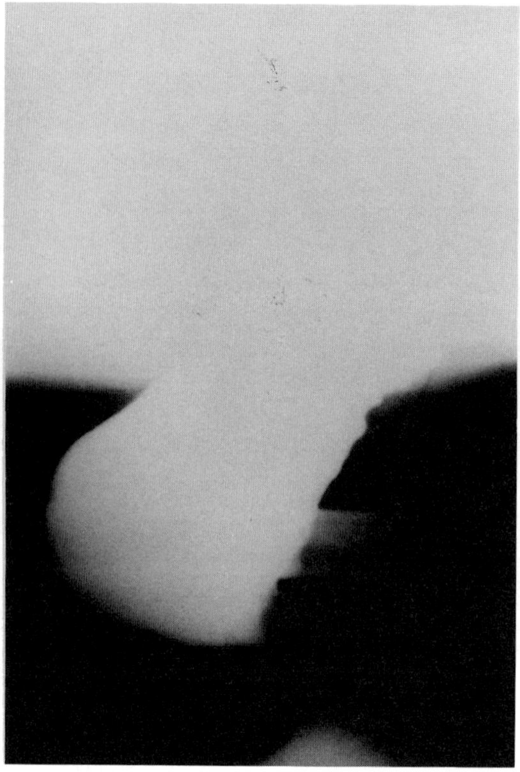

FIGURE 9.6 Moderately large rectocele projecting anteriorly during straining.

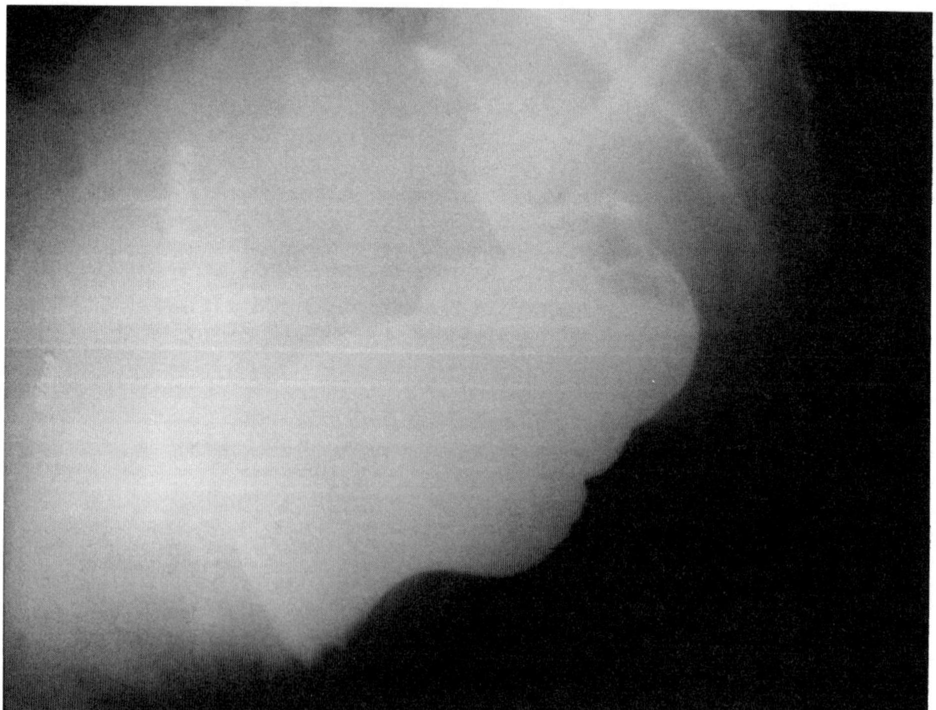

FIGURE 9.7 Anteriorly projecting rectocele and posteriorly projecting perineal hernia during straining.

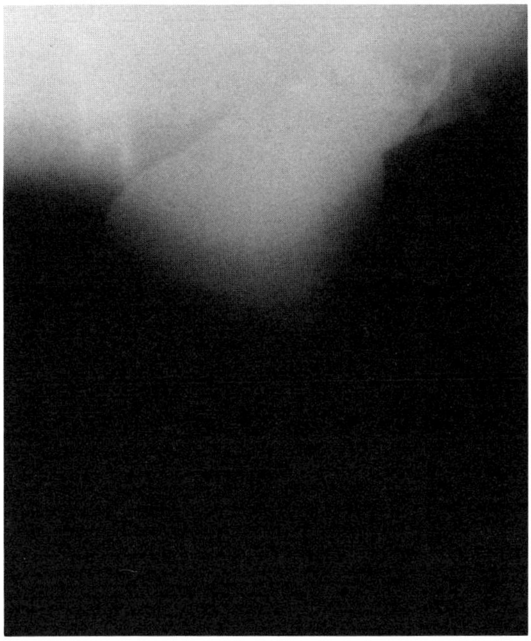

FIGURE 9.8 Large rectocele and perineal hernia. Notice the normal diameter of the rectum above the rectocele consistent with absence of megarectum.

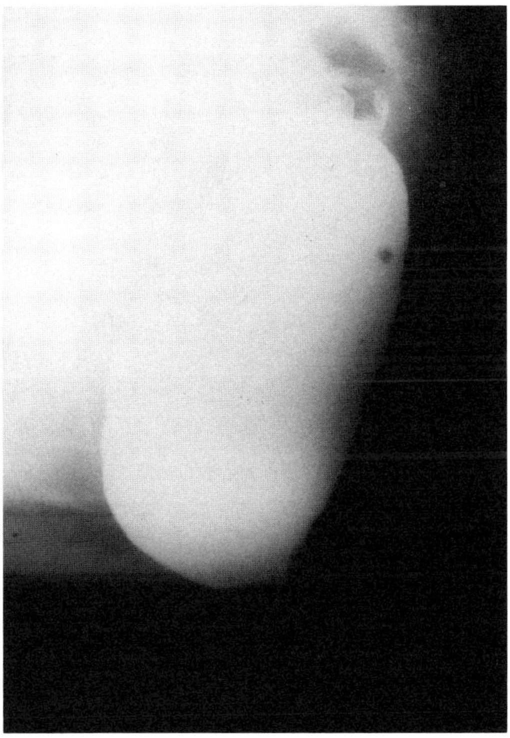

FIGURE 9.9 Megarectum with an 11-cm diameter of the rectum above the rectocele.

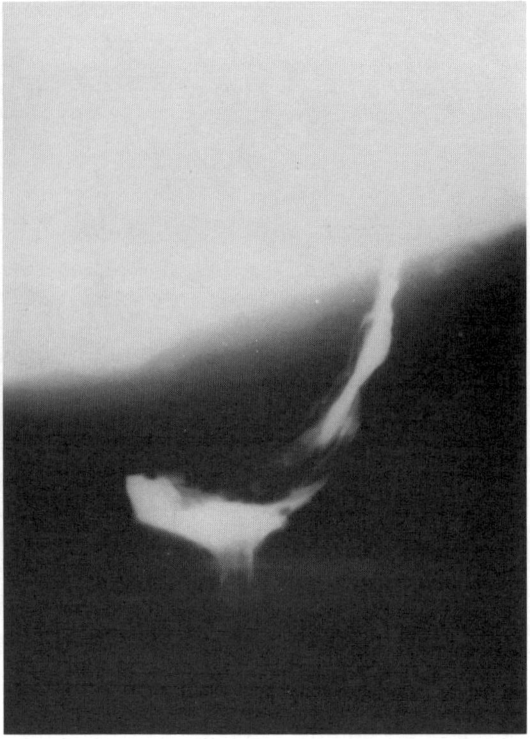

FIGURE 9.10 Impression of nonopacified small bowel on the superior surface of the rectum in this postevacuation image is diagnostic for an enterocele.

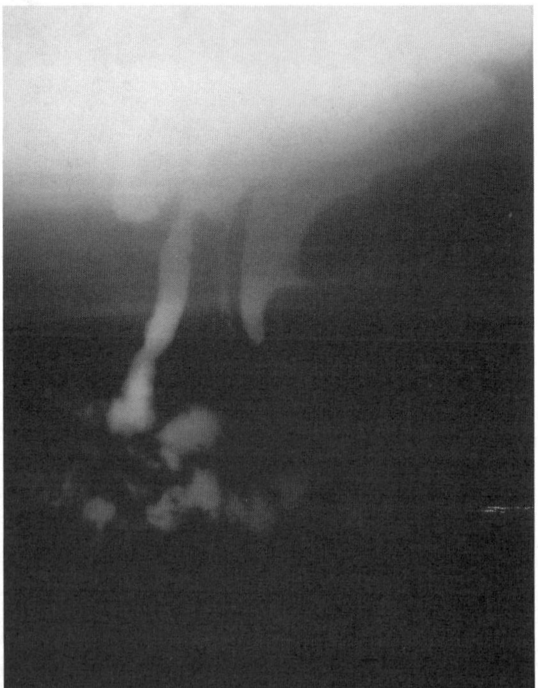

FIGURE 9.11 Large enterocele projecting anterior to and markedly below the rectum.

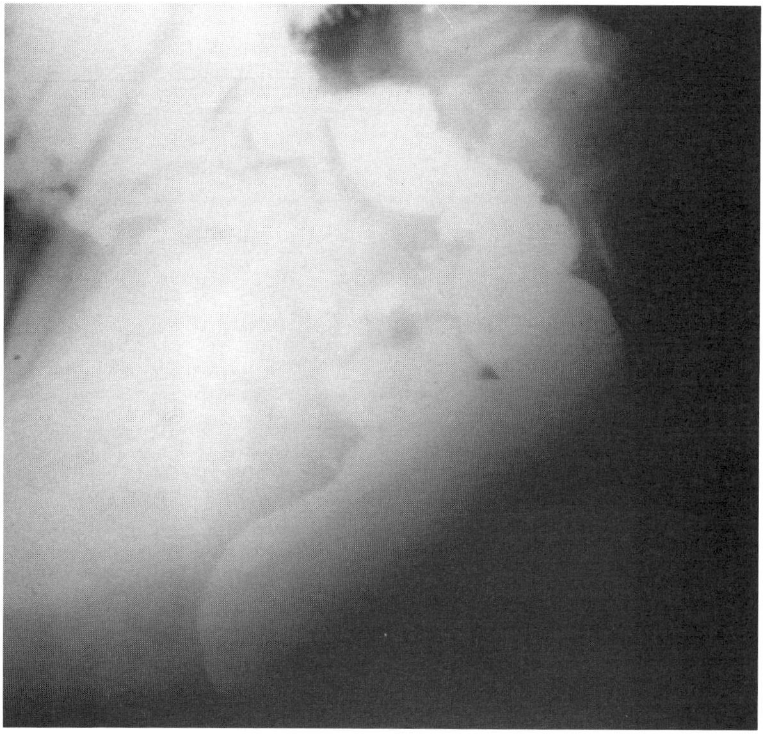

A

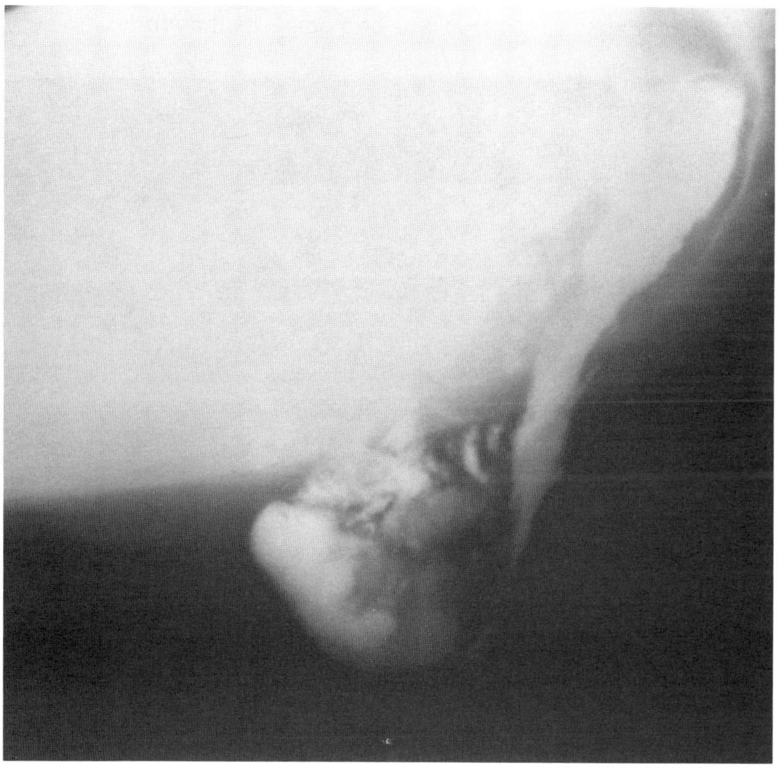

B

FIGURE 9.12 A Normal lateral view. **B** Postevacuation view showing a large enterocele. Often enteroceles are only seen on the postevacuation view.

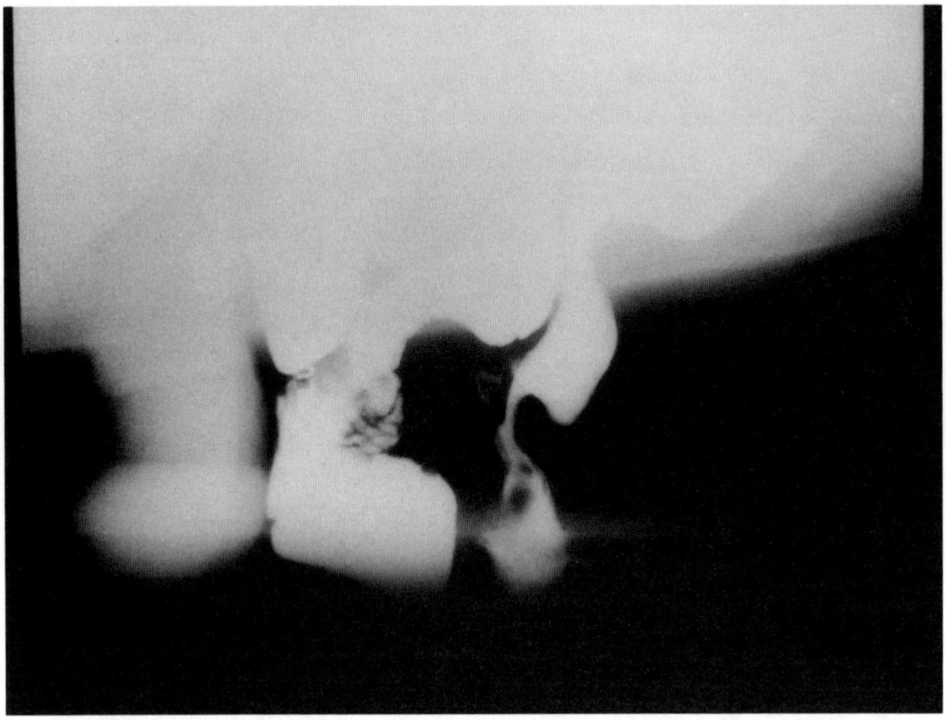

FIGURE 9.13 Diffuse pelvic floor relaxation with cystocele anteriorly, enterocele in the midposition, and rectal descent posteriorly. The bladder was filled with water-soluble iodinated contrast at the beginning of the study.

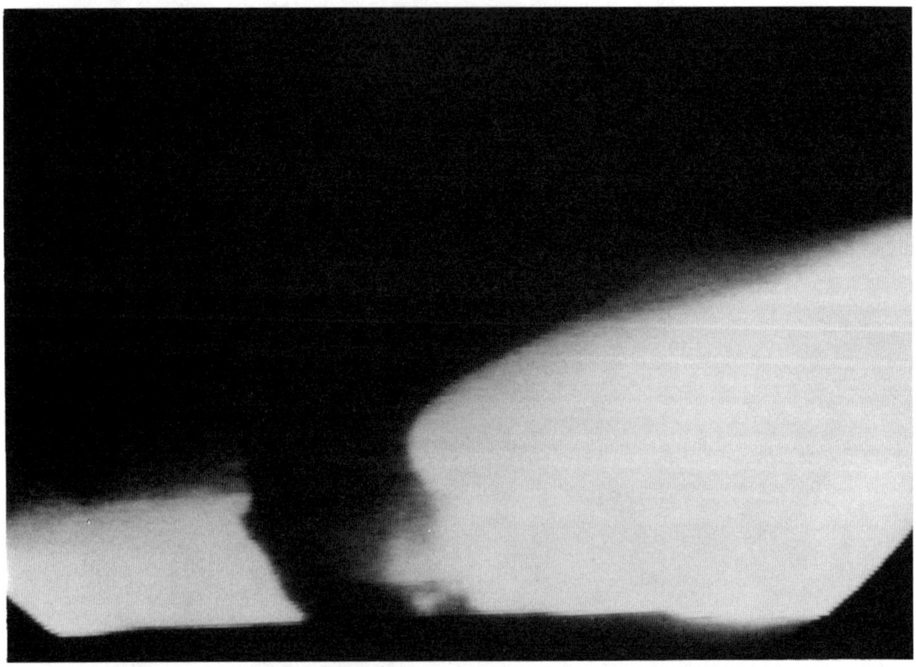

FIGURE 9.14 Image from videotape during defecation showing abnormally wide anal canal consistent with poor sphincter tone. Image of barium is black in this video image.

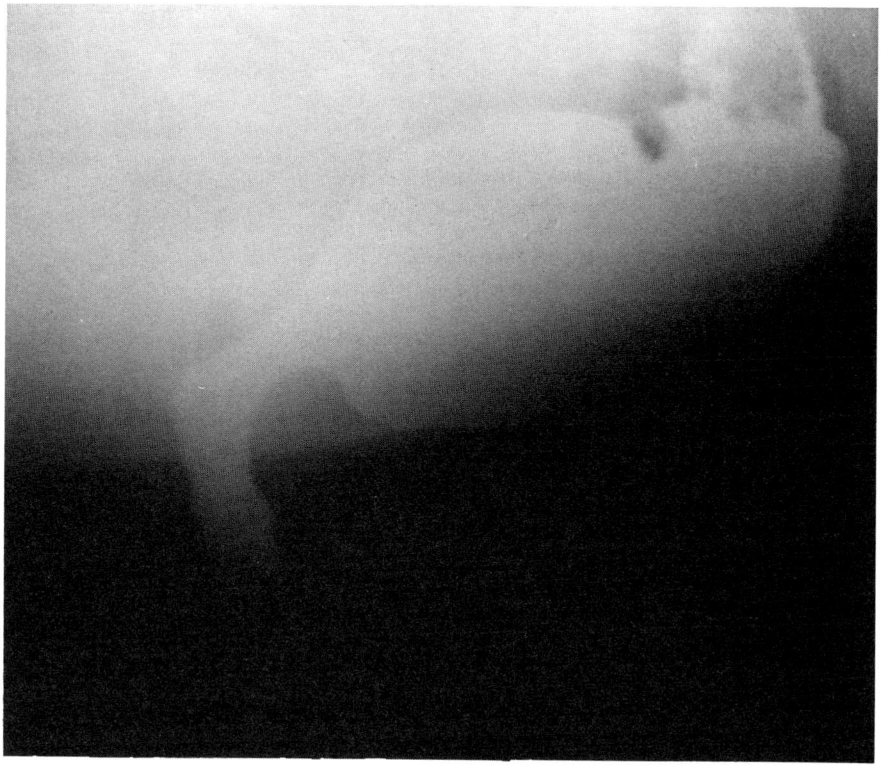

FIGURE 9.15 Prominent puborectalis impression on film during defecation diagnostic of nonrelaxation.

Excessive pelvic floor movement is diagnosable when movement of the anorectal junction is more than 4 cm, especially in the downward direction as occasionally a strong puborectalis can elevate the junction upward in a clinically irrelevant amount in excess of 4 cm.

Anal canal width is measured as the minimum diameter during maximum evacuation and is abnormal when greater than 2.5 cm. An abnormal result suggests a weak sphincter as does an open canal at rest.

The criteria for diagnosing megarectum combine both size and function. An anterior-posterior diameter of the rectum above 9 cm at the lower sacral level coupled with abnormal emptying is necessary. The abnormal emptying is evaluated using the first test done only, usually the scinitigraphic test. The added volume of the second contrast in addition to any remaining contrast from the first study may be enough to stimulate the megarectum to complete evacuation, thus giving the false impression of normal emptying.

Rectoceles and perineal hernias are diagnosed as anterior and posterior rectal outpouchings respectively. They are most prominent during maximal evacuation. Retention of barium in these hernias should be reported.

Enteroceles are diagnosed when the small bowel descends to or below the rectum. They may be seen only after the rectum empties, thus the postevacuation straining film is often critical for the diagnosis.

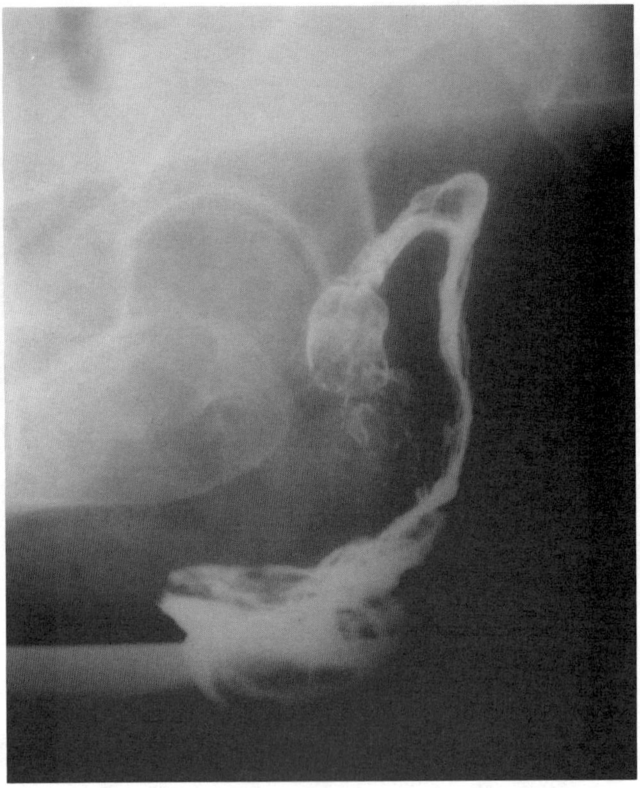

FIGURE 9.16 Internal procidentia seen prominently on the postevacuation view.

SUMMARY

Defecography is a valuable tool in the evaluation of anorectal disorders but its findings must be correlated with the results of other tests and the clinical symptomatology to be useful in treatment planning. The examination is quickly performed and can easily be done in most hospital or outpatient departments. The interpretation of the exams requires cooperation between the radiologist and knowledgeable clinicians or incorrect conclusions will be drawn, leading to inappropriate treatment. Radiologists should not fear the exam or the patients who arrive for it.

SUGGESTED READINGS

Finley IG, Bartolo DCC, Bartram CI, et al: Proctography. *Int J Colorect Dis* 3:67–89, 1988.

Kelvin FM, Maglinte DDT, Hornback JA, et al: Pelvic prolapse: Assessment with evacuation proctography (Defecography). *Radiology* 184:547–551, 1992.

Mahieu P, Pringot J, Bodart P: Defecography: I. Description of a new procedure and results in normal patients. *Gastrointest Radiol* 9:247–251, 1984.

Mahieu P, Pringot J, Bodart P: Defecography: II. Contribution to the diagnosis of defecation disorders. *Gastrointest Radiol* 9:253–261, 1984.

Rex DK, Lappas JC: Combined anorectal manometry and defecography in 50 consecutive adults with fecal incontinence. *Dis Colon Rectum* 35:1040–1045, 1992.

Shorvon PJ, McHugh S, Diamant NE, et al: Defecography in normal volunteers: results and implications. *Gut* 30:1737–1947, 1989.

CHAPTER 10

Digital Subtraction Defecography*

Luc P.A. Lesaffer

Digital subtraction defecography techniques provide rapid imaging and allow dynamic comparisons at different points in time during defecation. The superimposition of images defines movement of the anorectum, the pelvic floor, and the infoldings and herniations. Since 1990 we have made refinements in order to visualize the whole pelvic floor, achieving a "cysto-colpo-entero-defecography."

EQUIPMENT

1. A hollow, 16-cm-high toilet seat is filled with water, which permits equalization of penetration. This commercially available seat was created for older people to elevate the toilet seat. On the rear of the seat a ruler is created by sticking lead bars onto the back at 1-cm intervals.
2. A viscous paste to fill the rectosigmoid is made by mixing barium, water, and maizena. Three tubes of barium, each with a different consistency, are prepared: a tube with ordinary liquid barium, the second with a semisolid paste, and the third the most solid paste. The difference between tubes two and three is the different quantity of maizena.
3. A barium-soaked gauze compress is used to mark the vagina.
4. Water-soluble contrast is introduced into the bladder by a urethral catheter.

* This text is modified from: *Defecography—Update 1994: The Model of Expulsion. Digital Subtraction Cysto-colpo-entero-defecography. The Perineal Support Device.* Published by Luc P. A. Lesaffer, M. D., Radiologist. Aalst, Belgium. Distributed by J. Story-Scientia, Scientific Books, Ghent, Belgium.

5. An ice-cold mixture of $1/3$ water, $1/3$ liquid barium, and $1/3$ water-soluble contrast, diatrizoate meglumine (Gastrografin) is made to image the small bowel.
6. Barium paste is used to mark the perineal skin.
7. A digital subtraction arteriography apparatus is employed. During arteriography contrast is injected; however, during defecography, contrast is evacuated. Postprocessing of each image permits superimposition of images at different stages of defecation.

TECHNIQUE

The examination takes about 40 mins. The postprocessing takes at least 1 hr. No specific preparation of the anorectum is necessary. Solid food is discouraged just before the examination. The patient must not be pregnant.

The medical history is reviewed, the procedure is explained, and informed consent is obtained. Specifically, the vaginal barium marker, oral contrast, and urethral catheterization are described to the patient.

The patient drinks the ice-cold mixture of $1/3$ water, $1/3$ liquid barium, and $1/3$ water-soluble contrast. This water-soluble contrast is hyperosmolaric, resulting in an accelerated filling of the small bowel loops; thus the examination can be started in 20 mins. This mixture makes the small bowel loops less distinct than the densely filled rectosigmoid, permitting a good differentiation.

The patient is asked to urinate and, if necessary, defecate just before beginning the filling process. The bladder is filled with 200 cc of contrast. A compress soaked with liquid barium is placed in the vagina. In years past, we used a standard vaginal tampon, but it was too rigid. The skin of the perineum is marked with a barium paste.

Before introducing the barium into the rectum, a digital examination is important to instruct the patient in following commands: squeeze (close), relax (rest), and strain (push). Also we evaluate the movement, strength, and coordination of the puborectalis and anal sphincter muscle. The patient is cautioned not to use the gluteus muscles. The caulking gun fitted with an enema tip is employed to introduce the barium mixture. Usually we inject about 100 cc from each of the three tubes, starting with the most dilute tube. However, more is required in larger rectums.

The patient is placed on the defecography chair and the patient is asked to sit in a relaxed position which is termed as "at rest." Next the patient is asked to squeeze maximally. After rest and squeezing, the patient is permitted to defecate and urinate without making unnecessary movements. The images are taken at an interval of one image every 2 secs. The series can be stopped and restarted at any time to avoid unnecessary x-ray exposure. Since we also evaluate the micturition, there is often a need for more imaging. If micturition is difficult, we begin filming when the patient indicates micturition has started. Finally the patient is asked to strain unnaturally hard for a few seconds. This may show some extreme movements of the pelvic floor or a pathological descent of the small bowel or sigmoid.

Sometimes a few images are taken in an anterior-posterior view during straining and squeezing. This additional projection gives us a three-dimensional concept of the anatomy. An anterior-posterior view at the beginning of the examination is useful if there is a herniation in the pelvic floor; squeezing often exaggerates the hernia.

INTERPRETATION

We look at the stages of defecation: rest, squeeze, formation of the anorectal funnel, opening of the upper anal canal, the anal canal, relaxation of the puborectalis, the contour of the posterior perineum, the descent, anterior displacement, and the volume of the funnel. After expulsion, we note postevacuation and restoration. Anatomic features sought are the transverse fold, the peritoneal cul-de-sac, the fixation of the sacral part of the rectum, and the closure at the rectorectal level. The time and the effort from the patient, and the completeness of evacuation are then analyzed. Surrounding structures, such as sigmoid and small bowel, bladder, vagina and uterus, may be seen.

Good expulsion is predicated upon a balance between relaxation and a sufficient resistance. Remember that defecography shows only a part of defecation, giving information particularly at the moment of expulsion. Defecation also requires filling, sensation, resulting forces from above, and distal relaxation.

EXAMPLES OF DIGITAL SUBTRACTION DEFECOGRAPHY

A series of cases demonstrates the variety of combinations of pathology. The model of expulsion permits a more complete and dynamic evaluation of the whole pelvic floor. Cysto-colpo-entero-defecography in a single examination gives information useful also to the gynecologist and the urologist.

Case 1: This 49-year-old man had dyschezia, periods of diarrhea, and periods of constipation. He required much straining to evacuate; however, he had a normal defecogram. This case illustrates aspects of normal expulsion. The ampullary part of the rectum distended and collapsed with a peritoneal cul-de-sac at a high level after filling, but at a low level after expulsion (Fig. 10.1A). The funnel forms as the upper canal opens which fuses with the ampullary part of the rectum. The rectum descends from an upper to a lower level by inclination of the posterior perineum. During expulsion, the funnel is compressed. The transverse folds and the peritoneal cul-de-sac descend (Fig. 10.1B). At the end of expulsion the collapsing anorectum fits totally into the previously descended funnel (Fig. 10.1C). The rectorectal level of the closure (arrow A) and the free border (arrow B) are fairly visible. The lower part of the funnel, the upper anal canal, remains dilated with the formation of a pocket, while the ampullary part of the rectum collapsed (Fig. 10.1D). The sacral part of the rectum is fixed, and there is no enterocele.

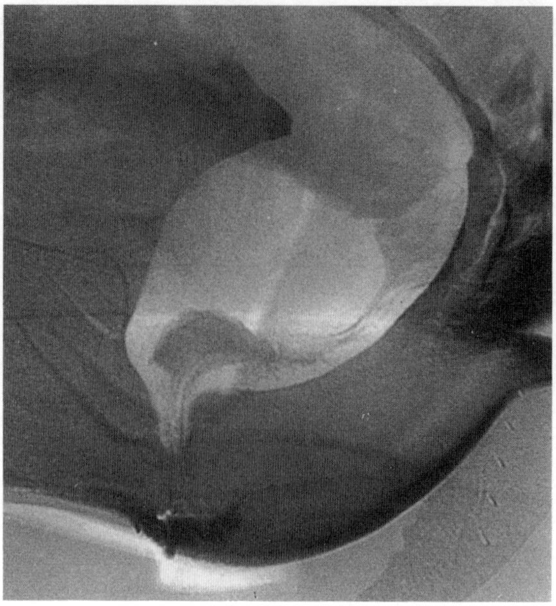

A

FIGURE 10.1 Normal defecogram. **A:** Filled rectum at rest, plus collapsed anorectum at the end of expulsion during squeezing. **B:** Filled funnel during straining, plus a stage during expulsion. **C:** Filled funnel during straining, plus collapsed anorectum at the end of expulsion during straining. **D:** Study of the folds of the collapsed anorectum during straining.

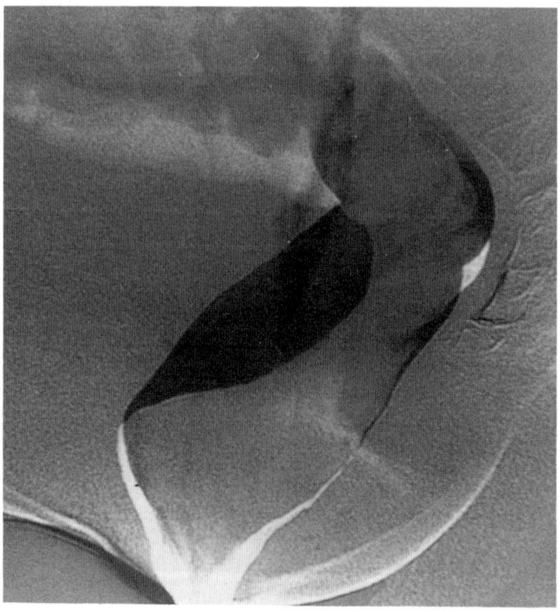

B

C

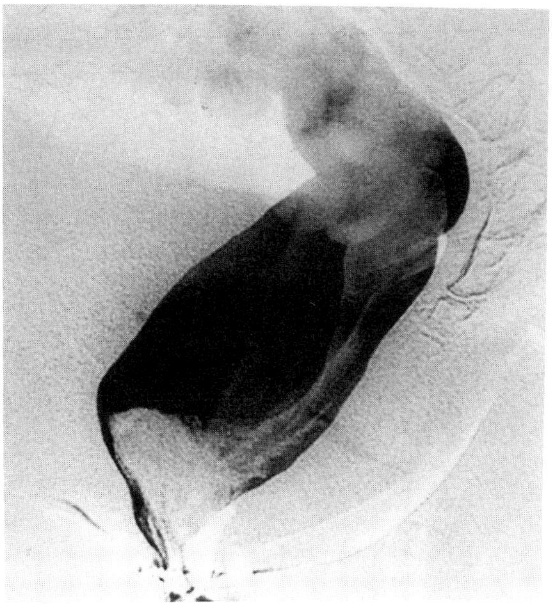

D

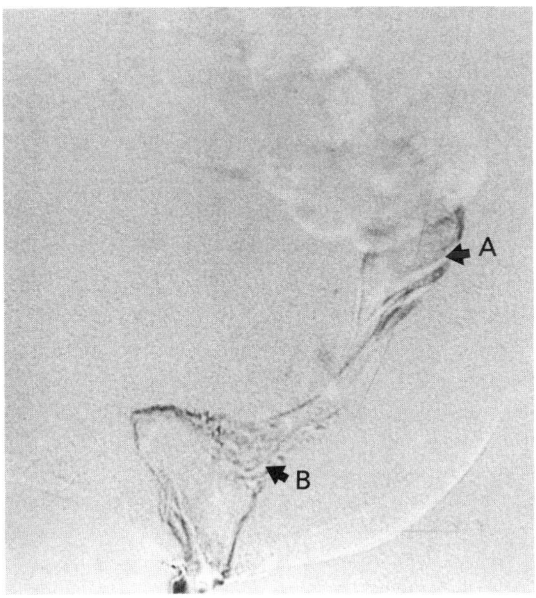

Case 2: This 32-year-old woman had a difficult delivery with her only child and was sterilized afterward. She was constipated, associated with hard straining, incomplete evacuation, and need for laxatives. During evacuation she felt pressure within the vagina. With these symptoms she avoided toilets away from her home. The signs of dyssynergia were present. There was only a minimal descent between rest position and formation of the funnel, with a pathological bulging of the posterior perineum and an anterior displacement of the anorectum (Fig. 10.2A, B).

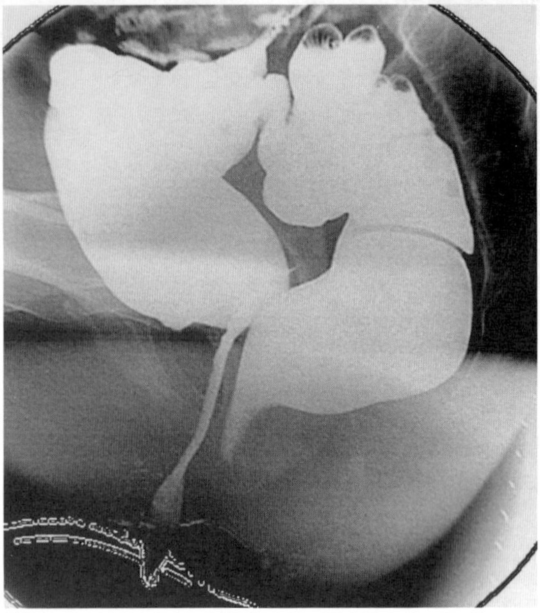

A

FIGURE 10.2 Moderate dyssynergia. **A:** At rest. **B:** At rest, plus during straining. **C:** During maximal straining and evacuation. **D:** After a second attempt. Stage of relaxation, plus stage of contraction of the puborectalis.

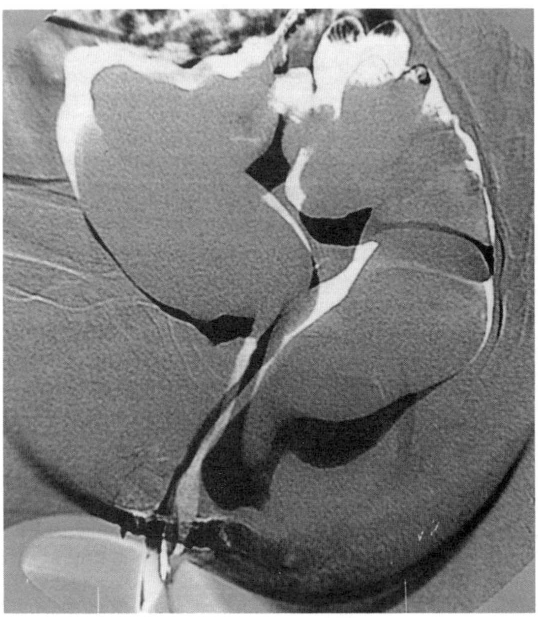

B

Despite hard straining, there was only a minimal evacuation and a persistent indentation by the puborectalis muscle (Fib. 10.2C). The series was stopped and restarted after a period of relaxation; the problem was explained to the patient; then a second attempt was tried with better evacuation, but again there was paradoxical contraction (Fig. 10.2D, small arrows). However, finally there was a closure at the normal rectorectal level and normal micturition.

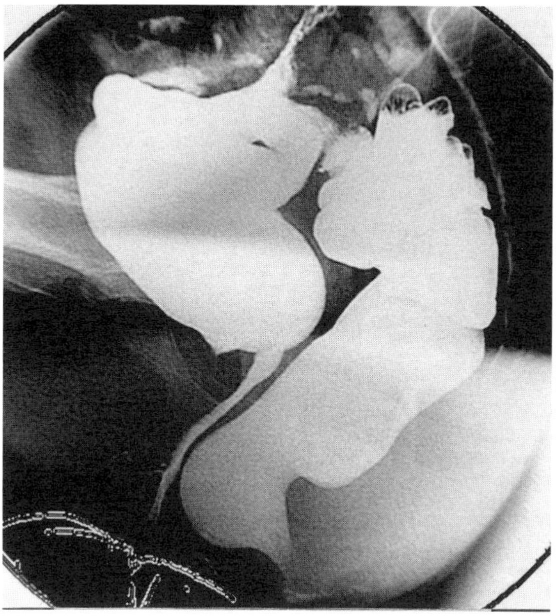

C

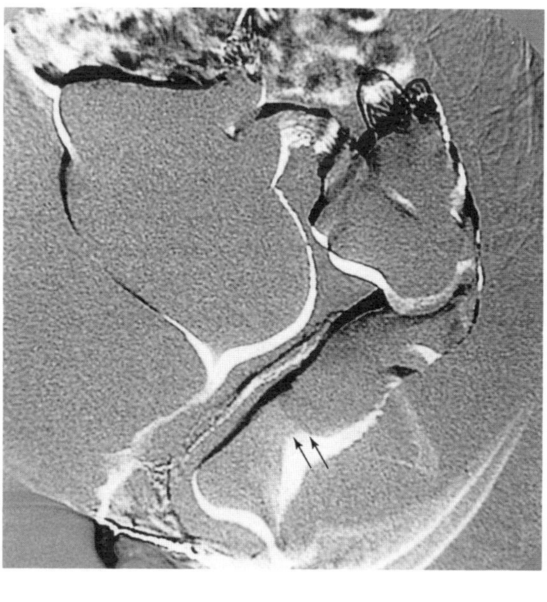

D

Case 3: This 59-year-old mother of two had a hysterectomy 18 years ago and a cystopexy 1 year ago. She has been constipated for many years, but worse during the past year. She has severe hemorrhoids secondary to hard straining. Digital examination reveals retained feces in the rectum and a rigid pelvic floor. There was minimal movement between rest position and the formation of the funnel, suggesting increased tone of the puborectalis and the levator ani muscles; there was a bulging anteriorly (Fig. 10.3A). During straining the perineum distended

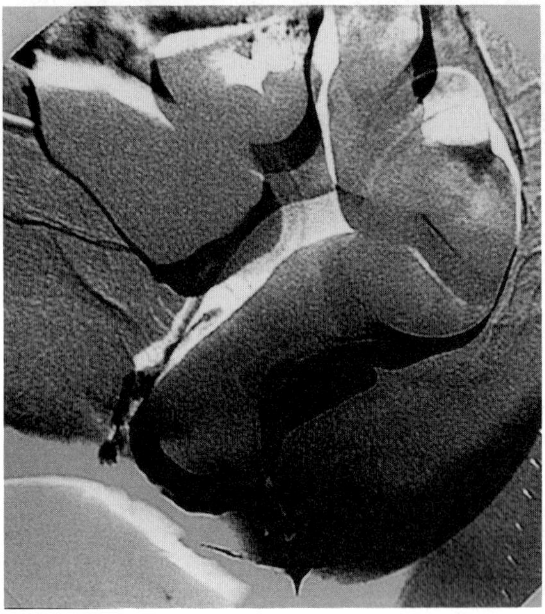

A

FIGURE 10.3 Transition of dyssynergia with rectocele and enterocele, evolving to a descending perineum. **A:** At rest, plus formation of the funnel during straining. **B:** Funnel during straining. **C:** The end of expulsion during straining. **D:** The end of expulsion during squeezing.

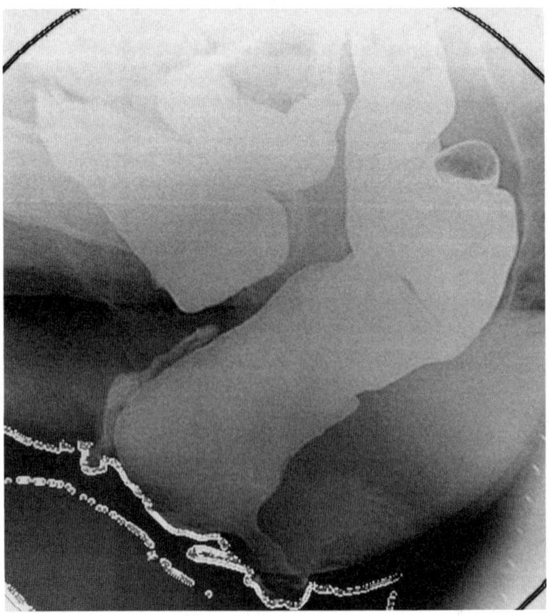

B

with formation of a large funnel (Fig. 10.3B). At the end of expulsion, the large rectocele was compressed by an enterocele (Fig. 10.3C). The rectocele became more evident during squeezing (Fig. 10.3D). There was a cystocele with an anteriorly located urethra. This case represents a transition of dyssynergia with rectocele evolving to a descending perineum syndrome. There are characteristics of both. Diluted contrast in the small bowel loops revealed the enterocele (Fig. 10.3C).

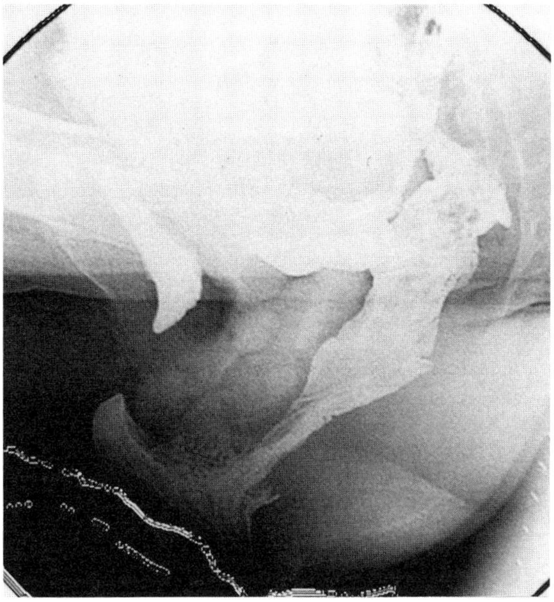

C

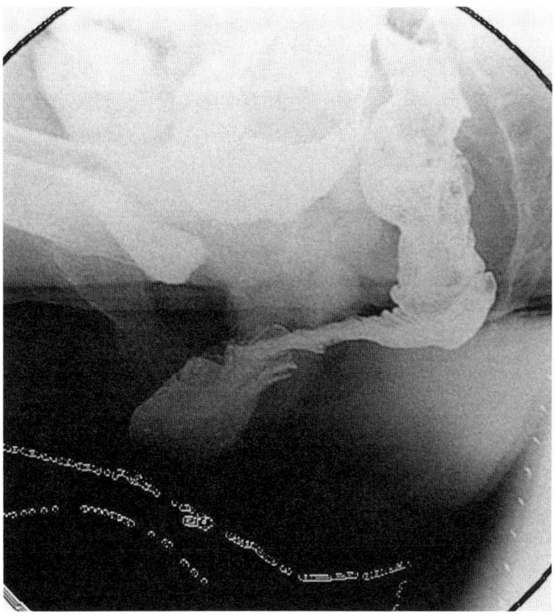

D

Case 4: This 34-year-old mother of two had severe constipation since age 20. She used glycerin suppositories and manually extracted stool. She had urine incontinence and vaginal infections. The image at rest and squeezing was normal, except for the anal canal, which was situated anteriorly (Fig. 10.4A). The puborectalis relaxed slowly, but once relaxed, there was a severe pelvic floor descent (Fig. 10.4B, C). There was a dramatic breakdown of the pelvic floor, with a rectocele

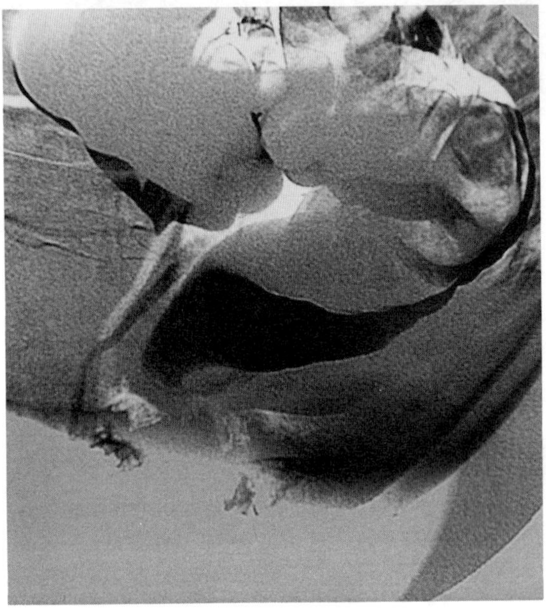

A

FIGURE 10.4 A descending perineum, rectocele, deep cul-de-sac, cystocele, and uterine prolapse. **A:** At rest, plus during squeezing. **B:** Formation of the funnel during straining. **C:** Squeezing, plus formation of the funnel during straining. **D:** At the end of expulsion.

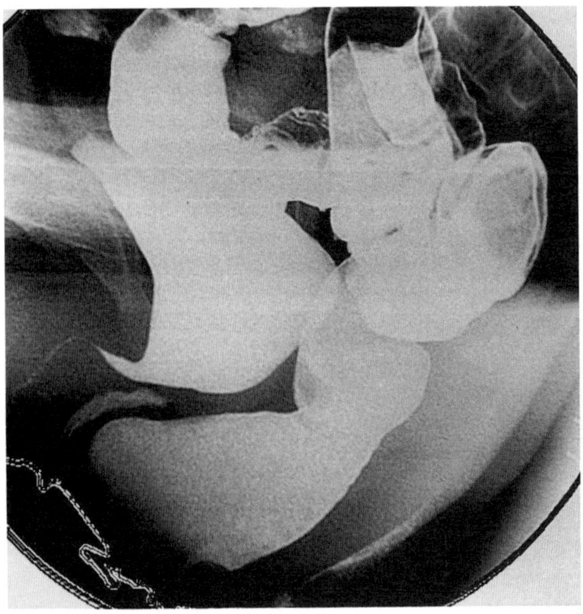

B

compressed by a cystocele. The anal canal was transposed beneath the pubic symphysis. The anococcygeal ligament probably lost its ability to maintain the anal canal posteriorly. The posterior perineum bulged. The impression of the retroflexed prolapsing uterus was visible on the anterior rectal wall. The sigmoid filled the cul-de-sac (Fig. 10.4D). The ligamental suspension apparatus was faulty.

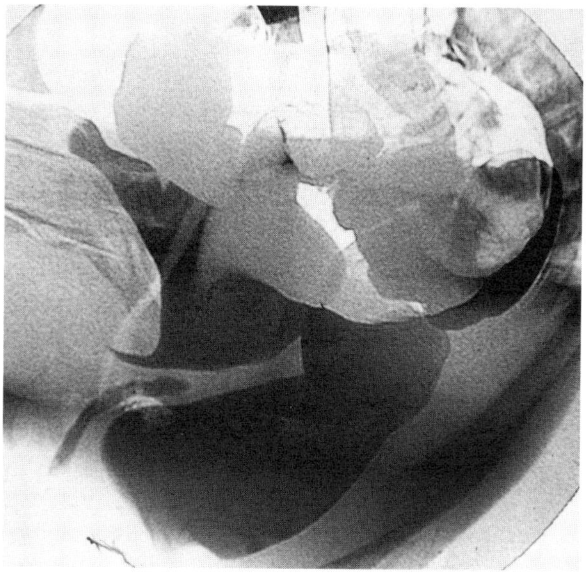

C

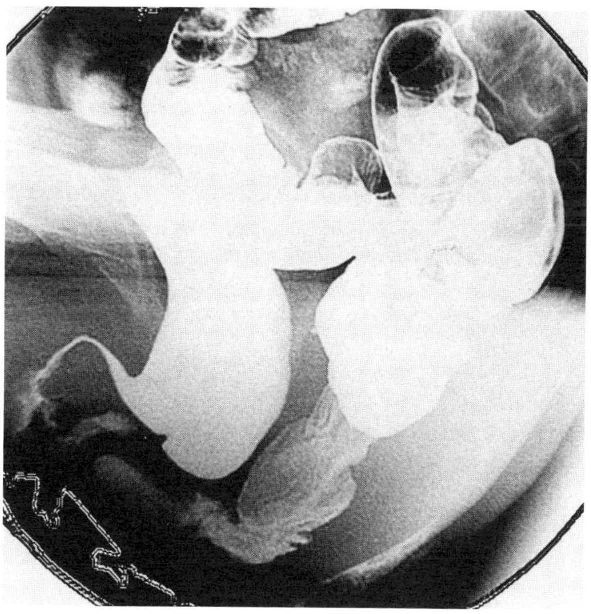

D

Case 5: This 36-year-old mother of two had a hysterectomy 6 years before for endometriosis. She had constipation with straining and a sense of a "ball" in the vagina during defecation. At rest there was squeezing to maintain continence and a horizontal position of the coccyx and the rectum (Fig. 10.5A). The funnel was large and descended (Fig. 10.5B). The rectorectal level closed and a rectocele and

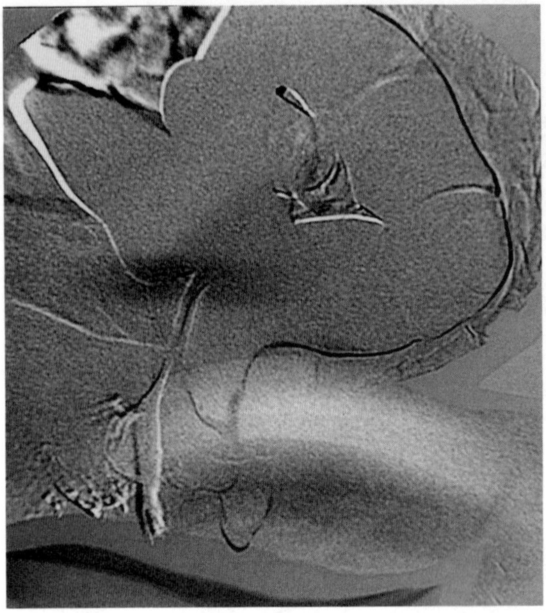

A

FIGURE 10.5 A descending perineum, rectocele, and intussusception. **A:** Study of the contours of the anorectum at rest. **B:** The formation of the funnel in the beginning of expulsion. **C:** At the end of expulsion during straining. **D:** Straining at the end of expulsion, plus squeezing at the end of expulsion. Black is squeezing and white is straining.

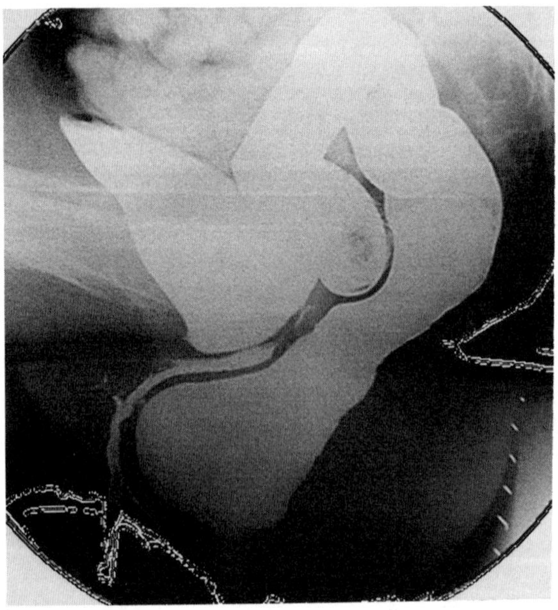

B

an intussusception formed (Fig. 10.5C). The sigmoid filled the cul-de-sac. A cystocele was present with voiding. There was some laxity of the fixation of the sacral part of the rectum. Between straining down and squeezing, there was too much movement (Fig. 10.5D). Note the movement of the coccyx (Fig. 10.5D).

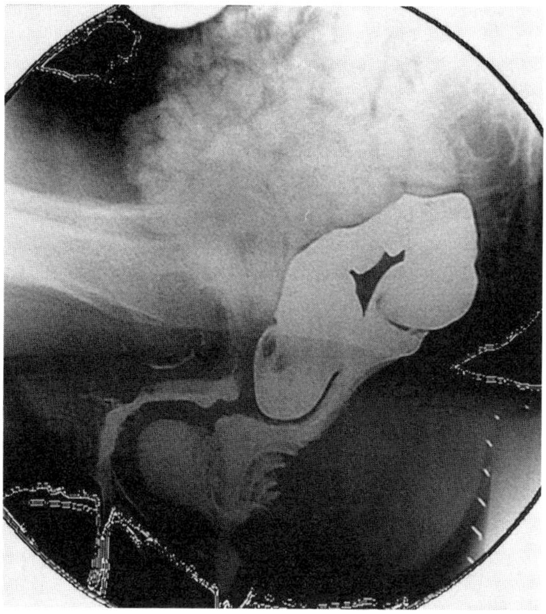

C

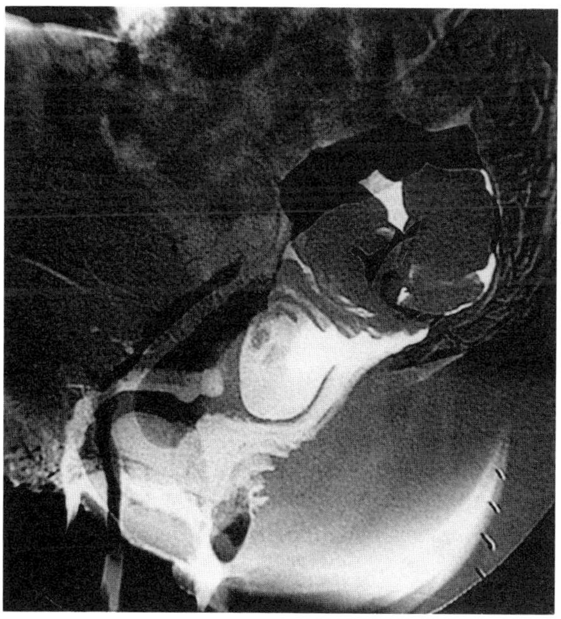

D

Case 6: This 59-year-old mother of two had a hysterectomy 8 years before. She had a sense of incomplete evacuation, but no constipation. She had pain of the coccyx and urinary stress incontinence. At rest this patient showed formation of the funnel; this was only partially reduced during squeezing. Once straining began, there was formation of a large funnel with bulging anteriorly and posteri-

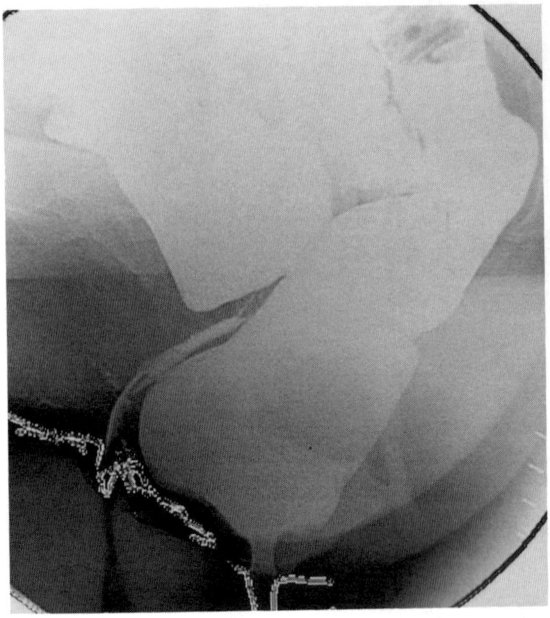

A

FIGURE 10.6 A descending perineum, rectocele, and large enterocele. **A:** The filled funnel during straining just before expulsion. **B:** At the end of expulsion and micturition during straining. **C:** Image of contours at the end of expulsion, during squeezing. **D:** Image of contours in an anteroposterior view at the end of expulsion and micturition, during straining.

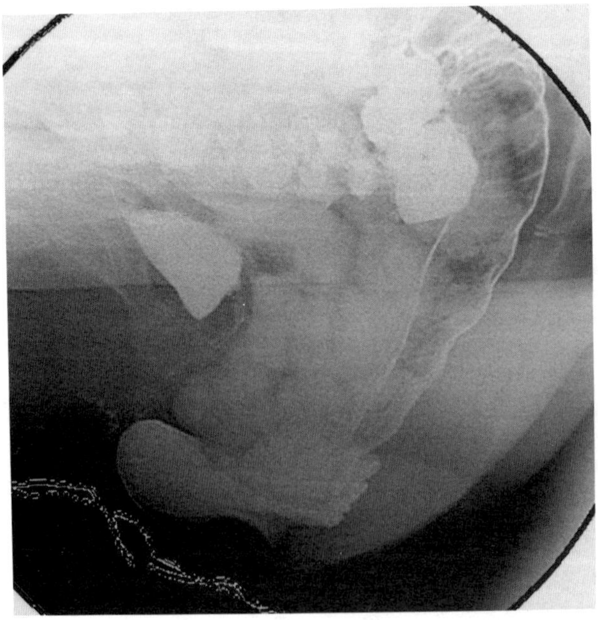

B

orly (Fig. 10.6A), a severe descent, and a short anatomical anal canal. During evacuation a large enterocele compressed the rectocele (Fig. 10.6B). The rectocele was more visible during squeezing (Fig. 10.6C). The small bowel loops filled with diluted contrast forming the enterocele were demonstrated in the anterior-posterior view (Fig. 10.6D).

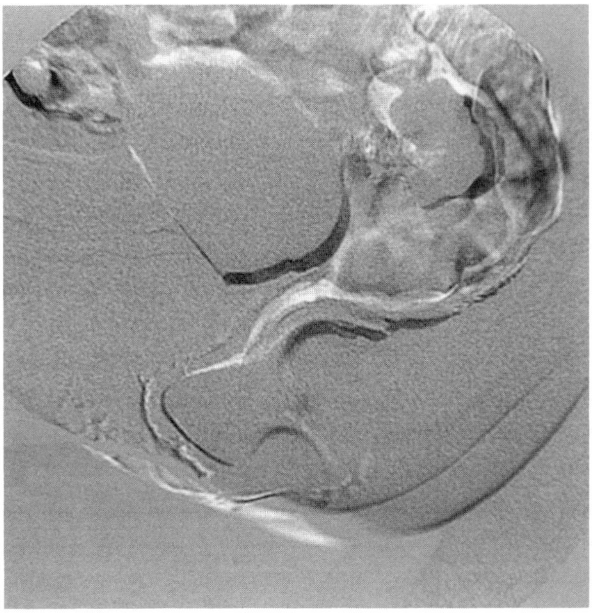

C

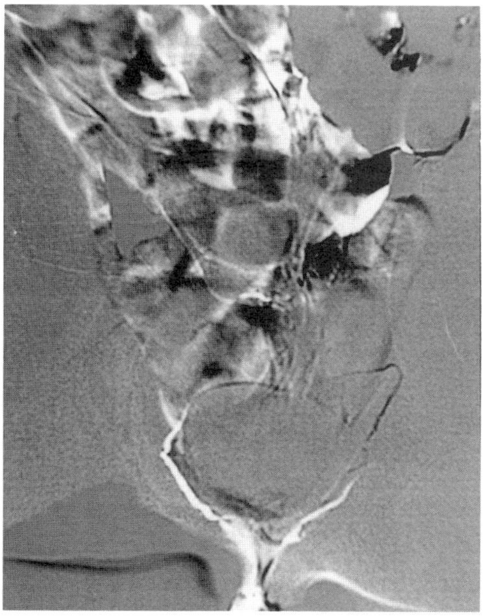

D

Case 7: A 51-year-old mother of one who had a recent hysterectomy developed a fecal outlet obstruction and urinary incontinence. The funnel was present at rest and did not reduce during squeezing; the puborectalis did not pull the posterior perineum into a horizontal position (Fig. 10.7A). The patient did not admit to fecal incontinence, but we expect that in time it will ensue. This example shows the need to study urological, gynecological, and proctological factors.

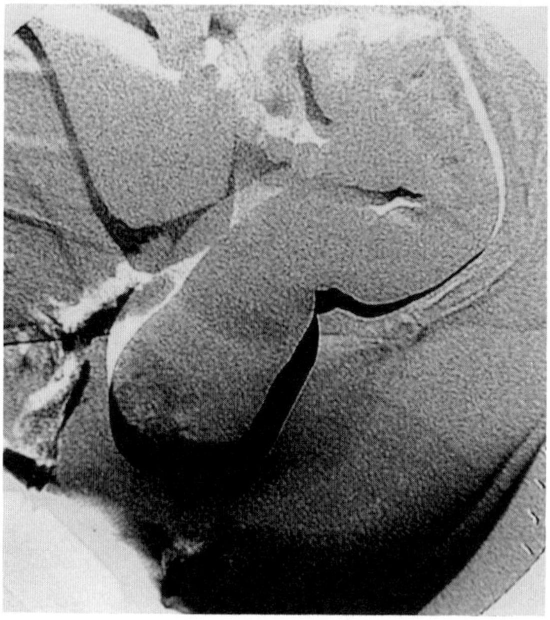

A

FIGURE 10.7 A severe descending perineum, large enterocele, and intussusception. **A:** The filled rectum at rest, plus during squeezing. **B:** During expulsion, transverse folds descent as the rectum collapses. **C:** The funnel filled during straining, plus the collapsed anorectum during straining. A large enterocele descends. **D:** Study of the folds and contour at the end of expulsion during straining.

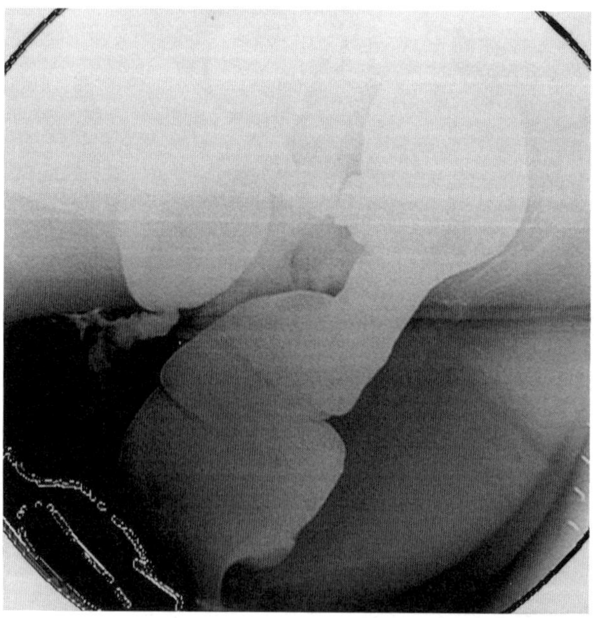

B

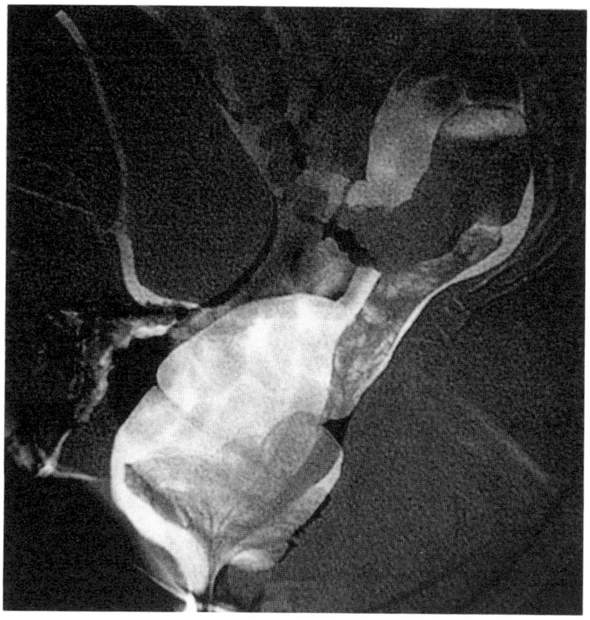

C

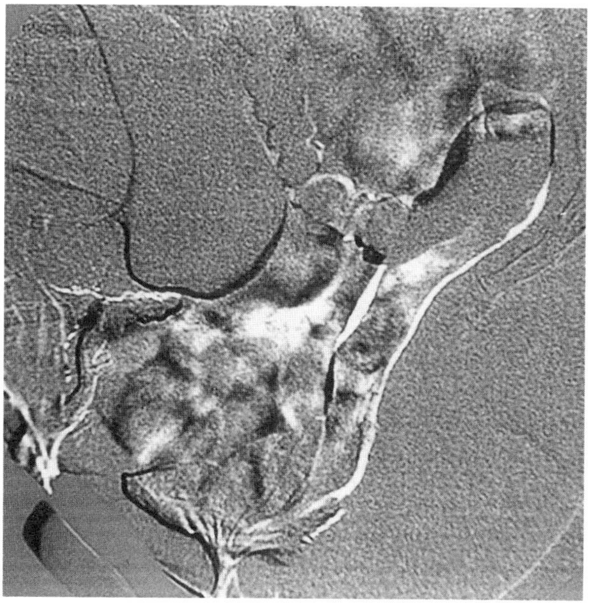

D

Case 8: This 58-year-old mother of two had a hysterectomy and a bladder suspension. A fissure, outlet obstruction, and urinary incontinence were associated. The digital examination showed a high resting tone of the anal canal. The funnel was present at rest with bulging anteriorly (Fig. 10.8A). During straining this bulging accentuated with descent of the transverse fold and pathological descent of the sacral part of the rectum (Fig. 10.A, B, C). At the end of expulsion there was

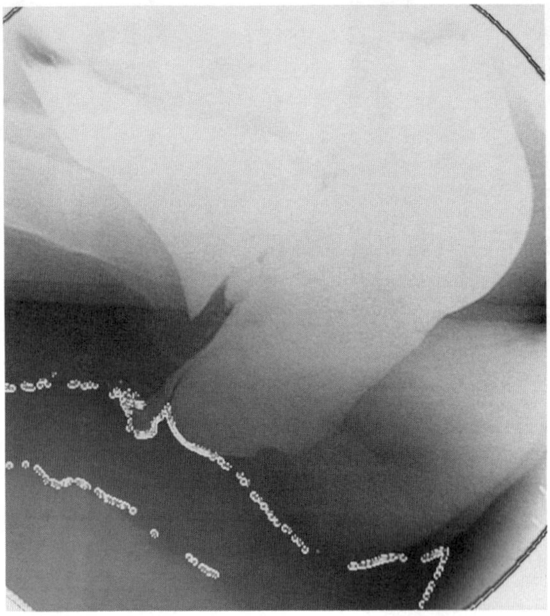

A

FIGURE 10.8 Descending perineum, rectocele, intussusception, enterocele, loosening of the sacral fixation and cystocele with partial herniation of the bladder into the cul-de-sac. **A:** The rectum filled at rest. **B:** Formation of the funnel with the beginning of expulsion. **C:** During expulsion with partial evacuation already. **D:** At the end of expulsion during straining.

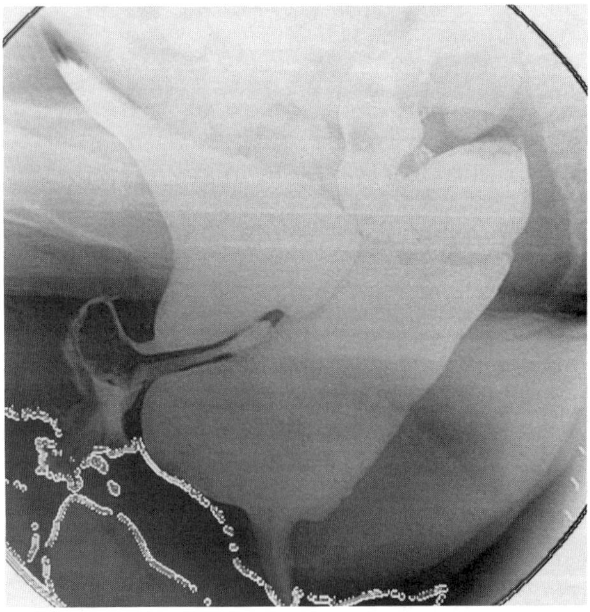

B

an intussusception and loosening from the sacral suspension, with a large enterocele (Fig. 10.8D). There were small bowel loops in both the enterocele and in the presacral space. The bladder presented with herniation of the enterocele. This very complex pathology could not be predicted on a clinical basis. There was a deficiency of the ligamental suspension apparatus of the pelvic floor.

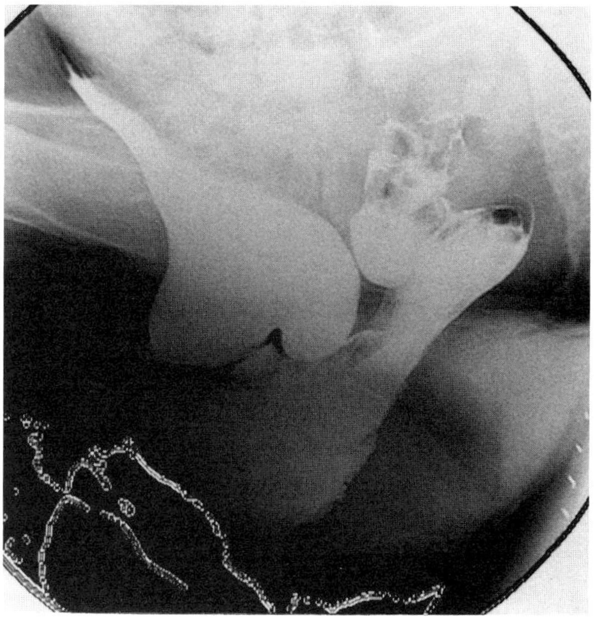

C

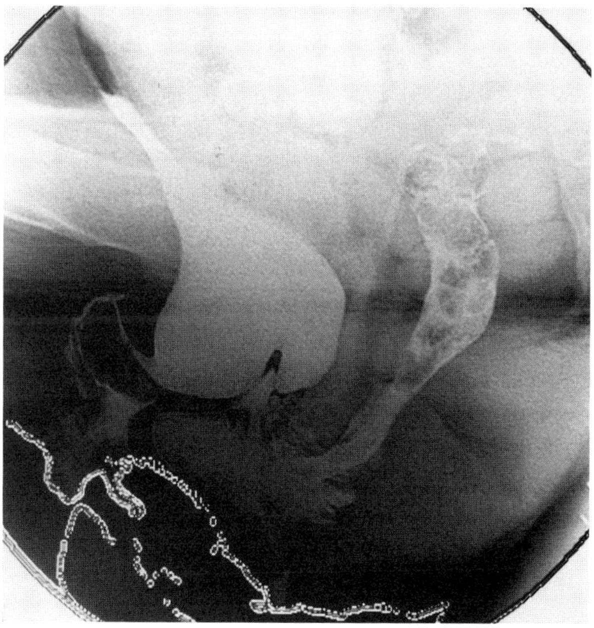

D

Case 9: A 34-year-old male who had been constipated since age 8, had perianal pain at night. A rectal ulcer was painful at proctoscopy. Manometry and an E.M.G. were normal. Digital examination revealed a hypertonic sphincter. The movement at rest and during formation of the funnel was normal (Fig. 10.9A). On the image depicting the contour of the wall at rest, we can delineate the ulcer (Fig. 10.9B), on

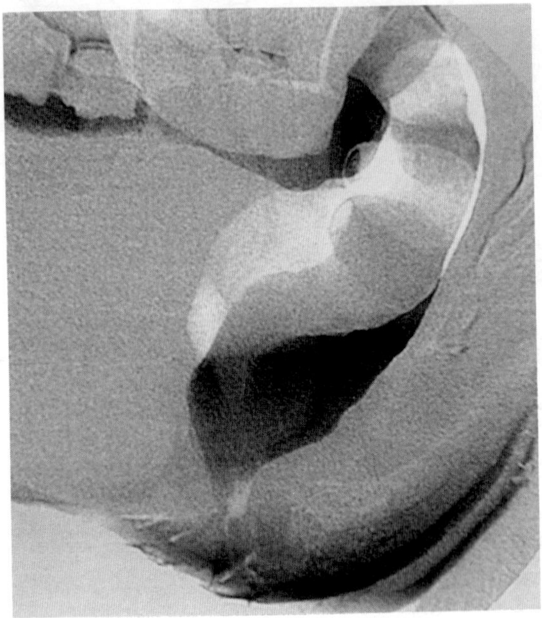

A

FIGURE 10.9 A solitary ulcer and intussusception with the onset of an external prolapse. **A:** At rest after filling, plus the formation of the funnel. **B:** Study of the contours, and folds at rest after filling. **C:** Superimposition of two stages during expulsion. **D:** At the end of expulsion during straining.

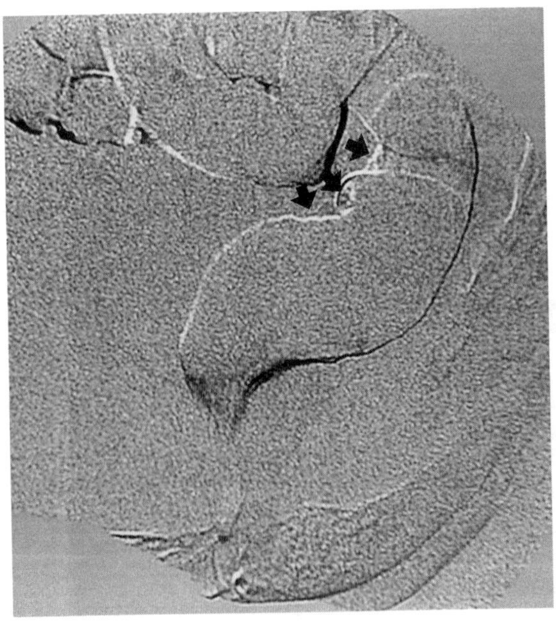

B

the anterior wall at the level of the transverse fold. This ulcer was delineated well (Fig. 10.9C) (*black arrows* indicate the ulcer), and showed the pathological descent of the transverse fold. At the end of expulsion we see an image of intussusception, which was protruding beyond the anal orifice (Fig. 10.9D). This represents the beginning of an external prolapse.

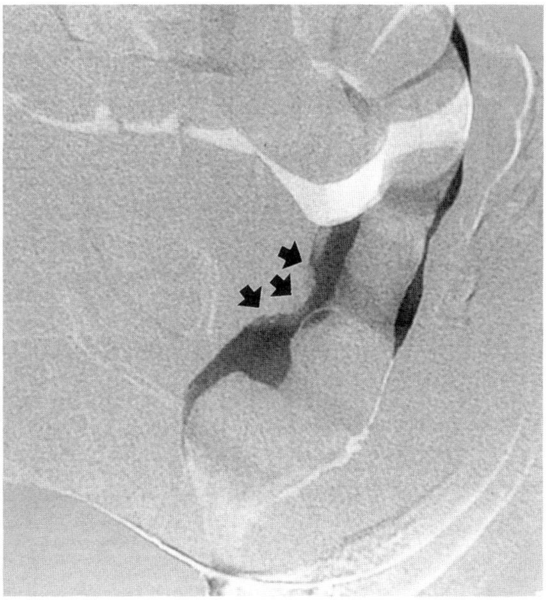

C

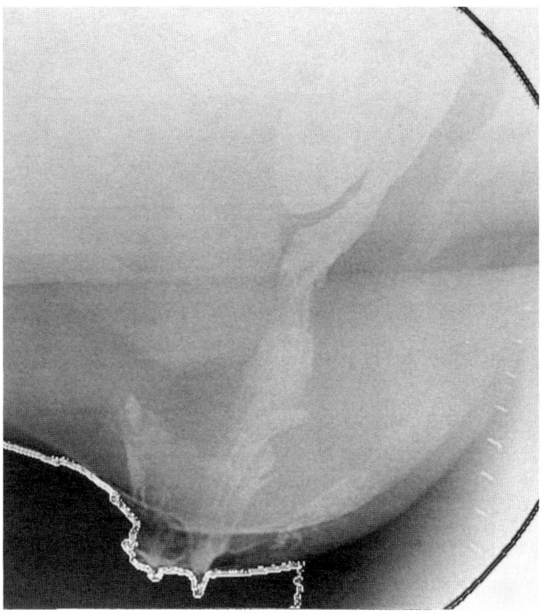

D

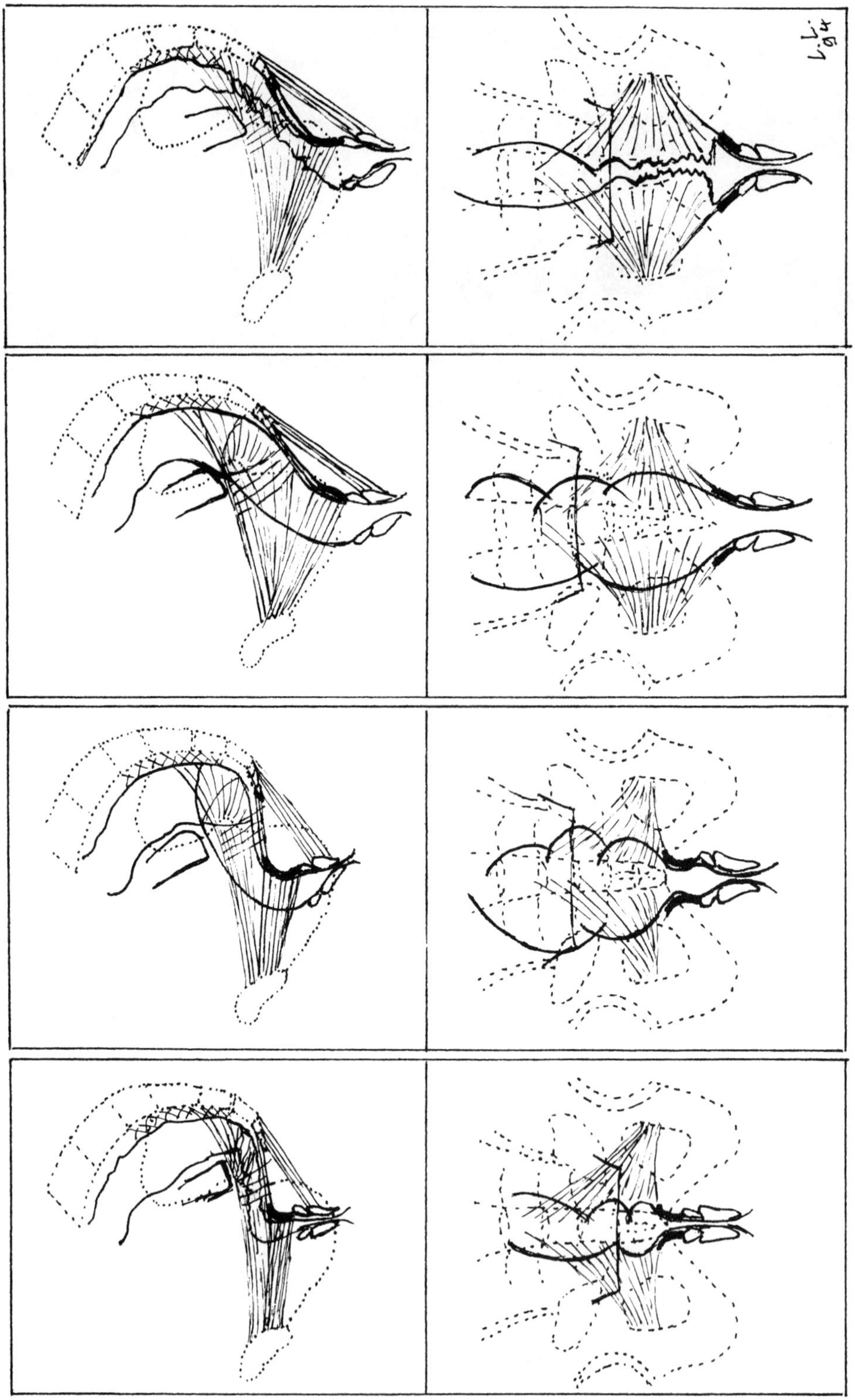

A B C D

FIGURE 10.10 THE MECHANISM OF EXPULSION, DICTATED BY THE FORMATION OF THE FUNNEL AND THE APPEARANCE OF A SUPERIOR RECTORECTAL LEVEL OF CLOSURE.

A: CONFIGURATION OF THE PELVIC FLOOR AT REST WITH CLOSED ANAL CANAL.
The ampullary part of the rectum is empty. The peritoneal cul-de-sac is at a low level with the transverse folds close together. As well, the upper anal canal as the anatomical anal canal are closed. Initial stage without call to stool.

B: FILLING OF THE SACRAL AND THE AMPULLARY PART OF THE RECTUM, WITH CONTRACTION OF THE PUBORECTALIS.
The filling of the ampullary part of the rectum requires propulsive forces coming from above and presupposes an upward movement of the cul-de-sac with a spreading out of the transverse folds. Opening of the upper anal canal by the rectal anal inhibitory relaxation reflex of the internal anal sphincter. There is no call to stool. The posterior perineum and the os coccyx are in a horizontal position with an anorectal and a rectorectal angle of about 90°. The anatomical anal canal is closed.

C: THE FORMATION OF THE FUNNEL WITH EXPULSION.
The relaxation of the puborectalis permits the inclination of the posterior perineum, with the ampullary part of the rectum coming from a higher horizontal to a lower more vertical level, providing a sliding effect. The dilated upper anal canal, being the lower part of the funnel, fuses with the distended ampullary part of the rectum with outfolding of the levator ani with the pelvic floor coming under tension. Once the anatomical anal canal opens, expulsion can start. At this moment there is no more movement at the anorectal junction, which is the lower part of the funnel. At the midrectal level, the cul-de-sac and the transverse folds descend, reducing the volume of the funnel and forcing evacuation.

D: THE END OF EXPULSION WHILE STRAINING.
The expulsion ends when closure appears at the superior, rectorectal level along the posterior border of the funnel. The cul-de-sac descends to a low level with the transverse folds approximating each other. The ampullary part of the rectum is sequestered and collapsed. Further straining is ineffective.

CONCLUSION

Our understanding of expulsion, including the role of the pelvic floor and the functional division of the rectum (Fig. 10.10), has directly influenced our method of performing the examination. In order to visualize more of the pelvic floor we extended the digital subtraction technique to a more complex cysto-colpo-entero-defecography. We have performed over 500 such examinations, and we believe that this approach directs the type of therapy. Our good results with the perineal support device, combined with biofeedback training, support the concept that a good expulsion requires a good function of the pelvic floor.

SUGGESTED READING

Lesaffer LPA: The mechanism of expulsion during defecation. *Colo-Proctology* 3:187–192, 1993.

CHAPTER 11

The Measurement of Perineal Descent

Michael Henry

INTRODUCTION

The concept of abnormal perineal descent was first advanced by Parks and colleagues who described a clinical condition of disordered defecation associated with abnormal degrees of descent of the pelvic floor as assessed by simple and unquantified clinical examination. Since the initial description of this abnormality, attempts have been made to assess the position of the pelvic floor objectively and to relate this to function and disorder. As discussed below, the relevance of the abnormality is based on the belief that abnormal pelvic floor descent is indicative of underlying denervation of the pelvic floor musculature. Abnormal pelvic floor descent is hence a feature in patients complaining of anal incontinence, urinary incontinence in addition to other pelvic floor disorders. The detection of perineal descent has important clinical implications. In a patient with perineal descent and pelvic floor denervation, anal continence may be largely dependent on normal internal anal sphincter function. To subject such a patient to lateral sphincterotomy or manual dilatation may render the patient fecally incontinent.

CLINICAL ASSESSMENT

Although this is nonphysiological, most patients are examined clinically in the left lateral position. Under these circumstances, in the normal state the plane of the perineum should lie above that of the ischial tuberosities in the resting state. During a straining effort the perineum descends 1–2 cm but should not extend below the ischial tuberosities. In patients with abnormal descent a marked "ballooning" of the perineum occurs during straining with descent well below the bony outlet. If the straining effort persists, such patients frequently display a complete or partial rectal prolapse.

In the environment of the outpatient clinic or "office" this clinical abnormality may be quantified very simply using the St. Mark's Perineometer (Fig. 11-1). The device consists of a steel frame with moveable struts which are placed on the ischial tuberosities of the patient who is examined in the left lateral position. A central latex cylinder is capable of free movement within the steel frame and is brought into contact with the perianal skin. By means of a centimeter scale inscribed on the cylinder, measurements of the perineal plane in relation to the plane of the body outlet of the pelvis (ischial tuberosities) are made in the resting state and during maximum straining.

Using this simple device, the measurements obtained in a normal population of more than 100 controls are shown in Figure 11.2. Hence in normal subjects the perineum occupies a position 2.5 cm (±0.6) above the ischial tuberosities in the resting state. During maximum straining, the perineum descends by a mean value of 1.6 cm to a position 0.9 cm above the ischial tuberosities (±1.0).

In patients with abnormal descent, the position of the perineum at rest is lower but remains above the ischial tuberosities. During straining, however, the perineum descends to a level of 1.2 cm *below* the level of the ischial tuberosities.

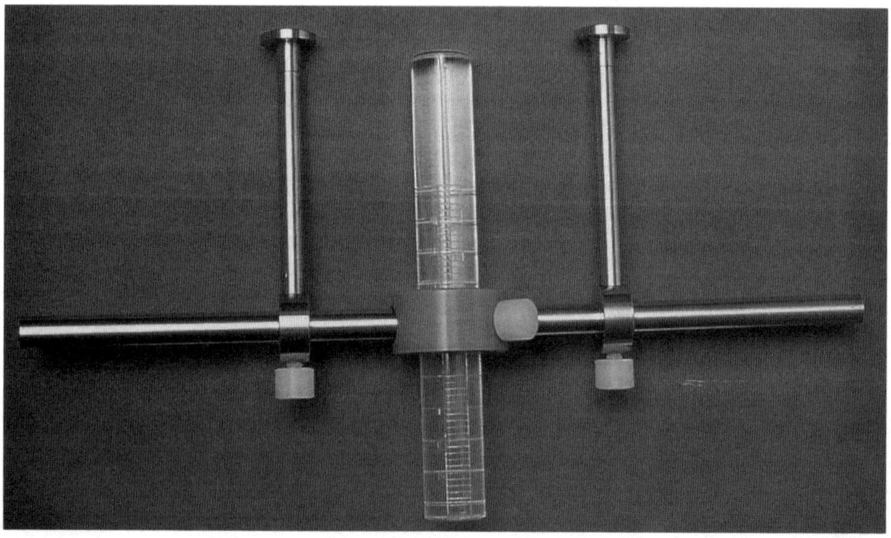

FIGURE 11.1 The St. Mark's perineometer.

FIGURE 11.2

Controls	Perineal Descent
* 2.5CM (+/−0.6) A	
	* 2.0CM (+/−1.0) A
* 0.9CM (+/−1.0) B	
	* 1.2CM (+/−0.8) B (p = .005)

RADIOLOGICAL METHODS

The plane of the perineum can be assessed along with other parameters (e.g., anorectal angle, anal canal length, presence of rectocele, time taken to evacuate) during the investigation of evacuation proctography. Many differing techniques have been described but the method described by Mahieu has found general favor. With this technique a barium water suspension is added to potato starch and the preparation is injected into the rectum. The patient is seated on a specially constructed commode and cineradiography is performed with the patient at rest and during evacuation of the contrast material.

The obvious advantage of this technique is that it permits accurate assessment of the perineum plane in the physiological position during defecation rather than in the nonphysiological state adopted with the patient lying in the left lateral position. The plane of the perineum is also accurately assessed during the act of defecation rather than just during "mock" defecation associated with straining. The major disadvantage, however, is that the technique involves irradiation to the pelvis frequently in women of childbearing age. Radiological doses are typically about 0.02–0.66 cGy to the right hip area with an ovarian dose of 0.036–0.053 cGy.

Measurement of perineal descent is usually based on comparison with the anorectal junction with some bony landmark. With larger films it is possible to use the pubococcygeal line (from the upper border of the pubic symphysis to the tip of the coccyx). With the restricted views provided by the use of cineradiography, the anorectal junction is usually related to the inferior plane of the ischial tuberosities.

In normal subjects, using radiological methods pelvic floor descent usually averages 2 to 3 cm and generally does not exceed 4.5 cm. The range in normals has been found to be extensive, however. It has further been shown that the extent of pelvic floor descent decreases in the elderly presumably because the resting position is lower in this age group.

COMPARISON OF THE TWO METHODS

Oettle and colleagues compared clinical with radiological methods and found that the perineometer underestimates movement of the pelvic floor by as much as 60%. However, although relatively inaccurate in comparison with radiological methods, the perineometer has the clear advantage of being cheap, safe, and portable and is hence ideal for use in the "office." On the other hand radiological methods are cumbersome and involve irradiation of the pelvis. Radiological techniques, however, do allow for measurement of other parameters (e.g., anorectal angle) and also provide visualization of the rectum to permit exclusion of rectocele and internal intussusception for example.

CLINICAL APPLICATIONS

As discussed above, the recognition of abnormal pelvic floor descent is of importance in that the physical sign is indicative of pelvic floor denervation. Jones and colleagues (8) demonstrated by use of the perineometer that there was a linear relationship between the degree of perineal descent and the degree of damage within the pudendal nerves. The latter was estimated by measurement of the pudendal nerve terminal motor latency. This study hence further indicated how accurate measurement of the perineal plane was an important indicator of pelvic floor function.

SUGGESTED READINGS

Henry MM, Parks AG, and Swash M: The pelvic floor musculature in the descending perineum syndrome. *Br J Surg* 69:470–472, 1982.

Jones PN, Lubowski DZ, Swash M, et al: Relation between perineal descent and pudendal nerve damage in idiopathic faecal incontinence. *Int J Colorect Dis* 2:93–95, 1987.

Kelvin FM, Stevenson GW: In Freeny PC, Stevenson GW (eds): *Alimentary Tract Radiology.* Mosby, 1994, pp 840–851.

Mahieu P, Pringot J, Bodart P: Defecography: 1. Description of a new procedure and results in normal patients. *Gastrointest Radiol* 9:247–251, 1984.

Oettle GJ, Roe AM, Bartolo DCC et al: What is the best way of measuring perineal descent? A comparison of radiographic and clinical methods. *Br J Surg* 72:999–1001, 1985.

Parks AG, Porter NH, Hardcastle JD: The syndrome of the descending perineum. *Proc R Soc Med* 59:477–482, 1966.

Pinho M, et al: The effect of age on pelvic floor dynamics. *Int J Colorect Dis* 5:207, 1990.

Shorvon PJ, McHugh S, Diamant NE, et al: Defecography in normal volunteers: results and implications. *Gut* 30:1737–1749, 1989.

CHAPTER 12

Scintigraphic Assessment of Pelvic Ileal Pouch Emptying

Paul Belliveau

INTRODUCTION

Since the first reports of restorative proctocolectomy with ileoanal reservoirs for ulcerative colitis or familial polyposis coli, functional results have been of great interest and concern to surgeons and physiologists. The degree of evacuation of these intestinal pouches has created a new and unnatural environment at the mucosal level leading to yet unknown long-term consequences. The technique, however, permits fecal continence in patients who otherwise would require a permanent ileostomy. One aspect of the functional assessment of these reservoirs can now be quantitated, using a simple, safe and reproducible method that allows the determination of the emptying capability of these reservoirs adding important information in their management and evolution. Problems of emptying may be implicated in the pathogenesis of fecal stasis and local inflammatory reactions of the mucosa (pouchitis).

INDICATIONS

1. Pelvic ileal reservoirs of *various configurations* can be assessed using this method to evaluate their comparability.
2. The adequacy of compliance of the reservoir, months or years after its creation, can be studied.
3. The *reflux* of material into the proximal small bowel may be demonstrated and its extent quantitated.
4. The significance of *outlet obstruction* on emptying function can be quantitated.

5. The presence or suspicion of *fecal stasis* in the reservoir can be demonstrated, and treatment directed at improving emptying can be undertaken.
6. Malabsorption with *stagnant loop* syndromes can be assessed before and after therapy.
7. *Diarrhea* can be related to reservoir dysfunction or proximal small bowel overactivity, and this study may indicate the level of dysfunction.
8. Evacuation parameters of defunctioned reservoirs, i.e., while loop ileostomy is still in place or has been reestablished.
9. Known cases of pouchitis may be assessed.

CONTRAINDICATIONS

1. A recent anastomosis, i.e., less than 2 to 3 months.
2. Uncooperative patient.
3. Incapacitating anal pain.
4. Significant stricture of the anastomosis preventing insertion of a catheter.
5. Presence of a reservoir fistula.
6. Small bowel obstruction.
7. Allergy to eggs or to milk.

PATIENTS AND SUBJECTS

Patients who have undergone a mucosal proctectomy with ileoanal anastomosis for chronic ulcerative colitis and familial polyposis coli are candidates for this examination. The examination could be used to assess certain defecation disorders accompanied by incomplete evacuation: outlet constipation, internal intussusception, perineal descent, mucosal prolapse, etc. The procedure should be explained carefully to the patient to ensure compliance with instructions. A negligible amount of radiation is involved. The procedure is done in the Department of Nuclear Medicine by a certified technician. The patients are warned that they may experience a sensation of fullness when the material is infused.

MATERIALS AND METHODS

The patient is asked to have a bowel movement before coming to the hospital for the examination. There is no specific preparation and specifically no period of fasting or enema is required. Two fresh eggs are beaten and ^{99m}Tc (1.0 mCi) sulfur colloid is added by the technician. The mixture is heated at a low setting until the

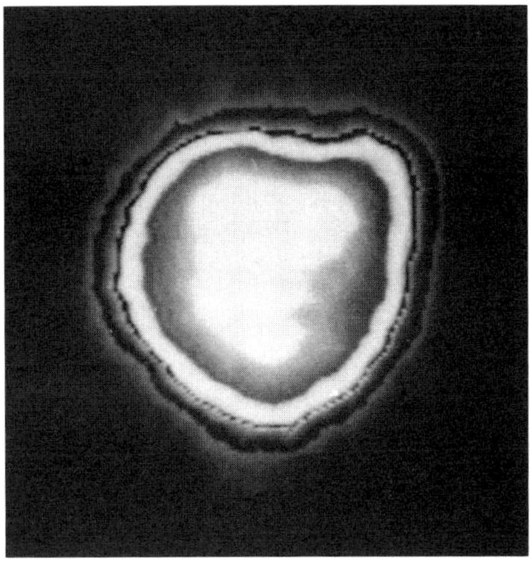

FIGURE 12.1 Initial scan following infusion.

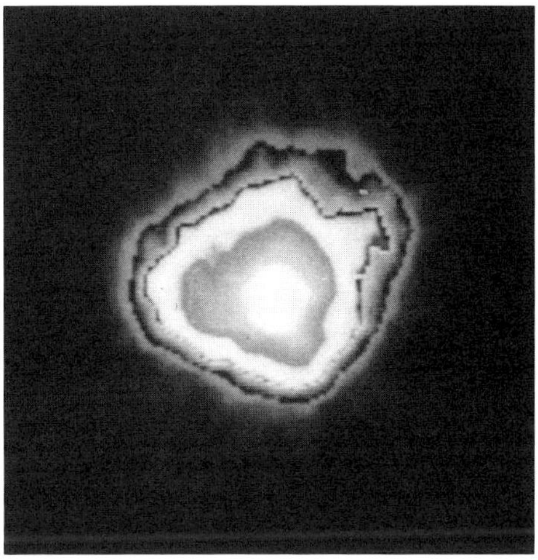

FIGURE 12.2 Postevacuation scan.

consistency resembles the individual's usual stool. Milk is added to the labeled cooked eggs to make a volume of 350 cc.

The patient is asked to lie on the examining table in the left lateral decubitus position with the right leg flexed. A size 24 Foley catheter is inserted gently about 10 cm into the anus, and the prepared material is injected slowly. The mixture is instilled using a large syringe until the set volume of 350 ml oral maximal sensory threshold is reached and the volume recorded. The catheter is withdrawn and the patient is asked to hold on to the mixture. The patient is placed prone and is scanned for 2 min (2-min acquisition time). Scintigraphic preevacuation image (posterior view) is obtained using a gamma camera with a parallel-holed, all-purpose collimator, interfaced with a computer (Fig. 12.1).

At the end of the acquisition (2 min), the patient is asked to walk around for 5 min and to evacuate the contents of the ileal reservoir in a private washroom. The patient is repositioned prone, and a 2-min acquisition time postevacuation image is then obtained (Fig. 12.2). Subsequent to the completion of the acquisition, a

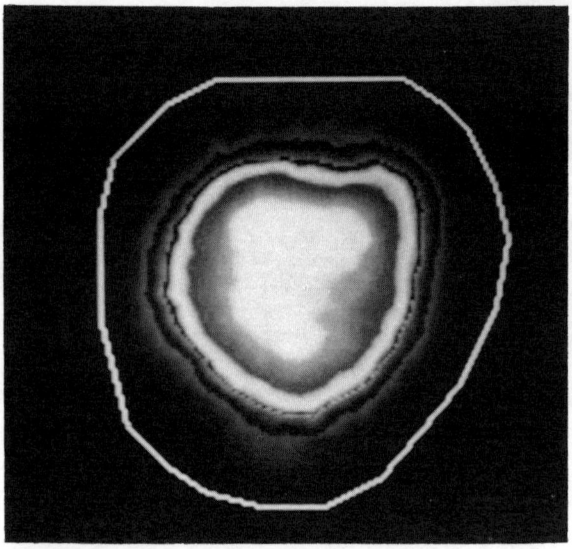

FIGURE 12.3 Preevacuation region of interest.

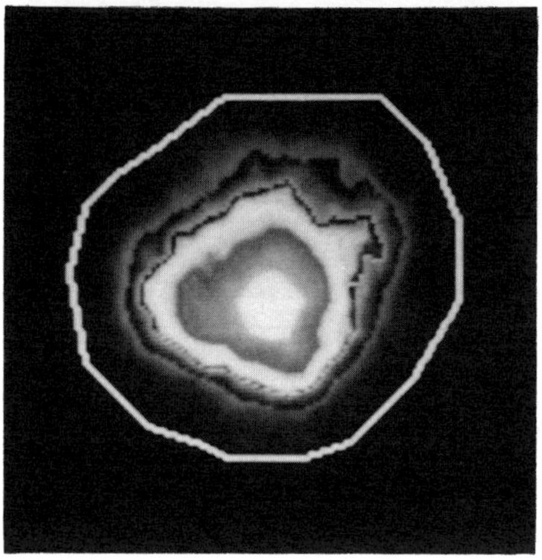

FIGURE 12.4 Postevacuation region of interest.

region of interest is drawn over the ileal reservoir display, and the evacuation fraction is calculated (Figs. 12.3 and 12.4):

$$\text{Evacuation fraction} = \frac{\text{Preevacuation counts} - \text{Postevacuation counts}}{\text{Preevacuation counts}}$$

INTERPRETATION OF RESULTS

A study can be considered normal if greater than 60% of the infused material is expelled during the bowel movement. In ten control subjects the percentage of emptying of the normal rectum was 90 + 3%. In patients with an emptying

TABLE 12.1 PATIENTS STUDIED

Number: 53
Mean age: 35.9 ± 10.8 (18–59)
Male: 38
Female: 15

TABLE 12.2 RESULTS

>60% Evacuation	<60% Evacuation
Number: 38	Number: 15
Male: 28	Male: 10
Female: 10	Female: 5
Range: 60–96%	Range: 0–51%
Mean %: 77.2 ± 10.9	Mean %: 29.1 ± 14.0

fraction of less than 30%, an assessment of the anal canal is indicated, and consideration should be given to a trial of self-intubation and the study repeated, using this method of evacuation. In a series of 53 patients studied, all having a diagnosis of ulcerative colitis and all having an S-shaped reservoir (Table 12.1), the results were as shown in Table 12.2.

In the follow-up of these patients the recording has proven very useful in sorting out the problems which they develop over the years. Specifically, those who develop evacuation difficulties and require straining more than others can be helped with specific advice about their situation, such as avoidance of prolonged useless forcing and consideration of intermittent intubation in periods of more intense difficulty.

Patients with diarrhea may show findings in the normal range, indicating that dysfunction is related to activity of the small intestine rather than to pouch obstruction. Pouchitis is being diagnosed with increasing frequency and this study may shed some light on the possible etiological factors responsible. Repeating the recording over time in certain cases is used to follow the evolution of the functional component of these neorectums.

SUGGESTED READINGS

Heppell J, Belliveau P, Taillefer R, et al: Quantitative assessment of pelvic ileal reservoir emptying with a semisolid radionuclide enema. A correlation with clinical outcome. *Dis Colon Rectum* 2:81–85, 1987.

O'Connell PR, Pemberton JH, Brown ML, et al: Determinants of stool frequency after ileal pouch-anal anastomosis. *Am J Surg* 153:157–164, 1987.

CHAPTER 13

Electromyographic Techniques

Ridzuan Farouk

THE MOTOR UNIT POTENTIAL

Electromyography (EMG) is one of the principal techniques used in the investigation of the internal and external sphincters as well as the pelvic floor muscles. Individual muscle fibers derived from a motor unit summate to form the motor unit action potential which can be recorded at a greater distance than the close proximity that is required to record activity of individual muscle fibers which have small action potentials of brief duration (fibrillation potentials). A motor unit consists of the anterior horn cell, its axon and terminal branches, and the muscle fibers it supplies. The number of muscle fibers innervated by each anterior horn cell varies between 10 and 200 dependent on whether the muscle is used for fine or coarse control of function. Each motor unit potential will have the characteristics of amplitude, duration, and characteristic shape of electrical response. Analysis of duration and shape is of physiological value.

The striated muscles of the pelvic floor and the external anal sphincter are continuously active. Injury to the afferent nerves results in fibrillation of the muscles which can be recorded. Investigation of the striated pelvic floor muscles has been directed at recording changes in motor unit potentials by concentric needle work, and alterations to single-fiber EMG patterns suggesting muscle reinnervation.

METHODOLOGY

A full explanation of the procedure is given and consent obtained. The patient is then placed in the left lateral position with a ground electrode placed. The anal skin is cleansed to remove moisture and reduce electrical "noise."

Concentric Needle EMG

Concentric needle electrodes are commonly used and consist of bare-tipped steel wire of 0.1 mm diameter with an insulating resin. The area of uptake of the electrode is small and any electrical activity recorded is that into which the electrode is inserted. Individual muscle fiber action potentials cannot however be identified reliably using concentric needle electrodes.

A conventional concentric needle electrode (Type 13149; Dantec, Copenhagen, Denmark) is inserted into the lateral aspect of the external anal sphincter and advanced parallel to the anal canal until it is 5 cm from the skin. Muscle potentials are recorded during advancement, and it often appears that the electrode passes out of one muscle into a silent area before entering a second striated muscle. In this position, it is assumed that the needle lies in the puborectalis muscle, having traversed the medial area of the ischiorectal fossa.

The Dantec Neuromatic 2000 (Fig. 13.1) (Dantec, Copenhagen, Denmark) is used to display and amplify recordings obtained. The settings of the amplifier are set as follows: gain at 0.2 mV/division or 0.5 mV/division, low-frequency filter at 20 Hz, high-frequency filter at 5 kHz. A time base of 5 to 10 msec/division was used. Trigger and delay facilities enable individual motor unit potentials to be identified and the stability of their components to be assessed.

The Neuromatic 2000 features a dedicated single-potential program with the capacity to store eight traces in memory. Having identified the potential, its duration is measured on the screen. A hard copy record may be stored on a personal computer hard disk or printed out (Hewlett-Packard 550C Color-Jet Printer).

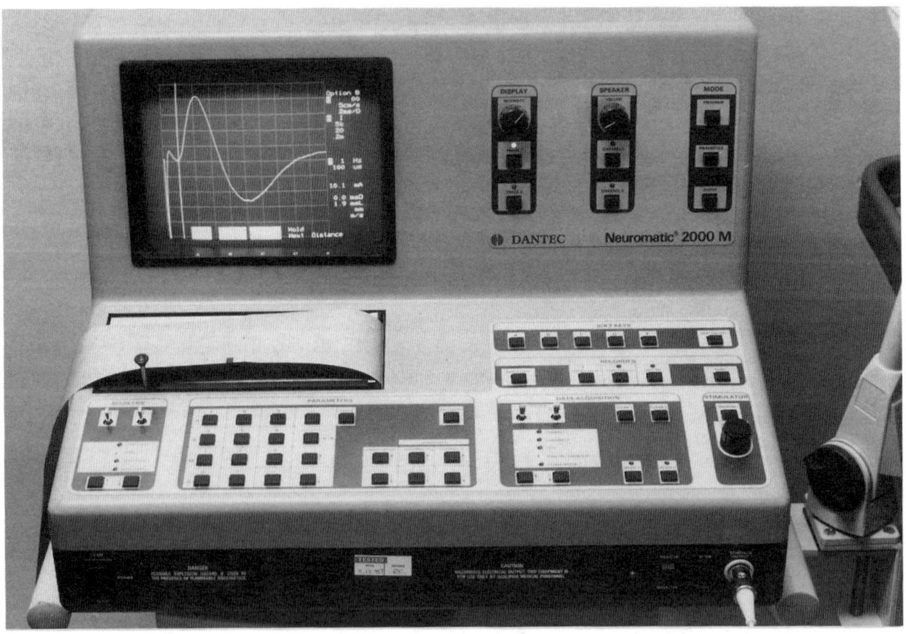

FIGURE 13.1 The Dantec Neuromatic 2000 M.

The duration of each motor unit potential is taken as the time interval from the departure of the sweep from the baseline at the onset of the potential to the return of the sweep to the baseline after the last component of the potential. Recordings are obtained from both lateral margins of the external anal sphincter and puborectalis. At least 20 motor unit potentials should be recorded from each of the four muscle sites. During recording, care should be taken to avoid repeatedly measuring the same motor unit potential. As the electrode is moved, the amplitude of the potential will increase or decrease in size as the electrode shifts toward or away from the motor unit. In a large complex motor unit, the various components will also vary in amplitude, but the overall duration will remain constant. Moreover, one component of the complex may increase while the other decreases.

Interpretation of the Motor Unit Potential

The amplitude of a motor unit potential depends on the number of fibers discharging synchronously. Amplitude also varies with the distance of the recording electrode from the motor unit. Reproducibility of recordings, however, may vary up to 40%. Amplitude of motor unit potentials therefore does not provide a useful index of comparison.

Duration of the motor unit potential provides a more reproducible means of comparative assessment. There is an increase in the mean duration of motor unit potentials from infancy to adulthood that is attributed to the growth in width of the end plate zone. In the biceps of the newborn the average width of the end-plate zone is 6 mm, as compared to 25 mm in adults. There is evidence that the duration of motor unit potentials of adults increases from 20 to 70 years of age. This increase does not appear to be attributable to decreased conduction velocity or changes in end-plate width. Grouped denervation atrophy resulting in polyphasic potentials of longer duration may contribute to this observation.

The evidence of age-related changes in motor unit potential duration of the human external anal sphincter is inconclusive. The more recent studies on this subject indicate that there is a significant correlation between age and motor unit potential duration in normal control subjects. Information about the controls used in these studies was limited, however.

The motor unit potential as recorded by a concentric needle electrode represents the algebraic summation of single-fiber action potentials. Most motor unit potentials are bi- or triphasic. Polyphasic potentials, which are defined as four or more phases, are also observed in normal skeletal muscle. The incidence of such polyphasic potential varies according to the type of muscle. It is usually no more than 12% in a sample of 20 to 40 motor unit potentials but may be as high as 25% in the deltoid muscle. The reported incidence of polyphasic potentials in the human external anal sphincter varies between 7 and 25%.

The duration of polyphasic potentials in relation to the mean duration of simple shaped potentials can be used to indicate underlying neurological dysfunction. Those of short duration suggest a myopathic disorder. Polyphasic potentials of prolonged duration represent a sign of muscle reinnervation. The prolonged duration represents delayed conduction along immature nerve fibers or nerve sprouts.

TABLE 13.1 MOTOR UNIT POTENTIAL DURATION IN HEALTH AND DISEASE

	Motor unit potential duration (msec)	
	Puborectalis	**External anal sphincter**
Normal controls	5.5 (4.1–7.1)	6.4 (4.0–8.8)
Constipation (continent)	6.3 (4.4–7.3)	7.8 (5.3–9.8)
Perineal descent (continent)	7.1 (4.8–14.7)	9.3 (5.1–15.4)
Incontinent single-fiber EMG	9.1 (5.4–15.1)	8.9 (6.0–13.2)

The single-fiber EMG electrode which has an uptake radius of 270 μM can record the activity of individual muscle fibers within a motor unit (Fig. 13.2). The electrode consists of a needle slightly narrower than 0.1 mm filled with resin. A central wire opens at the midshaft of the electrode through a 25-μM leading off surface. The cannula of the electrode represents the reference electrode and a separate ground electrode is also required. An amplifier with a 500-Hz low-frequency filter setting and a trigger delay line are required with the amplifier set at 2–5 msec per division. The mean duration of motor unit potentials consisting of more than one component recorded by this method is less than 8 msec.

METHOD. Right and left lateral stabs are made without anesthetic and 20 different recordings are taken from each muscle. The fiber density is assessed by counting the number of peaks recorded per stab. The 20 recordings are totalled and then averaged (Fig. 13.3). The potentials are recorded on the Dantec Neuromatic 2000 (Dantec, Copenhagen, Denmark).

Once again, care should be taken to avoid repeatedly measuring the same potential by using multiple insertions at different sites. It is advisable to keep hard copies for later analysis, with at least two for each discharge.

Single-fiber Density

The number of spikes or phases using single-fiber EMG forms the basis for the measurement of fiber density. In normal circumstances, only a small number of muscle fibers from a single motor unit lie within the uptake area of a single-fiber electrode. In normal subjects the fiber density of most muscles is less than two though this increases slightly with age. In reinnervated muscle, the number of fibers belonging to a single motor unit increases, leading to an increased number of recorded potentials being recorded at one electrode position (Fig. 13.4).

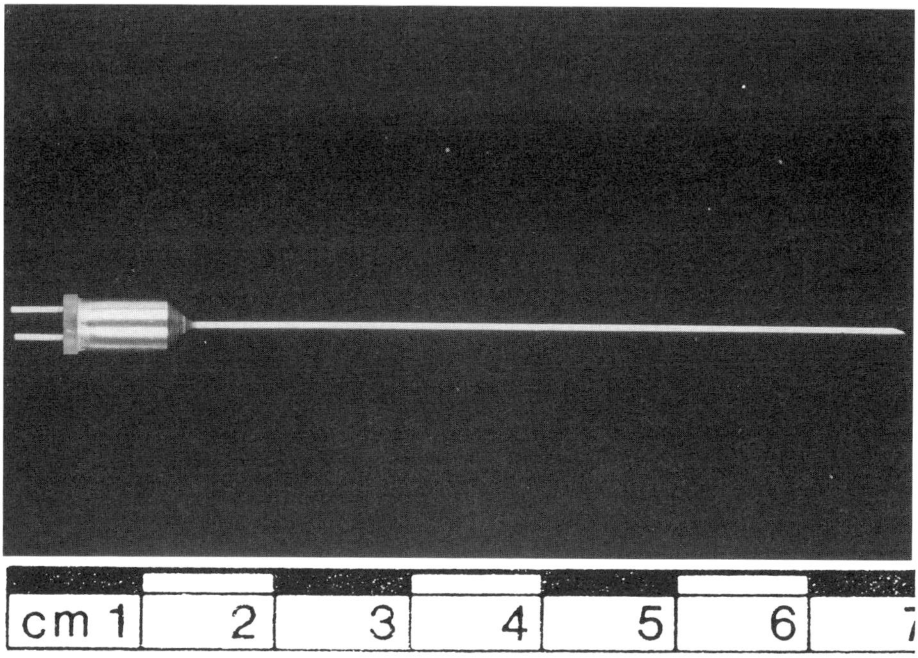

FIGURE 13.2 A single-fiber EMA electrode.

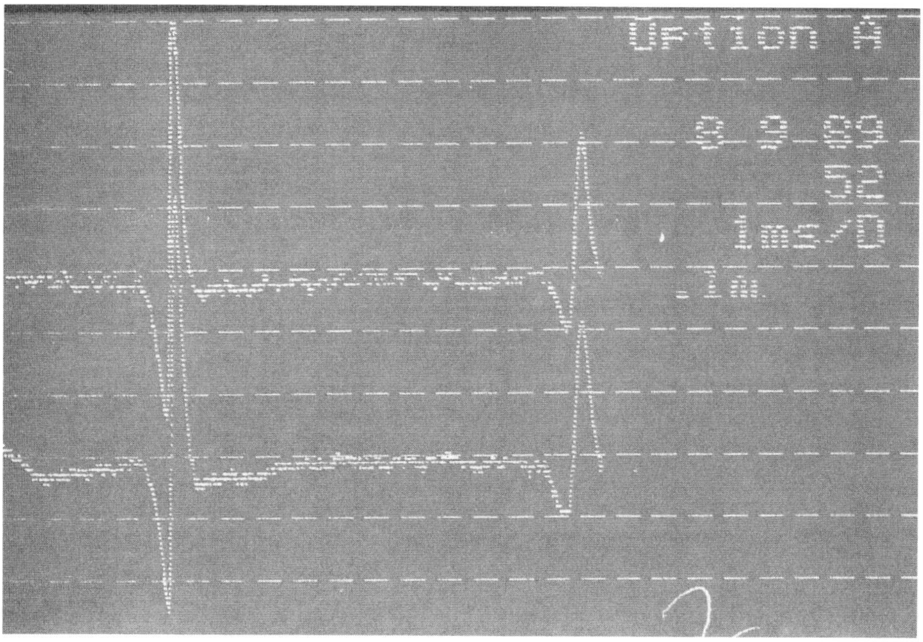

FIGURE 13.3 A normal single-fiber electronic microanalyzer (EMA) trace.

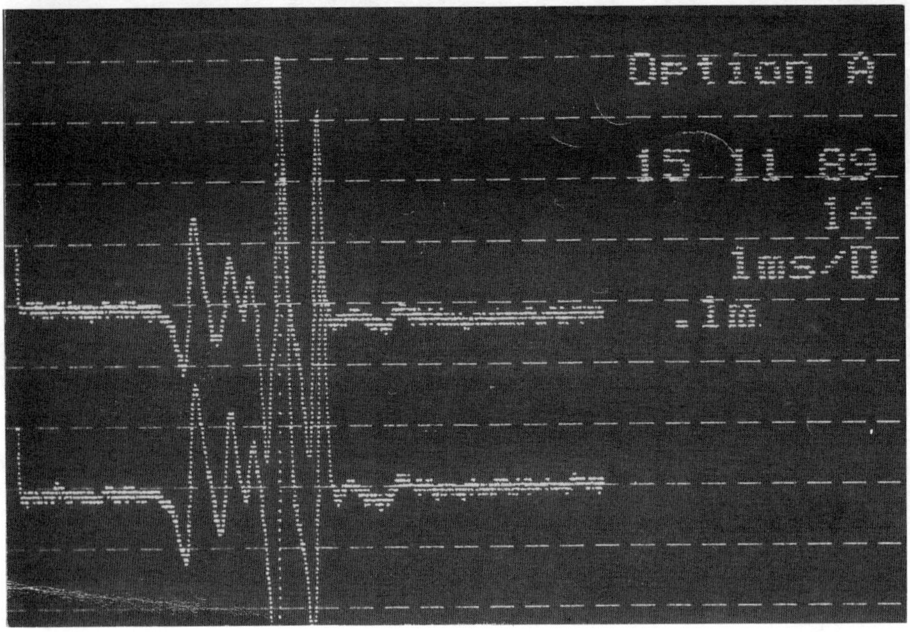

FIGURE 13.4 An example of polyphasic potentials from a single-fiber EMG recordings.

Neuromuscular Jitter

If a single-fiber EMG electrode is positioned so that it records from two fibers from the same motor unit, the time relationship at consecutive discharges will not be constant. This fluctuation is due to a variability in neuromuscular delay known as *jitter*. Jitter is increased in neurological disorders, such as myasthenia gravis and where there is peripheral nerve sprouting in reinnervation. Newly formed sprouts are not myelinated initially and do not transmit nerve impulses well.

ASSESSMENT OF SPHINCTER INTEGRITY

Traditional assessment of anal sphincter integrity following traumatic childbirth or anal surgery has relied on mapping the complete ring of the external anal sphincter using a concentric EMG needle. Insertion of the needle into areas of muscle disruption or scar tissue may possibly demonstrate electrical silence confirming disruption. The technique requires multiple insertions into tonically contracting anal sphincter muscle. This technique is somewhat painful and does not provide adequate assessment of the internal anal sphincter. Perhaps the most common indication for electromyographic mapping is the patient with a suspected obstetric injury. These women usually present with one of the following histories:

1. Difficult forceps delivery
2. Breech delivery
3. Extended episiotomy
4. Second- and third-degree tears
5. Baby weight in excess of 4 kg
6. Occipitoposterior presentation
7. Prolonged second stage of labor

The technique of EMG mapping of the external anal sphincter has largely been replaced by endoanal ultrasonography which provides superior imaging of the anal sphincter complex using a relatively painless technique.

A number of different centers have performed prolonged recordings of anorectal function. These have usually involved the use of pressure catheters as the primary tool of investigation. The use of surface electrodes to record external anal sphincter activity has also been reported. There have been few reports of studies assessing internal anal sphincter function however.

METHOD OF AMBULATORY ASSESSMENT OF ANAL SPHINCTER EMG ACTIVITY

Equipment

The ambulatory recorder used was the 7MPR recorder manufactured by Gaeltec Ltd., Isle of Skye. This recorder has a memory capacity of 512 kbytes and has the potential of displaying seven separate channels at any one time (Fig. 13.5). The recorder which is a digital system possesses an events marker and a clock facility. Three of the channels were used for the recording of electromyographic activity and the remaining channels were used for manometry. The recorder samples the information from each channel at a minimum rate of 8 times per second, sufficiently frequent to detect the low frequency of the internal anal sphincter which in humans is within the range of 0.1–0.6 Hz.

In essence, the recording program has the facility to scan the 7-channel recording on a second-to-second basis. If the recording value per channel remained constant in 1 sec, only the first and last points of the recording were stored and a presumption is made of a straight line recording between these points. Should there have been a change of values in that 1 sec, the recorder logs the intervening points to reconstruct the record. A value of 2 units was chosen as our predetermined recording accuracy, i.e., pressure channels accurate to within 2 cm H_2O and the EMG channels accurate to within 2 μV. The sensitivity of the recorder can be readjusted by entering the Eeprom of the recorder using the main program provided by Gaeltec and altering its sensitivity, e.g. to 5 units. Such readjustments do not affect real-time recordings but alter the accuracy of subsequent reproduction of the record.

An additional modification made possible by entry to the Eeprom was to alter the exponential settings of the recorder. This has the effect of altering the sensitivity of the recording. An increase in the exponential factor by one has the effect

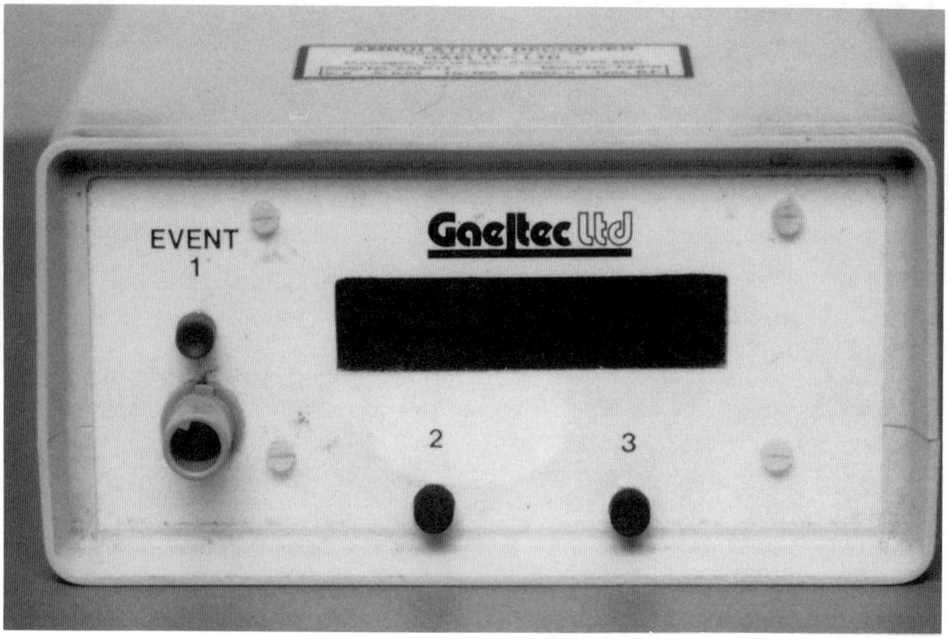

FIGURE 13.5 The Gaeltec 7MPR ambulatory recorder.

of halving the sensitivity of the unit recorded. For example, setting the EMG or the catheter header amplifiers to record 1 μV or 1 cm H_2O, respectively, would produce channels whose basic unit was 2 μV or 2 cm H_2O, and by consecutive increases in the linear factor, the units could be set to exponentially decrease the sensitivity i.e., to 1, 2, 4, 8, 16, then 32 units etc. These two options, although seemingly similar have major differences on recorder function. Changing the recorder accuracy does not in effect alter the real-time record, it simply alters the records accuracy of reproduction. Altering the exponentials alters not only the compressed but also the real-time record.

The replay parameters of the recording on a personal computer were alterable to suit the needs of the various studies possible. The default screen showed 1 min of recording per page but this could be altered by a factor of 2 to display up to 128 min per page on the screen, with 4 min per page being the most satisfactory display for analysis. The pressure channels displayed up to 200 cm H_2O between channel division lines and this was satisfactory but could have been varied between 25 and 800 cm H_2O. The EMG channels could be defaulted to 0.2 mV (200 μV) between the division lines. This could be increased up to 3.2 mV, and the values used depended on the individual subject level of activity. The range usually lay between 0.2 and 0.4 mV.

Hard records of the recordings are available on an Epson-compatible screen dump, a HP laser, or a colorjet dump. Copies of the recordings themselves can be retained on the hard disk or transferred to a 3.5'' floppy disk for storage and later retrieval.

The ambulatory recorder was dedicated to the Gaeltec range of microtransducer-pressure-sensitive catheters and two types have been used. A four-transducer pressure catheter had transducers mounted at 1, 2, 10, and 14 cm measured from the anal verge (type CTR4). The first two transducers were combined as a single built unit. This was the catheter in general use and had an outside diameter of 2.5 mm.

The 7-MPR recorder is not equipped with the suitable amplifiers for EMG recordings. Three header amplifiers were therefore constructed by Gaeltec for this purpose. The fine-wire method of EMG recoring was thought to be most appropriate as it allowed "clean" recordings of all the muscles assessed, and reduced the likelihood of dislocation.

Method of Wire Insertion

Each patient was invited to attempt defecation prior to wire insertion. Bowel preparation was never used. Topical lignocaine cream was then applied to the perineum for 1 hr. A pair of fine barbed, bared steel wires (diameter 0.13 mm) was then inserted into the internal anal sphincter, external anal sphincter, and puborectalis muscles (Fig. 13.6). The internal and external sphincter were identified digitally by palpation of the natural groove that exists between both muscles. Puborectalis was identified by digitally identifying the anorectal muscle, and then asking the patient to strain which results in pelvic floor descent. The wires were introduced with the aid of a 19-gauge hypodermic needle. The ends were barbed to allow retention within the muscle and offset by 1 mm to prevent short-circuiting. Once the pair of wires was inserted, the hypodermic needle was withdrawn, and the wires secured to the header amplifier board which is serially in contact in turn with the 7-MPR recorder. The wires and header amplifier board were taped securely to the patient to prevent dislodgement. Accurate positioning of the wires was determined by direct observation of the computer screen which allowed real-time recording of the traces concerned. Satisfactory positioning of the wire electrodes was based on obtaining the characteristic EMG traces of the muscle concerned. Accurate positioning of these wires could also be determined by performing endoanal ultrasound.

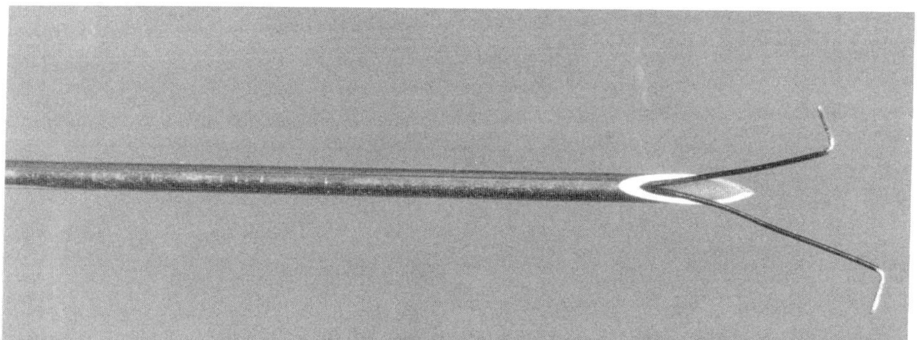

FIGURE 13.6 Baked steel wires 0.013 mm in diameter mounted on a 21-gauge hypodermic needle used for ambulatory electronic microanalyzer (EMA) recordings.

The manometer probe was then inserted in turn through a pediatric proctoscope. Accurate positioning of the transducers was determined by withdrawing the probe in a continuous pull-through method to align the "double" transducer unit within the zone of high pressure in the anal canal. This facility was again available because the procedure was performed with real-time recordings on a personal computer.

The Learning Curve

A total of 314 subjects were assessed using this technique. The method of ambulatory assessment was not entirely straightforward to learn, and there was an associated learning curve. The most difficult EMG recording to obtain was in fact

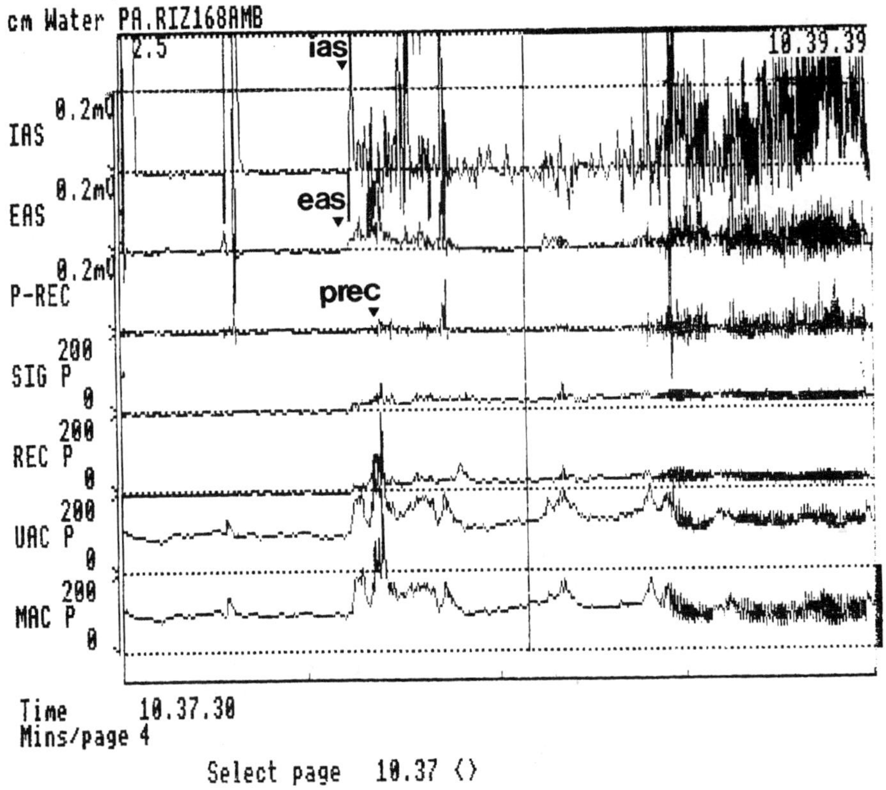

FIGURE 13.7 Identification of correct positioning of the EMG wires is carried out by observing for the characteristic EMG activity of the muscles concerned. In this illustration, the onset of activity of the individual EMGs which results from accurate positioning of the wires is indicated by arrow.

that of puborectalis. The first 28 recordings obtained were the least successful, with only one of the three EMG recordings regularly obtained. The next 17 recordings were hampered by equipment malfunction. The pressure transducers were damaged and required repair. Ambulatory recordings were therefore commenced with satisfactory traces from patient 46 onward. The only patients excluded from ambulatory recordings following this were those who were considered too frail or mentally confused.

Of the 268 ambulatory recordings that were considered to be technically satisfactory, 261 recordings of the internal anal sphincter EMG were obtained, 253 recordings of the external anal sphincter EMG was obtained, and 231 recordings of the puborectalis EMG were recorded. All of these recordings consisted of at least two simultaneous EMG recordings. This rate of successful recordings compares favorably with previous reports with this equipment.

Inter-observer Variation of Recordings

A comparison of observations made in 26 recordings was undertaken with another investigator with experience of such recordings. Internal anal sphincter EMG frequency (IAS EMG) and ambulatory anal pressures (ARP) were measured independently and compared. The recordings compared consisted of those from normal control subjects and 15 patients with slow transit constipation. These results are summarized in Table 13.2.

TABLE 13.2 INTER-OBSERVER COMPARISON OF RESULTS

	Observer 1	Observer 2
Internal sphincter EMG frequency	0.39 (0.25–0.55)	0.39 (0.25–0.55)*
Ambulatory anal pressure	80 (40–150)	80 (45–145)*

* $p > 0.5$, Mann-Whitney U test.

CONCLUSIONS

The advent of endoanal ultrasonography has cast some doubt as to whether sphincter denervation has any role in disorders of continence. Sphincter electromyography is painful and gradually is being replaced by endoanal ultrasound as a means of primary assessment of the sphincter complex. Proponents of this endoanal ultrasound have not, however, shown why patients who initially have good function after sphincter repair subsequently deteriorate with poor long-term outcome. It is likely that continuing denervation contributes to this process.

SUGGESTED READINGS

Bartolo DCC, Jarratt JA, Read NW: The use of conventional electromyography to external anal sphincter neuropathy in man. *J Neurol Neurosurg Psychiatry* 46:1115–1118, 1983.

Bartolo DCC, Read NW, Jarratt JA, et al: Differences in anal sphincter function and clinical presentation in patients with pelvic floor descent. *Gastroenterology* 85:68–75, 1983.

Bouvier M, Gonella J: Nervous control of the internal anal sphincter of the cat. *J Physiol* 310:457–469, 1981.

Buchtal F, Guld C, Rosenfalck P: Action potential parameters in normal human muscle and their dependence on physical variables. *Acta Physiol Scand* 32:200–218, 1954.

Buchtal F, Guld C, Rosenfalck P: Innervation zone and propagation velocity in human muscle. *Acta Physiol Scand* 35:174–190, 1955.

Buchtal F, Guld C, Rosenfalck P: Multi-electrode study of the territory of a motor unit. *Acta Physiol Scand* 39:83–104, 1957.

Buchtal F, Kamieniecka Z: The diagnostic yield of quantified electromyography and quantified muscle biopsy in neuromuscular disorders. *Muscle Nerve* 5:265–280, 1982.

Buchtal F, Pinelli P: Action potentials in muscular atrophy of neurogenic origin. *Neurology* 3:591–603, 1953.

Buchtal F, Pinelli P, Rosenfalck P: Action potential parameters in normal human muscle and their physiological determinants. *Acta Physiol Scand* 32:219–229, 1954.

Caruso G, Buchtal F: Refractory period of muscle and electromyographic findings in relatives of patients with muscular dystrophy. *Brain* 88:29–88, 1965.

Duthie GS, Miller R, Bartolo DCC: Internal sphincter electromyographic frequency is related to anal canal resting pressure. Both are reduced in idiopathic fecal incontinence. *Gut* 31:A619, 1990.

Duthie GS: Ambulatory monitoring in anorectal disease. M.D. Thesis, University of Aberdeen, 1993.

Ekstedt J: Human single fiber muscle potentials. *Acta Physiol Scand* 61:1–91, 1964.

Floyd W, Walls E: Electromyography of the sphincter ani externus in man. *J Physiol* 16:638–644, 1953.

Kerremans R: Morphological and physiological aspects of anal continence and defecation. Brussels, Editions Arscia, 1969.

Neill ME, Swash M: Increased motor unit fiber density in external sphincter muscle in anorectal incontinence: a single fiber EMG study. *J Neurol Neurosurg Psychiatry* 43:343–347, 1980.

Pennickx F: Morphological and physiological aspects of anal function. Leuven, Acco n.v., 1981.

Stalberg E, Thiele B: Motor unit fiber density in the extensor digitorum communis muscle. *J Neurol Neurosurg Psychiatry* 38:874–888, 1975.

Swash M: Idiopathic fecal incontinence: histopathological evidence of pathogenesis. In Wright R: *Recent Advances in Gastrointestinal Pathology*. Philadelphia, Saunders, 1985, pp 71–89.

Tomlinson BE, Walton JN, Rebeiz JJ: The effects of aging and cachexia upon skeletal muscle. A histopathological study. *J Neurol Sci* 9:321–346, 1969.

Ustach JT, Tobon F, Hambrecht T, et al: Electrophysiological aspects of human sphincter function. *J Clin Invest* 49:41–48, 1970.

CHAPTER 14

Anal Electrophysiological and Pudendal Nerve Evoked Potentials

Jeffrey L. Cole
Lester Gottesman

INTRODUCTION

When the rectal (or urinary) sphincter dysfunctions, the clinical description and physical examination can often be misleading. The neuromuscular control lesions can run the gamut from hypoactivity to selective or general spasticity, from muscle regulation deficits (directly in the muscle or anywhere along the efferent neural pathway) to unyielding scar formations in the sphincter muscle that can prevent activity or hinder proper closure. The evaluation, therefore, frequently requires appropriate diagnostic studies, such as: anorectal manometry; colonic transit studies; cinedefecography; urodynamic evaluations (uroflowmetry, cystometry, etc.); quantitative surface and/or needle electromyographic (EMG) information over the rectal sphincter, bladder neck, perineal floor, and puborectalis muscle; nocturnal penile tumescence; bethanechol chloride supersensitivity testing; and other manometry procedures. Each of these studies provides some information about the functional activity in the rectal (and/or urinary) sphincter. However, a sense of the functional deficit (or activity) as well as superior documentation of muscle and nerve pathologies underlying the clinical problems, can be established with the addition of a culled sequence of electrodiagnostic studies.

A comprehensive electrodiagnostic testing algorithm is crucial to avoid duplicate testing and precisely establish the site and/or etiology of the lesion. Studies that have been in use for decades include: lower extremity nerve conduction studies (NCS); qualitative rectal sphincter and perineal area muscle EMG; the electrically induced bulbocavernosus (BC) and clitoral BC reflex studies; penile or clitoral elicited reflex responses in the external urethral sphincter muscle and external anal sphincter muscles; distal motor latency studies; and pudendal nerve (PN) somatosensory evoked potential (SsEP) studies. The tests must be sequenced so that each result can be used to help correctly interpret the next in the series. Each problem requires meticulous interpretation as no two have exactly the same combination of etiologies; these combinations must be correctly elucidated so we can ultimately offer the most appropriate restorative strategy.

The PN-SsEP was originally introduced in 1982 for the evaluation of impotence but since that time clinical indications have been established in a myriad of other conditions. An *evoked potential* (EP) is the bioelectrical response of the neuromuscular system to a discrete stimulation. The peripheral neuromuscular responses can be elicited by sensory (afferent) nerve stimulation as in the electrical penile and/or clitoral *BC reflex* or by direct (efferent) motor nerve stimulation as the *pudendal* (or *perineal*) *nerve terminal motor latency* (PNTML). A scalp-recorded EP response may be elicited by almost any type of synchronizable (visual, auditory, or somatic nerve) stimulus. An EP represents the algebraic summation of the electrical activity seen across the scalp at a given time relative to a select stimulus delivered via a predetermined sensory pathway. Most commonly studied scalp EP recordings are shown by plotting the voltage changes at a fixed point on the scalp following a time-locked stimulus.

An SsEP is elicited by repetitive low-voltage electrical stimulation of a superficial peripheral (mixed) nerve. The early cortical peaks, 40 msec or less are produced from the afferent sensory impulses along the large-diameter, high-speed epicritic (tactile and kinesthetic information) sensory system fibers. This signal travels rostrally through the ipsilateral spinal dorsal columns synapsing at the cervicomedullary junction in the dorsal column nuclei. Second-order dorsal column nuclei cells give rise to fibers which continue rostral transmission crossing the internal arcuate fibers in the lower medulla and continue via the medial lemniscus to the ventroposterolateral thalamus. From the thalamus, third-order fibers conduct to the primary somatosensory cortex with this being organized in accordance with the classical homunculus. The 70 msec and later components embody the smaller-diameter peripheral nerve fibers that ascend via the anterolateral columns. The intermediate latency cortical components, between 40 and 70 msec, are an overlapping of the two pathways' signals. The lower extremity and pudendal nerves activate the medial regions of the contralateral hemisphere, producing its highest scalp-recorded amplitude just posterior to the scalp vertex.

Information derived by qualitative and mapping EMG or SsEP test is unique in that it is generally related to physiological function, transmission, and processing of information, not just gross anatomical changes. It is therefore complementary to imaging studies and adds insight into the cause of pressure and motility changes observed through other studies. The studies can help one appreciate the severity of a partial or unilateral nerve lesion.

INDICATIONS

Rectal sphincter dysfunction can accompany a myriad of other problems, including birth canal trauma during vaginal deliveries, spinal column pathologies, neuromuscular diseases, metabolic problems, or pelvic traumas. With more understanding of the etiologies and better surgical and conservative therapeutic choices, there is more impetus to investigate such problems.

Anal EMG and SsEP are easily applied procedures for the complete evaluation of fecal incontinence or constipation, and as outlined below, they are finding an expanding role in the workups with a wide variety of clinical indications already shown in the literature:

1. Symptomatic patient with reduced rectal manometric pressure with no obvious explanation; and/or
2. Idiopathic rectal (with or without urinary) incontinence patient with a negative workup; and/or
3. Abnormal workup without rectal anatomical explanation;
   Severe lower extremity pain or muscle spasms (algodystrophy).
4. Localizing the site of peripheral nervous system dysfunction:
   Diabetic peripheral polyneuropathy
   Other metabolic (poly) neuropathic conditions
   Toxic (poly) neuropathic conditions
   Radiculopathy or radiculomyelopathy
5. Central nervous system causes of anorectal dysfunction:
   Myelopathy (spinal stenosis) or radiculomyelopathy
   Spinal cord injury
   Amyotrophic lateral sclerosis, Shy-Drager syndrome
   Multiple sclerosis (upper and lower motor neuron damage)
   Impaired pyramidal tract function (detrusor-sphincter dyssynergia syndrome)
   Parkinson's disease and other motor control problems
   Cauda equina and conus medullaris syndromes
   Spina bifida occulta
   Cerebro-vascular accidents
   Traumatic brain injury
6. Localize and characterize neuromyopathic and myopathic dysfunction or diseases affecting continence.
7. Acute rectal sphincter trauma (with the possibility of concurrent pudendal nerve or pathway injury):
   Traumatic injury to rectum and/or surrounding area
   Prior anorectal surgery
8. Occult or protracted injury to the anorectal and pelvic floor neuromuscular structures:
   Rectocele with or without failure to relax the sphincter skeletal muscle during attempted defecation (anismus)
   Pelvic floor (muscular) dysfunction
   Nerve injury from excessive traction and stretching during perineal descent as the proximal part of the PN is bound or entrapped in connective tissue as it angulates around the ischial spine (Fig. 14.1A). Among the more common etiologies of recurrent/chronic traction (partial) injuries to the pudendal or perineal nerve distal motor branches (that innervate the perineum and anus) are: prolapse, anorectal dyschezia, multiparity, for-

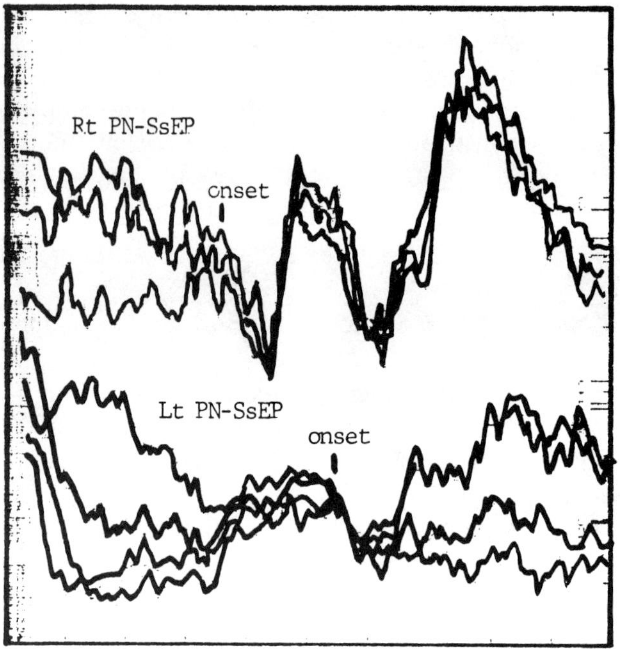

FIGURE 14.1A The traces shown are of a unilaterally delayed left PN (bottom) $P1_{(onset)}$ from a "stretch" injury due to birth canal trauma.

ceps delivery, increased duration of the second stage of labor, a third-degree perineal tear high-birth-weight children, prior pelvic surgery, chronic constipation straining and/or an anomalous accompaniment of aging.

9. Fecal incontinence that presented immediately following a vaginal delivery, incontinence in any woman who had forceps deliveries, or progressive incontinence with aging.

CONTRAINDICATIONS

The needle EMG examination of the anal sphincter, levator ani muscles, and adjacent perineal floor muscles can be uncomfortable to the patient and, as with any blind needling procedure, albeit relatively superficial, it carries a small risk of local infection and/or trauma to other structures in the area. Any active infection in the area to be examined should be treated prior to testing.

If prior surgery intervention or postepisiotomy scarring appears to be angulating or has displaced the rectum, the EMG needle cover can be lubricated and partially inserted into the rectum to ascertain the sphincter's alignment. This will reduce the possibility of needle entry into unanticipated structures.

There are no known risks or side effects of SsEP testing. Only slight discomfort may occur from the repetitive low-voltage electrical current which is applied to stimulate the nerves.

EQUIPMENT

Any electrodiagnostic equipment that has an electronic averager (to improve the signal-to-noise ratio) can be used to record the EP and any system that has sufficient and clear amplification can be used for the EMG studies. The machinery should be able to produce a hard-copy recording of the responses for proper documentation of the findings and further analysis, because a surgical decision will often be made on the basis of this data. Only one recording channel at a time is necessary, but multiple-channel machines usually also offer superior control of the recording and stimulating parameters. Such adjustments include: 2 to 5 microvolt (μV) amplifier gain; individual high-pass (10 Hz) and low-pass (2500 Hz) filter controls; stimulus repetition (0.8 to 1.2 stimuli per second) rate and pulse width (0.1 msec); stimulus voltage (or current) controls; and other parameters that may improve the recorded waveform and/or the patient's tolerance.

CONTROL DATA

Although fairly compatible published controls can be found in the literature for several lower-extremity nerve SsEP studies, PNTML values, electrospinogram (ESG) studies, and for the PN-SsEP (See Table 14.1) studies, each laboratory should establish its own controls for adults, based on height or height and age, using an age-matched volunteer plus a separate set of controls for children under 7 years old. This is necessary because seemingly slight variations in equipment, procedural techniques, and laboratory conditions can produce notable differences in the control data values.

PROCEDURES

Motor and Sensory Nerve Conduction Studies

The electrodiagnostic testing should be started with lower extremity NCS because it is necessary to rule in or out the presence of a (peripheral) neuropathic problem. If the patient's complaint suggests a predominantly motor control problem, at least two motor nerves and one sensory nerve should be tested. If the description suggests predominantly a sensory disruption is present, two sensory nerves and one motor nerve should be tested. If an unsuspected (poly) neuropathy is found, because of the enormous spectrum of possible associated problems, its impact can

TABLE 14.1 PUDENDAL NERVE SOMATOSENSORY EVOKED POTENTIAL AND ELECTROSPINOGRAM NORMAL LATENCY DATA

Height		Tibial Nerve Electrospinogram	Pudendal Nerve SsEP Peak Latencies					
in.	cm	Ankle->L1	$P1_{(onset)}$	$P1_{(peak)}$	N1	P2	N2	P3
59	149.9	15.5	—	—	—	—	—	—
60	152.4	15.9	28.36	35.40	45.65	58.32	73.40	91.16
61	154.9	16.2	28.88	35.97	46.20	58.80	73.84	91.89
62	157.5	16.6	29.39	36.55	46.77	59.27	74.28	92.63
63	160.0	17.0	29.90	37.12	47.33	59.74	74.71	93.36
64	162.6	17.3	30.42	37.70	47.89	60.22	75.15	94.09
65	165.1	17.7	30.93	38.28	48.45	60.69	75.59	94.82
66	167.6	18.1	31.44	38.85	49.00	61.16	76.03	95.55
67	170.2	18.5	31.95	39.43	49.57	61.64	76.46	96.28
68	172.7	18.8	32.47	40.00	50.13	62.11	76.90	97.00
69	175.3	19.2	32.98	40.58	50.69	62.59	77.33	97.74
70	177.8	19.6	33.50	41.16	51.25	63.06	77.77	98.47
71	180.3	19.9	34.01	41.73	51.81	63.54	78.21	99.20
72	182.9	20.3	34.52	42.31	52.37	64.01	78.65	99.93
73	185.4	20.7	35.04	42.89	52.93	64.50	79.09	100.66
74	188.0	21.0	—	—	—	—	—	—
75	190.5	21.4	—	—	—	—	—	—
Standard deviations								
Within each height group		2.10	2.73	2.72	2.97	3.58	5.14	7.91
Side to side		1.05	—	—	—	—	—	—

Source: Modified from Cole and Ducommun (1987) with permission.
Note: Mean latency values (in milliseconds) based on height. Early reports of latency differences by gender most likely reflect average height differences between the sexes.

not be ignored regardless of what else is found. Just as important, an unrecognized peripheral conduction slowing would preclude the correct interpretation of any subsequent abnormal (BC reflex, pudendal nerve SsEP, ESG, PNTML, etc.) studies.

Bulbocavernosus Reflex Studies

The electrically evoked BC reflex latency studies in men have shown an excellent correlation with sacral level neuropathies, Parkinsonism, and spinal column pathologies that can produce incontinence and sexual impotence. The electrical BC reflex is elicited from surface stimulation of the dorsal nerves at the penile base or glands[7] and is recorded through a concentric intramuscular needle electrode in the BC muscle or the external anal sphincter muscle. As it is the latency that gives the highest correlation with pathologies, the stimulus intensity is just brought up to a level sufficient to produce a clearly reproducible response. The reflex onset latency is typically in the range of 25 to 38 msec range from stimulation at the penile base and 28 to 42 msec from the glands area. These ranges only varying slightly with age and height.

The BC muscle EMG should be examined at its (electrically quiet) resting state, with differing volitional contraction activities, and in response to a Valsalva (coughing) maneuver while the intramuscular electrode is in place.

Pudendal Nerve SsEP Studies

In women, the right and left PN-SsEP studies were performed from stimulation of each nerve individually (See Figure 14–3). The person is placed in supine position with the legs in a gentle "frog" position (knees bent 90 degrees and the hips abducted and flexed) with a bolster under the knees. Disposable surface stimulating bipolar plastic bar electrodes are used bilaterally with the anodes placed close to the clitoris level in the sulcus between the labia majora and minora. The bars are placed vertically, so that the cathodes will end up more dorsally and slightly more lateral than the anodes. In this testing position, the (mixed motor and sensory) dorsal nerve of the clitoris is the primary afferent branch utilized with the inferior hemorrhoidal and perineal nerves being secondary.

In men, the right and left PN-SsEP studies are performed from simultaneous stimulation of both nerves using sterilized flexible ring electrodes which are lightly coated with a conductive gel (Fig. 14.1B). The cathode is positioned around the penile shaft base with the anode positioned 2–3 cm distally. Underneath the stimulating electrodes, a gauze pad is placed to isolate the stimulus to the penis.

For all pudendal and tibial nerve SsEP studies the active scalp-recording electrode is applied 1 cm behind the Cz site, designated as Cz′ (a slight modification of the International Ten-Twenty System). The reference electrode is usually placed between the Fp and Fz sites. For reliable recordings, patients are always advised to wash their scalp and hair the morning of the test and not to apply any conditioners, sprays, lotions, or other hair dressings.

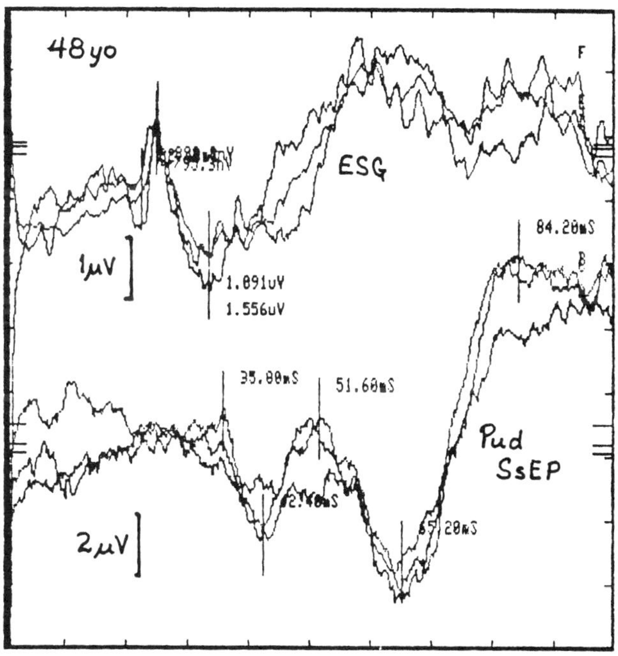

FIGURE 14.1B A normal T12-L1 ESG and (bilateral) PN-SsEP study in a man.

The stimulus intensity threshold is established and then doubled for the data collection runs. The responses are recorded using electronic averaging on the scalp midline (from Cz′ to Fpz) with a chin placement ground. Each averaged trace is recorded from normalizing summation of 100 to 200 individual responses. Three serial recordings are superimposed for confirmation of the latency, amplitude, and waveform morphology data.

Because the vast majority of people studied have pathology, it is prudent to establish a PN-SsEP internal control using the posterior tibial nerve. In normal subjects, the averaged cortical tibial and pudendal nerve SsEP waveform configurations are similar; in addition, the PN $P1_{(onset)}$ latency is in the same range as the $Pl_{(onset)}$ for the posterior tibial nerve SsEP response from ankle level stimulation. This tibial nerve SsEP correlation allows for an excellent internal control that is more sensitive than just "mean" height data alone.

The scalp recorded SsEP response amplitude is the result of a "central amplification" effect[6] produced by triggering multiple nerves at each synapse as the afferent neurogram progresses. The normal PN (early waveform components') amplitude should not be less than 50% of that obtained from a concurrent lower extremity study recorded at the same electrode set and, in women, a side-to-side difference that exceeded 50%, from the identical mid-line scalp electrodes, would be considered abnormal.

Anal Electromyography

The internal and external rectal sphincter, puborectalis and levator ani muscles can be examined using a concentric intramuscular needle electrode using essentially the same qualitative techniques that are employed in studying an extremity muscle. This would give information about the muscle activity at rest to look at baseline tone and presence of denervation potentials; with submaximal contraction activities to show graded recruitment sequences and motor responses to Valsalva maneuvers; and at maximal volitional effort showing the total motor unit capacity. When the volitional and/or reflexive motor unit recruitment is diminished in the 30–50% range, clinically significant weakness will be present in that sphincter muscle area. The rectal sphincter normal motor units duration of 4 to 8 msec can change in a variety of conditions and diseases. Also, rectal sphincter muscle activity and scar formations can be mapped in the external and internal sphincters segmentally utilizing volitional recruitment and Valsalva response differences in motor unit density in addition to electrode depth. Such a mapping is shown in Figure 14.2 and the topic is reviewed in detail in Chapter 13.

Pudendal Nerve Terminal Motor Latency Studies

Pudendal and perineal nerve terminal motor latency studies can be performed by intrarectal stimulation of the right and left PN at the level of the ischial spines and the evoked response recorded from the external and sphincter muscle. (See Chapter 15 for details.) Other methods have been described, such as transcutaneous stimulation spinal and direct PN stimulation across the perineum with the responses recorded at the rectal or periurethral sphincter musculature. Notwithstanding debates about technique differences and their accuracy, the one

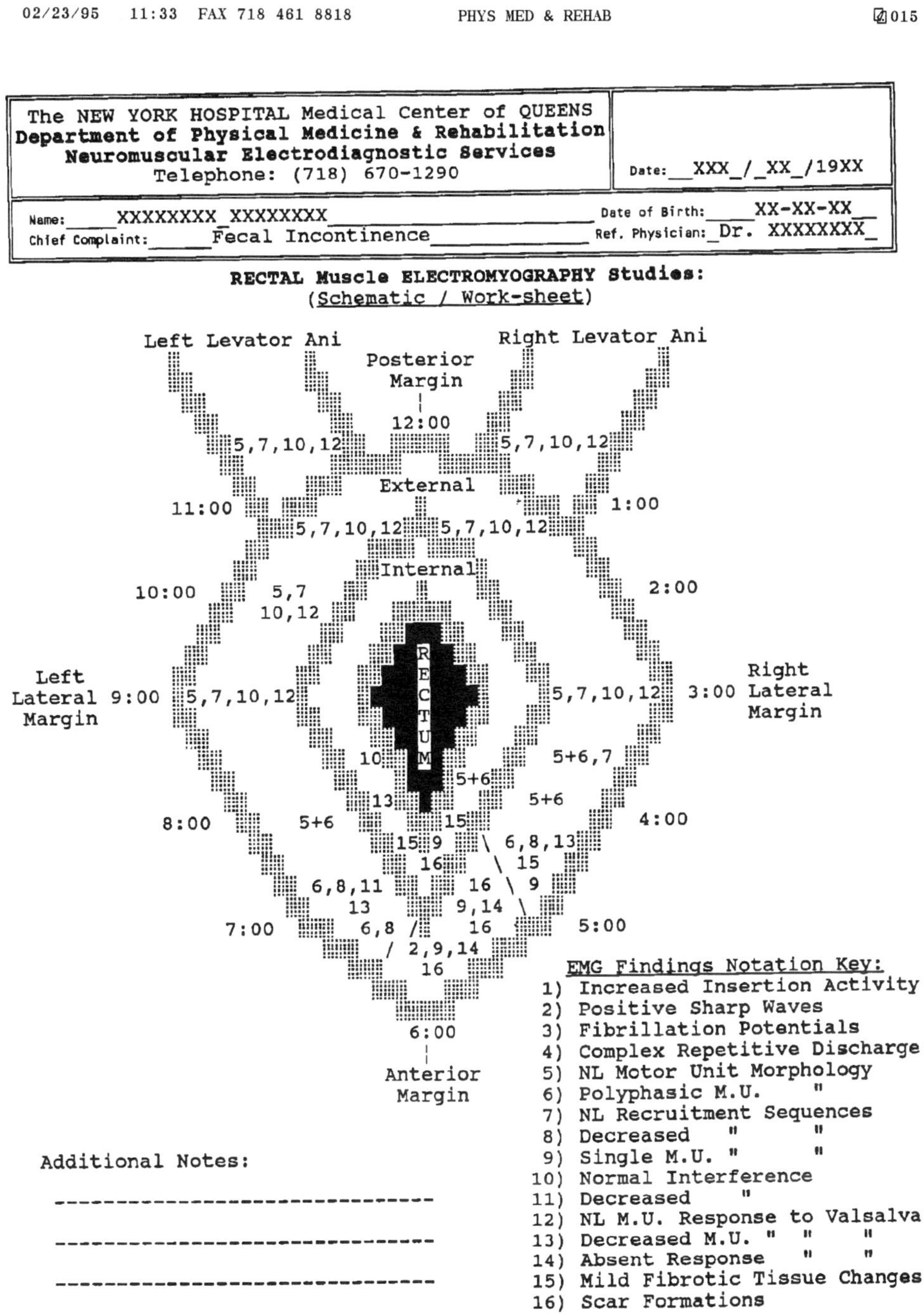
02/23/95 11:33 FAX 718 461 8818 PHYS MED & REHAB 015

The NEW YORK HOSPITAL Medical Center of QUEENS
Department of Physical Medicine & Rehabilitation
Neuromuscular Electrodiagnostic Services
Telephone: (718) 670-1290

Date:__XXX_/_XX_/19XX

Name:____XXXXXXXX_XXXXXXXX____________ Date of Birth:____XX-XX-XX__
Chief Complaint:_____Fecal Incontinence____________ Ref. Physician:_Dr. XXXXXXXX_

RECTAL Muscle ELECTROMYOGRAPHY Studies:
(Schematic / Work-sheet)

EMG Findings Notation Key:
1) Increased Insertion Activity
2) Positive Sharp Waves
3) Fibrillation Potentials
4) Complex Repetitive Discharge
5) NL Motor Unit Morphology
6) Polyphasic M.U. "
7) NL Recruitment Sequences
8) Decreased " "
9) Single M.U. " "
10) Normal Interference
11) Decreased "
12) NL M.U. Response to Valsalva
13) Decreased M.U. " " "
14) Absent Response " "
15) Mild Fibrotic Tissue Changes
16) Scar Formations

Additional Notes:

FIGURE 14.2 Example of an Anal Muscle "Mapping" Report.

consistent finding within each procedure is that the latency shows prolongation in neurogenic injury patients. The PNTML correlates well with rectal sphincter and perineal floor muscle EMG changes and it is more markedly increased in patients with fecal and urinary incontinence than with fecal incontinence alone.

Other Electrodiagnostic Studies

To offer a complete electrophysiological answer, the examining physician must also look for the possibility of other unforeseen and coincidental neuromuscular conditions (i.e., neuropathy, myopathy, radiculopathy, etc.) contributing to the presenting problem. Therefore, we are obligated to perform any other electrodiagnostic test (i.e., perineal floor EMG, a more complete extremity EMG/NCS, H-reflex latency studies, integrated EMG proctography, visual EP, repetitive stimulation studies, brainstem auditory evoked response, etc.) that may be necessary to define a concurrent disease or lesion.

ESG potentials from PN stimulation may also be recorded as an afferent volley over the spinal cord using a mono-polar electrode placed in the T12–L1 interspinous ligament which, in an average height adult, represents the nerve root entry level (from the intracolumn peripheral nerve) into the caudal spinal cord or conus medullaris. The latency difference between the spinal and scalp responses can yield a central conduction time calculation for the spinal cord to amplify intracolumn pathologies.

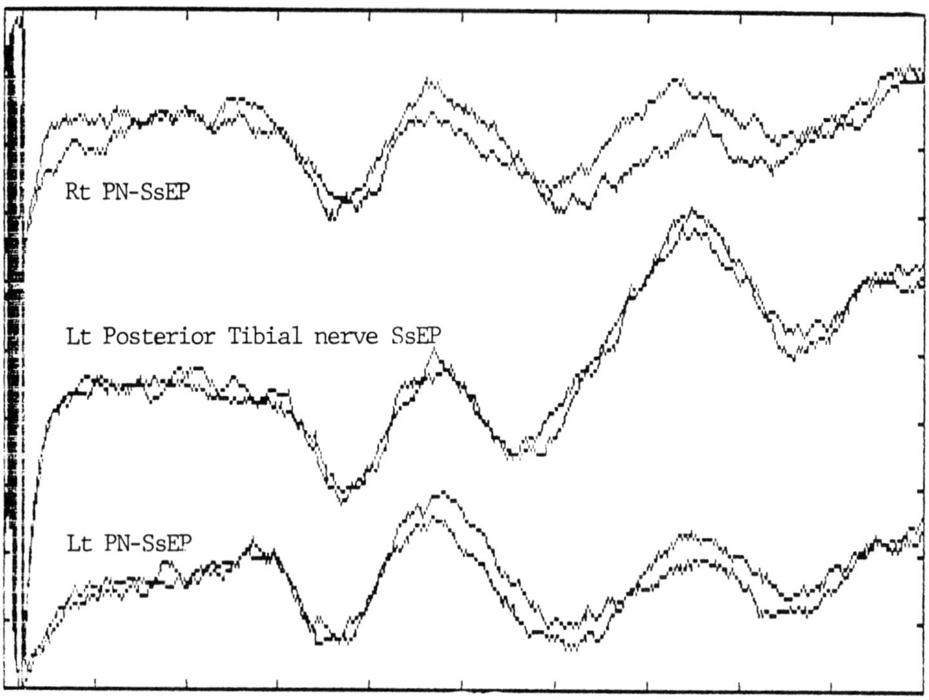

FIGURE 14.3 Normal right (top) and left (bottom) PN-SsEP and left tibial nerve (middle) SsEP studies recorded at 10 msec and 2 uV / division in a women.

Electrical and magnetic cortical evoked (peripheral) motor responses can easily be roused and its potential application has raised extensive interest. However, it is still regarded as primarily investigational. Basic technique reviews of motor cortex stimulation to the external urethral and anal sphincters, pelvic floor, and lower limb muscles have been reported[18] but specific applications have not yet been established.

Conduction velocity calculations of the dorsal nerves of the penis can be studied by multiple site percutaneous stimulation and by use of the latency differential of glands and penile base level stimulated BC reflexes. However, the velocity calculation is fairly unreliable due to the relatively short (in some) variable-length segment being studied. These potential errors generally make it too inaccurate to establish a neuropathic diagnosis with confidence and the velocities from different techniques cannot directly be compared to each other. Additionally, other more conventional and reliable reflex and peripheral conduction studies are readily available for this purpose.

INTERPRETATION

As the rectum and bladder share a common derivation and often work in synchrony, any lesion producing pelvic floor dysfunction can be the antecedent of both rectal and urinary symptoms. Anal EMG, PN-SsEP, and relative electrodiagnostic studies are easily applied procedure for the evaluation and clarification of numerous problems related to anorectal, urinary, and sexual dysfunctions.

The general strategy for SsEP interpretation is to look for the major components at each level in the pathway and to evaluate the conduction times between these major peaks (See Figures 14.1A, 14.1B, 14.3, 14.4, and 14.5).[5] The absolute and interpeak latencies from a single channel's traces may be compared to standardized data, and "internal control" study, or an uninvolved contralateral equivalent study. These approaches can be used to localize a problem which produces either a conduction block (as a loss or dispersion of the specific peak components), or a significant conduction delay in a pathway segment as evidenced by abnormal delay between components which are still recordable. SsEP abnormalities can thus be due to loss of expected components, prolonged central conduction times (within one trace or between traces of serial levels), abnormal latency differences between sides, or abnormal amplitude ratios. Peripheral conduction velocity must always be measured if the SsEP response is abnormally slow delayed or dispersed, the peripheral nerve conduction data must be known to be normal before the delay can be ascribed to a central pathway pathology. The SsEP can help uncover various peripheral nerve disorders, such as: demyelinating diseases (it is one of the most useful test for detection of subclinical lesions in multiple sclerosis, radiculopathies, chronic villous arthritis (CVA), traumatic brain injury (TBI) sequelae, spinal cord injury (SCI), spinal stenosis, and other myelopathies that present with anal sphincter dysfunction.

Along with the SsEP and other diagnostic studies that can document sensory disruptions, the EMG can be used to evaluate and document conus medullaris and cauda equina injuries producing sphincter motor disruptions, neuropathies, myo-

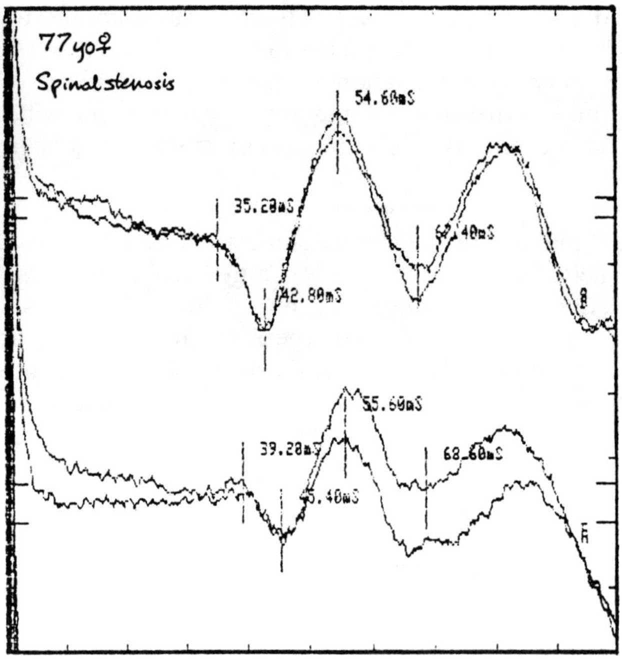

FIGURE 14.4 Bilateral delay of Pn-SsEP onset due to spinal stenosis (in a 154cm tall woman).

pathies, pseudomyotonia, and scarred muscle areas. The best study to prove fiber density increases, as proof of postinjury reinnervation, is the single-fiber EMG technique. This is without question the gold standard but it makes for an arduous test. The rectal sphincter muscle motor unit duration is shorter when recorded with a concentric needle electrode, normally less than 8 to 9 msec, so it is not difficult to define longer-duration polyphasic motor unit changes during a routine clinical examination which would also indicate reinnervation.

The electrical BC reflex latency delay gives a fine correlation with diminished perineal sensation, polyneuropathies, and perineal floor neuropathies. In upper motor neuron problems (spinal tumors, spinal stenosis, myelopathies, CVA, motor neuron diseases, etc.) the latency is usually normal, except in multiple sclerosis, where it can be prolonged. Its absence is often seen with cauda equina lesions. The electrical BC reflex can demonstrate above-normal amplitudes in hypertonic conditions from "spastic" recruitment.

Vaginal deliveries of large babies, need of forceps delivery, and/or prolonged second stage of childbirth can produce anterior rectal dehiscence and scar formation and partial (incomplete) perineal or pudendal nerve stretch injuries from excessive traction on one or both of the distal motor branches of the PN that innervate the perineum and anus (Fig. 14.1A and 14.2). This can also occur with excessive recurrent rectal descent during defecation straining. The anal sphincter and perineal floor EMG and PNTML studies are good procedures for documenting such injuries and defining the severity of involvement by showing the chronic

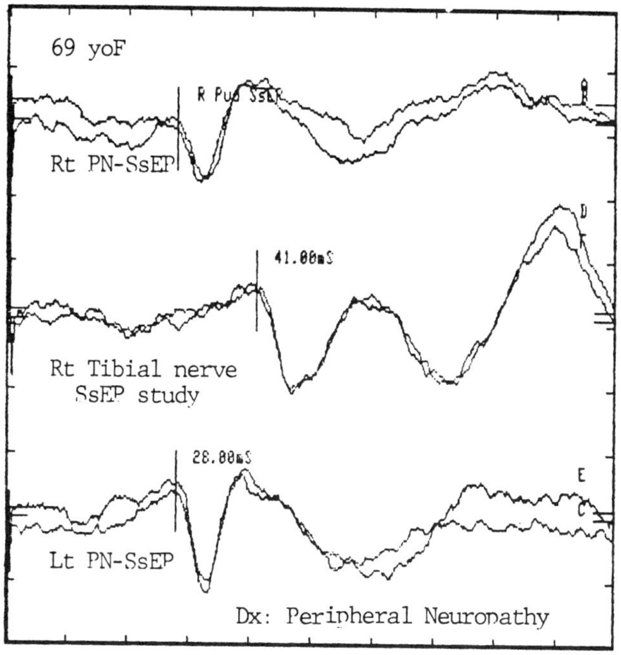

FIGURE 14.5 A relatively delayed tibial nerve SsEP study due to an unsuspected peripheral neuropathy.

(increased polyphasic motor units or muscle fiber densities) reinnervation or diminished motor unit recruitment and by showing chronic reorganization of peripheral nerves with a slowed terminal motor latency. In women, although the nerve damage is often initiated by childbirth, the muscle weakness can progress very slowly and typically does not appear for decades.

Normal detrusor-sphincter functioning dictates quiescence of the urethra EMG and pelvic floor muscles during detrusor contraction. If motor sequencing or control problems are suspected, the diagnosis of a detrusor-sphincter dyssynergia can be helpful. It demands the observation of dysreflexia or hyperreflexia instead of the anticipated relaxation in the pelvic floor muscles during attempted voiding or during Valsalva maneuvers. The abnormal coordination is usually found with patients with concurrent urinary complaints in upper motor neuron diseases or lesion of the central nervous system.

These are a few of the more common procedures and the pathologies that they can document. These test results can provide direct electrophysiological evidence of (partial denervation) damage to the innervation of the pelvic floor and rectal sphincter musculature in idiopathic fecal and/or double incontinence or they can delineate focal changes in a damaged or scarred rectal sphincter. The perineal nerve latency studies can further define idiopathic urinary stress incontinence due to similar causes. Of at least equal importance is the ability of the electrodiagnostic testing algorithm to show other, nonpelvic area pathologies that can affect fecal continence.

SUGGESTED READINGS

Abramson AS, Roussan MS, Boyarsky S, et al: The role of smooth and striated muscle in the dynamics of voiding: a method of study by combined cystometry and electromyography. Proceedings of 11th Annual Spinal Cord Injury Conference of the Veterans Administration. U.S. Government Printing Office, 1962, pp. 107–117.

Allen RE, Hosker GL, Smith ARB, et al: Pelvic floor damage and childbirth: a neurophysiological study. *Br J Obstet Gynaecol* 97:770–779, 1990.

Andersen JT, Bradley WE: The syndrome of detrusor-sphincter dyssynergia. *J Urol* 116(4):493–495, 1976.

Bump RC, Hunt WG, Fantl JA, et al: Assessment of Kegel pelvic muscle exercise performance after brief verbal instruction. *Am J Obstet Gynecol,* 322–329, 1991.

Cole JL, Ducommun EJ: Electrospinograms: evolution and application as a clinical tool. *Clin Evoked Poten* 5(2):21–26, 1987.

Cole JL, Pease WT: Central nervous system electrodiagnostics. In Delisa (ed): *Rehabilitation Medicine: Principles and Practice,* ed 2. Philadelphia, J.B. Lippincott, 1993.

Haldeman S, Bradley WR, Bhatia N, et al: Pudendal evoked responses. *Arch Neurol* 39:280–283, 1982.

Haldeman S, Bradley WR, Bhatia NN, et al: Cortical evoked potentials on stimulation of pudendal nerve in women. *Urology* 21:590–593, 1983.

Jacobs PPM, Scheur M, Kuipers JHC, et al: Obstetric fecal incontinence: role of pelvic floor denervation and results of delayed sphincter repair. *Dis Colon Rectum* 33:494–497, 1990.

Kamm M: Obstetric damage and faecal incontinence. *Lancet* 344:730–733, 1994.

Kegel AH: Progressive resistance exercises in the functional restoration of the perineal muscles. *Am J Obstet Gynecol* 56:238–248, 1948.

Kiff E, Swash M: Slowed conduction in the pudendal nerves in idiopathic (neurogenic) faecal incontinence. *Br J Surg* 71:614–616.

O'Donnell PD: Pitfalls of urodynamic testing. *Urol Clinics North Am* 18(2):257–268, 1991.

Simpson RK, Blackburn JG, Martin HF, et al: Peripheral nerve fiber and spinal cord pathway contributions to the somatosensory evoked potential. *Exp Neurol* 73:700–715, 1981.

Smith ARB, Hosker GL, Warrell DW: The role of partial denervation of the pelvic floor in the aetiology of genito-urinary prolapse and stress incontinence of urine. *Br J Obstet Gynaecol* 96:24–, 1989.

Snooks SJ, Badenoch DF, Tiptaft RC, et al: Perineal nerve damage in genuine stress urinary incontinence. An electrophysiological study. *Br J Urol* 57(4):422–426, 1985.

Snooks SJ, Barnes PR, Swash M: Damage to the innervation of the voluntary anal and periurethral sphincter musculature in incontinence: an electrophysiological study. *J Neurol Neurosurg Psychiatry* 47(12):1969–73, 1984.

Snooks SJ, Swash M: Abnormalities of the innervation of the urethral striated sphincter musculature in incontinence. *Br J Urol* 56(4):401–405, 1984.

Snooks SJ, Swash M, Henry MM, et al: Risk factors in childbirth causing damage to the pelvic floor innervation. *Int J Colorect Dis* 1(1):20–24, 1986.

Toglia MR, DeLancey JOL: Anal incontinence and the obstetrician-gynecologist. *Obstet Gynecol* 84(4), Part 2: 731–740, 1994.

CHAPTER 15

Determination of Pudendal Nerve Terminal Motor Latency

James W. Fleshman

GENERAL CONSIDERATIONS

The external anal sphincter muscle is innervated by the pudendal nerve. Pudendal nerve stimulation was first described for measuring distal pudendal nerve terminal motor latencies by Kiff and Swash in 1984. This technique allows objective quantitation of the neuromuscular function of the anal sphincter in the setting of incontinence. The majority of patients with idiopathic anal incontinence have prolonged pudendal nerve latencies. Determination of the pudendal nerve terminal motor latency should be used in conjunction with manometry as well as single-fiber and concentric needle electromyography. Pudendal nerve studies have a clinical role in localizing the cause of anal incontinence as well as a research role in helping to define the function of the pelvic floor.

INDICATIONS

1. To define the neuromuscular component of sphincter dysfunction in patients with anal incontinence, thereby aiding in therapeutic decision-making.
2. To evaluate the neurological damage done to the pudendal nerve and anal sphincter during childbirth in attempting to predict sphincter function after future vaginal deliveries or after sphincter reconstruction.
3. To assess the neuromuscular function of the anal sphincter before repair of rectal prolapse.

4. To assess the neuromuscular function of the anal sphincter in patients with a long history of constipation and straining prior to a rectal resection in an attempt to predict the possibility of incontinence.
5. To indirectly assess perineal nerve function in patients with urethral incontinence by measuring pudendal nerve terminal motor latency.

CONTRAINDICATIONS

1. Acute inflammation or ulceration of the rectal mucosa or anal canal.
2. Active infection of the perineum.
3. Anal stenosis.
4. Noncooperative patient.

PATIENT EVALUATION AND PREPARATION

1. Explain the procedure and enlist the patient's cooperation.
2. The patient should have a small enema before arrival.
3. Examine the patient for evidence of local inflammation or ulceration and anal stenosis.

PERSONNEL AND EQUIPMENT

1. A physician or a nurse/technician skilled in identifying the pudendal nerve in its course through the pelvis.
2. An assistant capable of assembling the equipment and assisting the patient and examiner during the study.
3. Electromyographic equipment capable of delivering a square wave 50-V stimulus lasting 0.1 msec and recording the motor unit action potential generated by the external anal sphincter (e.g., Dantec Neuromatic 2000 EMG apparatus).
4. Pudendal nerve stimulating and recording device (Fig. 15.1). The Dantec St. Mark's pudendal nerve is a thin strip of paper with tape backing with two metal stimulating electrodes 1 cm apart longitudinally at the tip (anode 4 mm in diameter, cathode 2 mm in diameter) (Fig. 15.2). At the base, 4 cm from the anode are two metal recording electrodes 7 mm in diameter and 1 cm apart on either side of the midline. The paper strip is placed on the examiner's gloved index finger on the volar surface with the stimulating electrodes at the tip and the recording electrodes at the proximal phalanx.

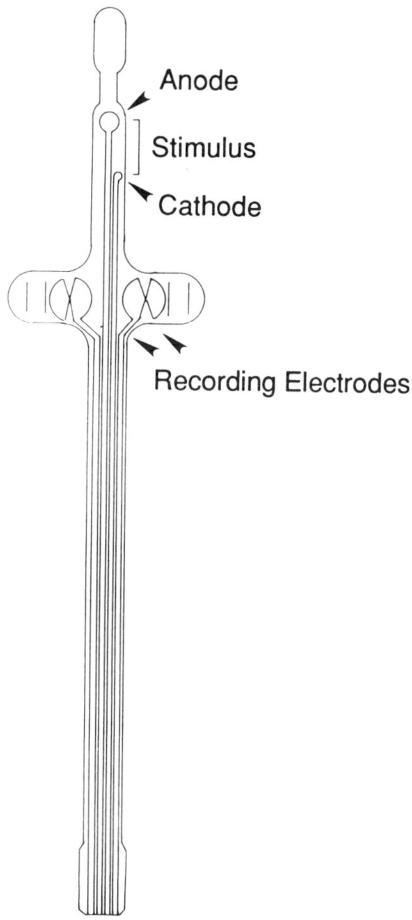

FIGURE 22.1 Pudendal nerve stimulating device (Dantec).

5. Electrode gel.
6. Grounding electrode. A saline-soaked contact band placed around the patient's upper arm and connected to the equipment will suffice.

TECHNIQUE

1. Position the patient in the left laterial decubitus position with knees flexed and hips pushed to the edge of the stretcher.
2. Connect the stimulating electrode lines to a stimulating source capable of delivering a square wave stimulus 0.1 msec in duration and 50 V either in 1-sec intervals or with manual control. The stimulus current should be limited to between 8 and 10 mA.

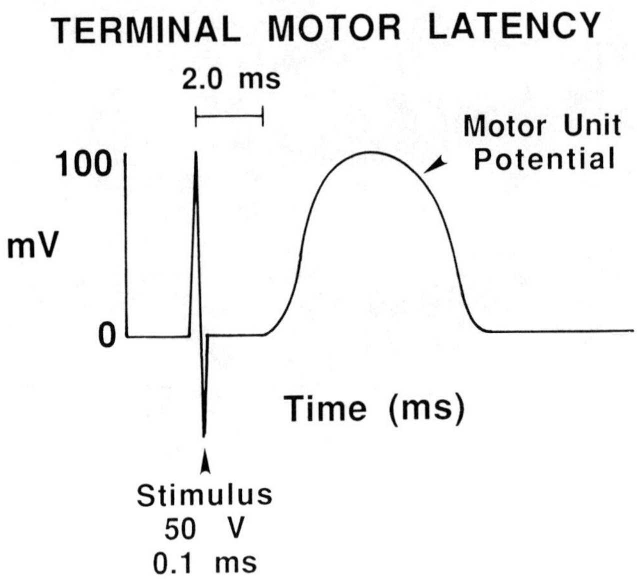

FIGURE 15.2 Pudendal nerve stimulating device and electromyography equipment (Dantec).

3. The recording electrode lines should be connected to the usual recording input channel. (If using the Dantec 2000M Neuromatic equipment, the program should be set to nerve conduction velocities with filters of 20 Hz and 5000 Hz, a sweep speed of 2 msec/division, gain at 200 mV/division.)
4. The device mounted on the examiner's gloved index finger is then inserted into the rectum. Electrode gel must coat the electrodes prior to insertion. Water-soluble lubricant can be used on the dorsal surface of the glove to facilitate insertion. Lubricant must be prevented from entering the outer glove to avoid false recording secondary to grounding.
5. The left ischial spine is palpated just above the pelvic floor musculature. Stimuli are then given either manually, or at continuous 1-sec intervals, as the tip of the finger is moved slowly across the pelvic wall. The desired response is a firm contraction of the external sphincter around the base of the finger and a maximal amplitude motor unit potential on the oscilloscope of the EMG apparatus (Fig. 15.3). These should coincide and be reproducible with each stimulus. A paper recording is obtained. If the equipment allows, two-channel recording facilitates localization of the point of maximal response over the nerve. The latency of response may be displayed directly on the screen before a paper readout is created.
6. The right pudendal nerve is similarly studied by rotating the device in the anal canal over the right ischial spine. It may occasionally be necessary to reposition the patient in the right lateral decubitus position to examine the right ischial spine.

INTERPRETATION OF RESULTS

The normal pudendal nerve terminal motor latency has been shown to be 2.0 ± 0.2 msec (SD). The latency of response is measured from the onset of the stimulus to the onset of the response in the external anal sphincter (Fig. 15.3). The right and left nerve latencies may be different but tend to vary only slightly from the mean.

In patients with idiopathic fecal incontinence pudendal nerve terminal motor latencies have been shown to be prolonged to a mean of 3.0 ± 0.9 msec. There is also a correlation between the degree of perineal descent and the pudendal nerve terminal motor latency.

Patients with a single normal pudendal nerve should notice improvement after anal sphincter reconstruction. However, bilateral nerve injury as indicated by abnormal pudendal nerve latencies will prevent recovery of anal sphincter function after repair.

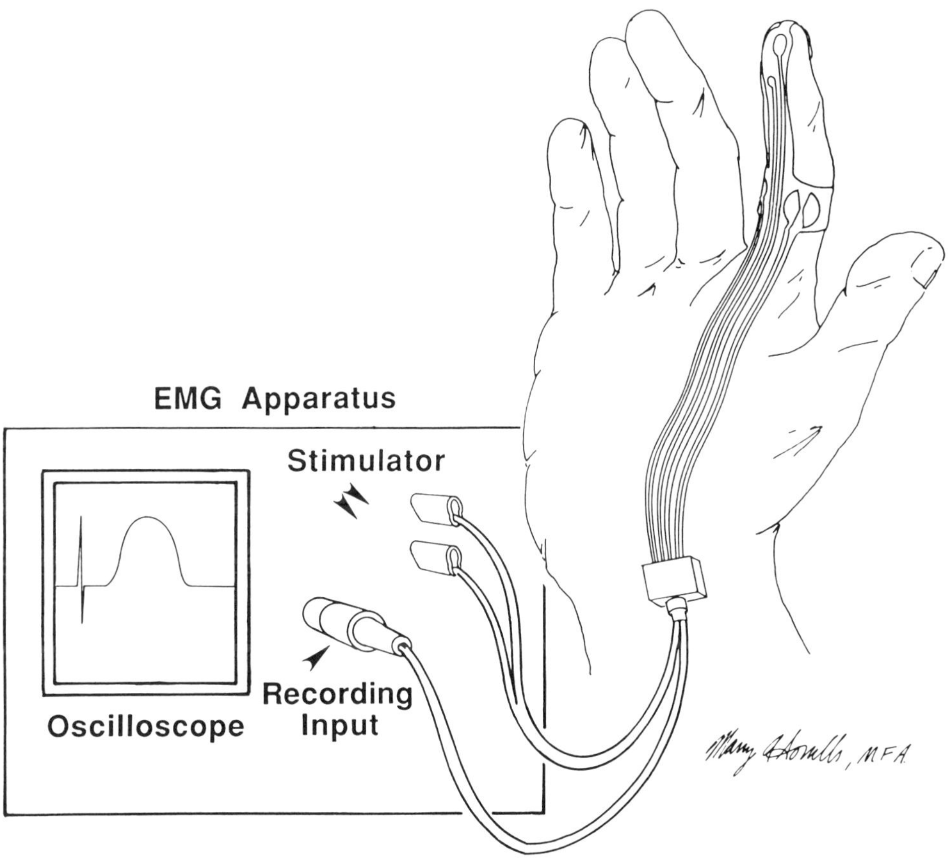

FIGURE 15.3 Pudendal nerve terminal motor nerve latency. Oscilloscope tracing showing method of determining terminal motor latency.

The terminal motor latency is the measurement of the fastest response in the pudendal nerve-external sphincter mechanism. A normal latency does not indicate absence of nerve damage. Neither does an abnormal latency indicate abnormal muscle function. Muscle reinnervation as documented by single-fiber densities on single-fiber EMG is necessary to quantitate damage.

SUGGESTED READINGS

Kiff E, Swash M: Slowed conduction in the pudendal nerves in idiopathic (neurogenic) fecal incontinence. *Br J Surg* 74:614–616, 1984.

Snooks SJ, Barnes RPH, Swash M: Damage to the voluntary anal and urinary sphincter musculative in incontinence. *J Neurol Neurosurg Psychiatry* 47:1269–1273, 1984.

Snooks SJ, Swash M: Nerve stimulation techniques. In Henry MM, Swash M: *Coloproctology and the Pelvic Floor: Pathophysiology and Management,* Chapter 7. London, Butterworths, 1985.

Kiff ES, Barnes RPH, Swash M: Evidence of pudendal nerve neuropathy in patients with perineal descent and chronic straining at stool. *Gut* 25:1279–1282, 1984.

Jones PN, Lubowski DZ, Swash M, et al.: Relation between perineal descent and pudendal nerve damage in idiopathic fecal incontinence, *Int J Colorectal Dis* 2:93–95, 1987.

CHAPTER 16

Rectal Compliance

Patrick Brillant
John H. Pemberton

The rectum in healthy people acts as a fecal reservoir to maintain continence. It accommodates passively to distension, facilitating low intraluminal pressures while the volume increases. Rectal compliance is defined as the change in pressure divided by the change in pressure. However, many authors choose single values to calculate compliance, and these vary greatly. These parameters include (1) rectal volume at first sensation, (2) volume at first urge, (3) volume at constant urge, and (4) maximal tolerable volume. In the overly compliant rectum, large changes in rectal volume occur with minimal changes in rectal pressures. Conversely, in a poorly compliant rectum only small changes in volume are accompanied by large changes in rectal pressure. Investigators using different techniques and a variety of multichanneled air and water perfused catheters have defined normal compliance in healthy subjects to vary between 5.0 and 18 ml/cm of H_2O or 2 to 6 ml/mm Hg. At Mayo, it is approximately 18 ml/cm of water.

This chapter details first the techniques we use to determine rectal compliance statically, that is, in the classic way. Its use in the evaluation of patients with disorders of anorectal function is next evaluated, and finally, newer methods which measure the compliance of the rectum (or of the colon or ileal pouch) dynamically are explored.

TECHNIQUES

A simple latex condom balloon is simply attached securely to intravenous tubing using suture material. A syringe is used to inflat the condom balloon via a pressure transducer. The length of the inflated balloon is about 10 to 11 cm. It is, of course, necessary to determine the compliance of the balloon itself. This is done by placing the balloon in a warm water bath at body temperature (37° C) and inflating the balloon in 10–20 ml increments. The corresponding pressure recording at each increment of volume is subtracted from the reading when the balloon is

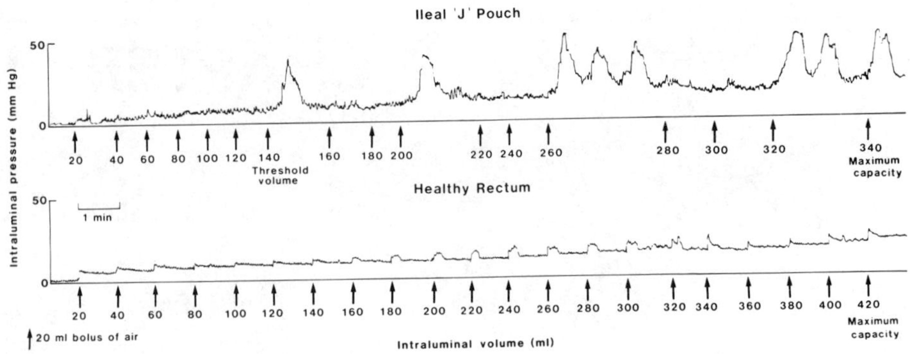

FIGURE 16.1 Effect of distension on intraluminal pressure and motility in ileal "J" pouch and healthy rectum. (Reprinted with permission from O'Connell PR, Pemberton JH, Brown ML, et al: Determinants of Stool Frequency After Ileal Pouch Anal Anastomosis, *Am J Surg* 1987, 153:157–164.)

placed into the rectum of the patient in order to determine the actual pressure reading. For instance, if at 100 ml of insufflation the internal pressure within the balloon is 50 cm of water, then that 50 cm of water is subtracted from whatever the pressure reading is when the balloon is actually inside the patient.

Next, all air is removed from the balloon and the lubricated assembly placed into the rectum such that the suture anchoring the balloon onto the tubing is seen at the top of the anal canal. The patients are then placed in the left lateral decubitus position for comfort. The balloon is inflated in 10–20 ml increments in stepwise fashion and the resulting pressure at each step is recorded. A 30-second accommodation period is provided at each step interval. Infusion is stopped at maximal tolerable volume. During infusion, the first and last urge to defecate are recorded. Of course, compliance can also be determined using continuous flow technique (ramp insufflation). A tracing of a normal rectum using the stepwise insufflation technique is shown in Figure 16.1 (lower half). The upper half (Figure 16.1) shows a tracing recorded during compliance testing in an ileal pouch.

DEFINITION OF COMPLIANCE

The *compliance* of the rectum is defined as 1/slope of $\Delta P/\Delta V$. This means that compliance describes the curve of the entire response of the rectum, from minimal to maximal insufflation, to volume infusion. If the volume in the balloon which is resting in the rectum increases a lot, but the resulting increase in pressure is small, then the rectum is described as being "highly compliant." If on the other hand, small increases in volume cause large changes in pressure, then the rectum is described as being poorly compliant (or of having a low compliance). It is important to understand that compliance determined in this way is a static measurement even if many individual measurements are made. One number is obtained and it describes the behavior of the rectum to the challenge of increasing volumes. If the rectum is stiff, as if it were inflamed (by chronic ulcerative colitis) or fibrosed (by radiation) or occupied (by a tumor or rectal prolapse), then each volume increase is met by a rectal wall that will not "comply." Such a wall is unable to accommodate to increasing volume and its compliance is thus low.

One can also conceptualize compliance by thinking of the rectal wall as being in a certain "state of contraction." The "contractile state" of the rectal wall is its *tone,* which is both a static and dynamic concept. The tone of the rectal wall can be described by the simple number derived from 1/slope of $\Delta P/\Delta V$ measurements, and thus, its static status enumerated. The contractile state of the rectal wall can also be measured dynamically, but another device is needed to do this and is experimental. Nonetheless, it is interesting and so we will discuss this later.

Therefore, static compliance can be measured in a straightforward way and a number for compliance derived. It is essential that each laboratory establish normal values in their patient populations, values to which the compliance of patients with symptoms of anorectal dysfunction can be compared.

USEFULNESS OF MEASURING COMPLIANCE

There is no single disease process for which determination of rectal compliance is invaluable. However, it is an additional tool in the armamentarium of colon and rectal surgeons to evaluate the pathophysiology of anorectal disease. A survey conducted recently showed that a measurement of rectal compliance was the ninth most common test performed in the evaluation of patients with colorectal complaints.

Fecal Incontinence

Rectal compliance likely plays a significant role in patients with fecal incontinence. In a large number of studies, patients with fecal incontinence have been shown to have "lower compliance" than normal controls. In most patients, the etiology for the low compliance is unknown. This, together with the nearly universal complaint of patients that they "cannot feel anything," leads to the speculation that there is a physiologic or learned abnormality of rectal sensation in patients with fecal incontinence. The common denominator in patients who complain of fecal urgency and leakage and who have inflammatory bowel disease, radiation, prolapse, or idiopathic fecal incontinence is likely low compliance.

Often the reasons for fecal leakage are not apparent if only anal manometry is performed. For instance, among patients with quiescent colitis and controls, resting and squeeze pressures are the same, but compliance in colitis patients was 10-fold less than in controls.

Irritable bowel syndrome (IBS) plagues the western world. In patients with diarrhea-predominant IBS, compliance was found in one study to be significantly lower than in patients with constipation-predominant IBS. Other studies contradict this finding, and indeed, show no difference in rectal compliance across the spectrum of IBS. Furthermore, compliance is of no help in evaluating problems that are caused primarily by pelvic floor muscular dysfunction, such as pudendal neuropathy, complete and occult rectal prolapse, and sphincter disruption.

Low compliance is implicated as a contributing factor to incontinence in patients after low anterior resection or coloanal anastomosis, radiation, Hirschsprung's disease, anorectal malformation, rectopexy, and anismus.

A mechanism that may mediate this effect is the rectoanal sphincter inhibition response (RASIR). In response to rectal distension, the anal canal relaxes in order to either sample the contents in the rectum or in anticipation of defecation. If the compliance of the rectal wall is high, then the response is triggered with little rectal distension. This causes urgency and leakage.

In an effort to determine the cause of fecal incontinence after ileoanal anastomosis, we have looked several times at pouch compliance as a possible factor. We have noted that in patients after ileoanal anastomosis, compliance was little different from controls (14.7 ± 1.4 ml/cm of H_2O versus 18.6 ± 2 ml/cm of H_2O). However, pouch compliance was not related to good result (16.2 ± 2.5 ml/mm of Hg, good result verus 13.4 ± 1.6 ml/mm of Hg, fair result). These studies did tell us that the pouch appeared to possess characteristics of a true reservoir; that is, passive accommodation to increasing volumes with concomitant small increases in intraluminal pressure.

Constipation

Studies on patients with constipation have failed to define a link between static measurements of compliance and altered function consistently. However, we have measured both colonic and rectal tone dynamically using an investigational device, the electromechanical barostat (Fig. 16.2).

By maintaining constant intraluminal pressures, the barostat measures changes in volume within an infinitely compliant intraluminal "bag." When the wall relaxes (decreases its tone), air is injected into the bag and the intraluminal volume increases. If the wall contracts (increases its tone), air is withdrawn from the bag and its volume decreases. In this way, dynamic changes in muscular wall tone can be measured. In our first studies in healthy volunteers, we documented that fast (phasic) as well as slow (tonic) changes in intraluminal bag volume (hence changes in wall tone) occurred and could be measured by the device when they could not be measured by simple manometric techniques alone. In response to feeding, the tone of the rectal wall increased such that intraluminal volumes in many instances decreased to zero, recovering to baseline only over time (Fig. 16.3). Neostigmine (which contracts smooth muscle) caused similar increases in rectal wall tone, while glucagon (which relaxes smooth muscle) decreased tone.

Next, we investigated in what manner these characteristic changes in tone of the rectal muscular wall may be affected in patients with constipation. We found profound differences in the contractile state of the rectal wall in patients with constipation compared to controls. Whereas in health, feeding decreased intrabag volumes by 65 ± 7% in patients with constipation, only a 35 ± 8% decrease occurred ($p < 0.05$). Neostigmine produced a 58 ± 6% decrease in intraluminal volume in health, but only a 39 ± 6% decrease in constipated patients. Glucagon caused a 64 ± 18% increase in volume in health, but only 28 ± 6% in patients with constipation.

Thus, the magnitude of changes in rectal volume (tone) was significantly less in constipated patients compared to controls. Response to these pertubations

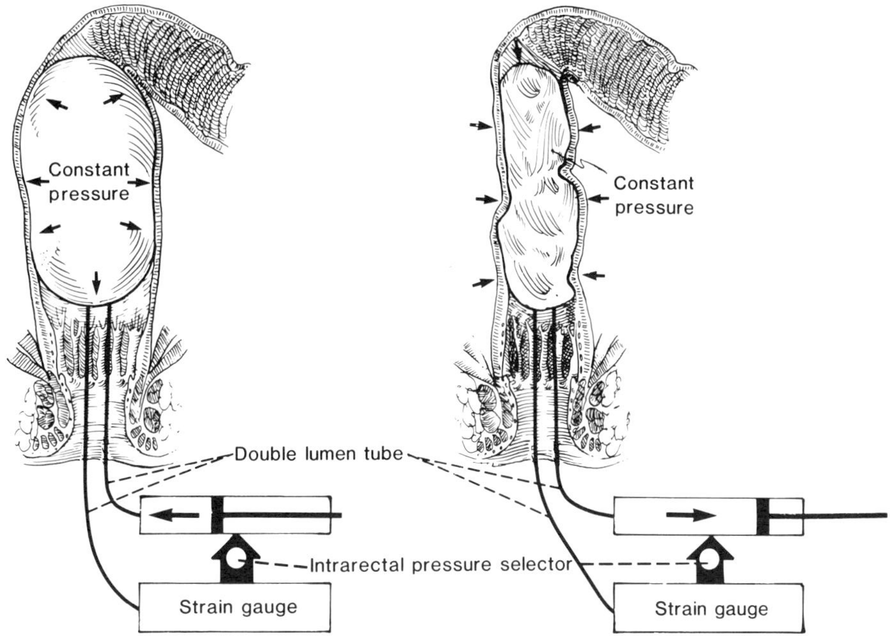

FIGURE 16.2 Diagram of barostat balloon within the rectum. The device maintains constant pressure within an infinitely compliant intraluminal bag. When the rectum relaxes, the barostat injects air (*left*); when the rectum contracts, air is aspirated (*right*). (From Bell A, Pemberton JH, Hanson R, et al: Variations in muscle tone of the human rectum: recordings with an electromechanical barostat. American Physiological Society, G17–G25, 1991.)

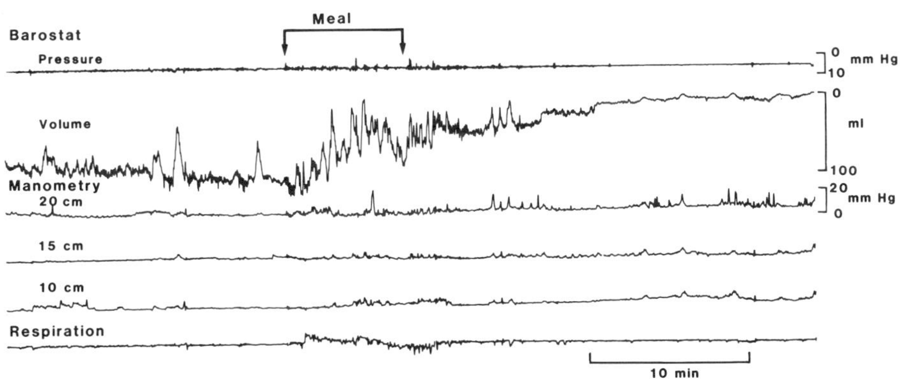

FIGURE 16.3 From top to bottom, barostat pressure and volume channels, 3 perfused manometric channels, and a respiratory trace in a volunteer before, during, and after feeding. Barostat volume tracing shows progressive reduction in barostat bag volume in response to meal, starting with the meal itself; this decrease continued until volume was zero. (From Bell A, Pemberton JH, Hanson R, et al: Variations in muscle tone of the human rectum: recordings with an electromechanical barostat. American Physiological Society, G17–G25, 1991.)

seemed almost blunted such that the rectal wall of patients with constipation could not be stimulated to increase or decrease its tone. In further experiments in which the barostat was placed more proximally, tracings are nearly identical to those shown here.

If the rectum fails to increase its tone after feeding, then rectal filling pressures will be low, the rectoanal sphincter inhibitory response will fail to occur, the sensation of filling will be blunted, and the call to stool will not be present. This would, of course, favor retention of content and constipation.

Have these observations led to practical tools for evaluating patients with constipation? At Mayo, we have begun to use the barostat in our evaluation of constipated patients with complex and sometimes contradictory findings. Indeed, in a patient with borderline transit studies (90–100 hr—7 day technique) and symptoms suggesting severe irritable bowel syndrome (pain, bloating, pressure), if the barostat study confirms characteristic blunting of the response to feeding, then the patient is diagnosed as having slow transit constipation and if unresponsive to aggressive medical management, offered abdominal colectomy and ileorectostomy.

COMMENT

Patients with disorders of anorectal function need to be evaluated logically using tools designed to quantify the dysfunction. Patients with constipation or incontinence are members of incredibly heterogeneous groups; no one etiology suffices to explain abnormalities in all the patients in each group. Measuring compliance statically (using simple balloon insufflation) measures the capacity of the rectum and its viscoelastic properties. If the capacity is tiny and the compliance high, the rectum could be characterized as a "lead pipe" connecting the colon to the anus; fecal urgency, frequency, and incontinence are the result. If the rectum is hugely capacious and compliance is low, it will overfill, there would be no "call to stool," and the patient is unable to stool spontaneously. If the colon and rectum fail to respond to feeding or perturbations that act to constrict or relax its muscular wall, as determined by dynamic measuring of changes in rectal wall tone with the barostat, then the patient has "constipation."

Although perhaps at first glance compliance seems an overly academic construct, it is in reality a very straightforward and easy-to-measure physiologic parameter, the determination of which is essential to the understanding, evaluation, and management of disordered anorectal function.

SUGGESTED READINGS

Akervall S, Fasth S, Nordgren S. et al: Rectal reservoir and sensory studied by graded isobaric distension in normal man. *Gut* 30:496–502, 1989.

Ambroze WL, Pemberton JH, Bell AM, et al: The effect of stool consistency on rectal and neorectal emptying. *Dis Colon Rectum* 34:1–7, 1991.

Batignani G, Monaci I, Ficari F, et al: What affects continence after resection of the rectum? *Dis Colon Rectum* 34:329–335, 1991.

Bell A, Pemberton JH, Hanson R, et al: Variations in muscle tone of the human rectum: recordings with an electromechanical barostat. *Am Physiol Soc.* G17–G25, 1991.

Christiansen J, Sorensen M, Rasmussen O, et al: Anorectal physiology measurements. *Eur Surg-Suppl* 564:73–74, 1991.

Devroede G, Vobecky S, Masse S, et al: Ischemic fecal incontinence and rectal angina. *Gastroenterology* 83:970–980, 1982.

Grotz R, Pemberton JH, Levin K, et al: Rectal wall contractility in health subjects and in patients with chronic severe constipation. *Ann Surg* 218:761–768, 1993.

Heppell J, Kelly K, Phillips S, et al: Physiologic aspects of continence after colectomy, mucosal proctocolectomy, and endorectal ileo-anal anastomosis. *Ann Surg* 195:435–443, 1982.

Ishihara M, Morita K: Continence and reflex pressure profile after surgery to correct the imperforate anus. *Prog Pediatr Surg* 24:86–96, 1989.

Jorge J, Wexner S: Anorectal manometry: techniques and clinical applications. *South Med J* 86 (8):924–931, 1993.

Karulf R, Coller J, Bartolo D, et al: Anorectal physiology testing—a survey of availability and use. *Dis Colon Rectum* 34(6):464–468, 1991.

Leighton J, Valdovinos M, Pemberton JH, et al: Anorectal dysfunction and rectal prolapse in progressive systemic sclerosis. *Dis Colon Rectum* 36(2):182–185, 1983.

Lester B, Penninckx F, Kerremans R: Biofeedback defaecation training for anismus. *Int J Colorect Dis* 6:202–207, 1991.

Loening-Baucke V, Metcalf A, Shirazi S: Anorectal manometry in active and quiescent ulcerative colitis. *Am Gastroenterol* 84(8):892–897, 1989.

Madoff R, Orrom W, Rothenberger D, et al: Rectal compliance: a critical reappraisal. *Int J Colorect Dis* 5:37–40, 1990.

McKee R, Lauder J, Poon F, et al: A prospective randomized study of abdominal rectopexy with and without sigmoidectomy in rectal prolapse. *Surg Gynecol Obstet* 174:145–148, 1992.

Meunier P: Physiologic study of the terminal digestive tract in chronic painful constipation. *Gut* 27:1018–1024, 1986.

Mollard P, Meunier P, Mouriquand P, et al: High and intermediate imperforate anus: functional results and postoperative manometric assessment. *Eur J Pediatr Surg* 1:282–286, 1991.

Musial F, Enck P, et al: The effect of loperamide on anorectal function in normal healthy men. *J Clin Gastroenterol* 15(4):321–324, 1992.

Nagashima M, Iwai N, Yanagihara J, et al: Motility and sensation of the rectosigmoid and the rectum in patients with anorectal malformations. *J Pediatr Surg* 27(10:1273–1277, 1992.

Pedersen I, Christiansen J: A study of the physiological variation in anal manometry. *Br J Surg* 76:69–71, 1989.

Penninckx F, Lestar B, Kerremans R: A new balloon-retraining test for evaluation of anorectal function in incontinent patients. *Dis Colon Rectum* 32(3):202–205, 1989.

Prior A, Colgan S, Whorwell P: Changes in rectal sensitivity after hypnotherapy in patients with irritable bowel syndrome. *Gut* 31:896–898, 1990.

Prior A, Maxton D, Whorwell P: Anorectal manometry in irritable bowel syndrome: differences between diarrhea and constipation predominant subjects. *Gut* 31:458–462, 1990.

Prior A, Read N: Reduction of rectal sensitivity and post-prandial motility by granisetron, a 5 HT_3 - receptor antagonist, in patients with irritable bowel syndrome. *Aliment Pharmacol Ther* 7:175–180, 1993.

Rao S, Read N: Gastrointestinal motility in patients with ulcerative colitis. *Scand J Gastroenterol Suppl* 172:22–28, 1990.

Rasmussen O, Christensen B, Sorensen M, et al: Rectal compliance in the assessment of patient with fecal incontinence. *Dis Colon Rectum* 33(8):650–653, 1990.

Rasmussen O, Sorensen M. Tezschner T, et al: Dynamic anal manomettry: physiological variations and pathophysiological findings in fecal incontinence. *Gastroenterology* 103(1):103–113, 1992.

Read N, Haynes W, Bartolo D, et al: Use of anorectal manometry during rectal infusion of saline to investigate sphincter function in incontinent patients. *Gastroenterology* 85:105–113, 1983.

Sagar P, Holdsworth P, Johnsonton D: Correlation between laboratory findings and clinical outcome after restorative proctocolectomy: serial studies in 20 patients with end-to-end pouch-anal anastomosis. *Br J Surg* 78:67–70, 1991.

Scott N, Pemberton JH, Barkel D, et al: Anal and ileal pouch manometric measurements before ileostomy closure are related to functional outcome after ileal pouch-anal anastomosis. *Br J. Surg* 76:613–616, 1989.

Sorensen M, Rasmussen, Tetzschner T, et al: Physiological variation in rectal compliance. *Br J Surg* 79(10):1106–1108, 1992.

Sorensen M, Tetzschner T, Rasmussen O, et al: Viscous fluid retention: a new method for evaluating anorectal function. *Dis Colon Rectum* 35(4):357–361, 1992.

Speakman C, Kamm M: Abnormal visceral autonomic innervation in neurogenic faecal incontinence. *Gut* 34:215–221, 1993.

Tuckson W, Faxio V: Functional comparison between double and triple ileal loop pouches. *Dis Colon Rectum* 34:17–21, 1991.

Tuckson W, McNamara M, Fazio V, et al: Impact of anal manipulation and pouch design on ileal pouch function. *J Natl Med Assoc* 83:1089–1092, 1991.

Wald A, Caruana B, Freimanis M, et al: Contribution of evacuation proctography and anorectal manometry to evaluation of adults with constipation and defecatory difficulty. *Dig Dis Sci* 35(4):481–487, 1990.

Wald A, Hinds J, Caruana B: Psychological and physiological characteristics of patients with severe idiopathic constipation. *Gastroenterology* 97:(4):932–937, 1989.

Wald A, Tunuguntla K: Anorectal sensorimotor dysfunction in fecal incontinence and diabetes mellitus—modification with biofeedback therapy. *N Engl J Med* 310:1282–1287, 1984.

Whitehead W, Engel B, Schuster M: Irritable bowel syndrome—physiological and psychological differences between diarrhea-predominant and constipation-predominant patients. *Dig Dis Sci* 25(6):404–413, 1980.

Yoshioka K, Matsui Y, Yamada O, et al: Physiologic and anatomic assessment of patients with rectocele. *Dis Colon Rectum* 34:704–708, 1991.

CHAPTER 17

Anal Sensation

Davinder Kumar

The anal canal has a rich sensory innervation consisting of free nerve endings and sensory organs. The free nerve endings are particularly abundant in the region of the anal valves and also throughout the anal transition zone above the valves (Duthie & Gairns, 1960). The anal epithelium is sensitive to pain, temperature, touch, and movement within the anal canal (Duthie & Gairns, 1960) and the appreciation of pain is most acute in the region of the anal valves. The highest level of pain sensation is between 0.5 and 1.5 cm above the valves, approximately 0.5 cm higher than the level for touch (Rogers, 1992) which extends from the anal verge to a level between 0.25 and 0.75 cm above the anal valves (Rogers, 1992). Temperature sensation also extends above the level of the anal valves. In contrast to the sensation for pain, temperature, and touch, where the anal canal is more sensitive compared to the perianal skin, movement of an object within the anal canal is perceived to the same degree as movement perceived by the perianal skin. In the perianal skin there are no organized nerve endings but intraepithelial free nerve endings are present. There is profuse innervation of hair follicles and this network of nerves forms a cylindrical arrangement around the sheath of each hair follicle. In the anal canal the anal margin contains very few hair follicles but the innervation is similar to that of the perianal skin. In addition there are organized nerve endings similar to Krause end-bulbs in close relatinship to hair follicles. This feature distinguishes the anal margin from perianal skin.

The innervation of the anal canal consists of free nerve endings beneath the epithelium, Meissner's corpuscles, Krause end-bulbs, Golgi-Mazzoni bodies, genital corpuscles, and pacinian corpuscles. Some of the nerve bundles go directly toward the epithelial surface before they branch to form free nerve endings beneath the epithelium. Others send branches into the epithelium where they terminate in discrete sensory organs. Meissner's corpuscles provide touch sensation and lie in the dermal papillae close to the epithelial margin. Krause end-bulbs lie deep in the dermis and respond to temperature stimuli. Golgi-Mazzoni bodies respond to pressure changes within the anal canal and are supposed to lie deep to the Meissner's corpuscles but superficial to the pacinian corpuscles. Genital corpuscles on the other hand lie at varying depth in the dermis but the majority lie close to the epithelium in the dermal papillae. Pacinian corpuscles are the deepest of all receptors and lie in close proximity to the internal anal sphincter. Like Golgi-Mazzoni bodies, pacinian corpuscles respond to pressure changes in the anal canal. In the area of the anal crypts and valves, free nerve endings become the most common modality of anal sensation. Sensation from the anal canal is carried to the sacral roots of S2, S3, and S4 by the inferior hemorrhoidal branches of the pudendal nerve.

RECTAL SENSATION

The rectum is insensitive to painful stimuli. It is, however, sensitive to distension of its lumen and the sensory response is perceived as a feeling of fullness in the rectum itself or sometimes referred to the sacral area (Goligher & Hughes, 1951). In healthy normal subjects, the rectum can perceive as little as 10 ml of air and 1 ml of water (Scharli & Kiesswetter, 1970). The precise mechanism of rectal sensation is not known. The free and organized nerve endings seen in the anal canal cease abruptly at the anorectal junction. It has been suggested that the rectal sensation arises from stimulation of the pelvic floor musculature and receptors in adjacent pelvic structures (Goligher and Hughes, 1951; Lane & Parks, 1977). The sympathetic nerve supply to the rectum is derived from the lower six thoracic and upper two lumber spinal segments (Gask & Ross, 1937). The parasympathetic supply is derived from the second, third, and fourth sacral segments. Rectal sensation is completely abolished following spinal anesthesia whereas colonic sensation is unaffected. Similarly, following inferior hemorrhoidal nerve block, the pressure threshold to produce colonic and rectal sensation is reduced. However, following bilateral sympathectomy, rectal sensation is preserved (Goligher & Hughes, 1951). This suggests that the sensation to volume distension of the rectum travels with the parasympathetic system to S2, S3, and S4 whereas the sensation to colonic distension travels via the sympathetic system.

MEASUREMENT OF SENSATION

Anal Sensation

Duthie & Gairns (1960) measured anal sensation using a Von Frey hair, pinprick, and metal plates at different temperatures. Such techniques are crude and provide only qualitative data. More recently two methods, namely, mucosal electrosensitivity and temperature sensation have been described (Miller et al., 1987; Roe et al., 1986). These provide a more objective and qualitative assessment of anal sensation.

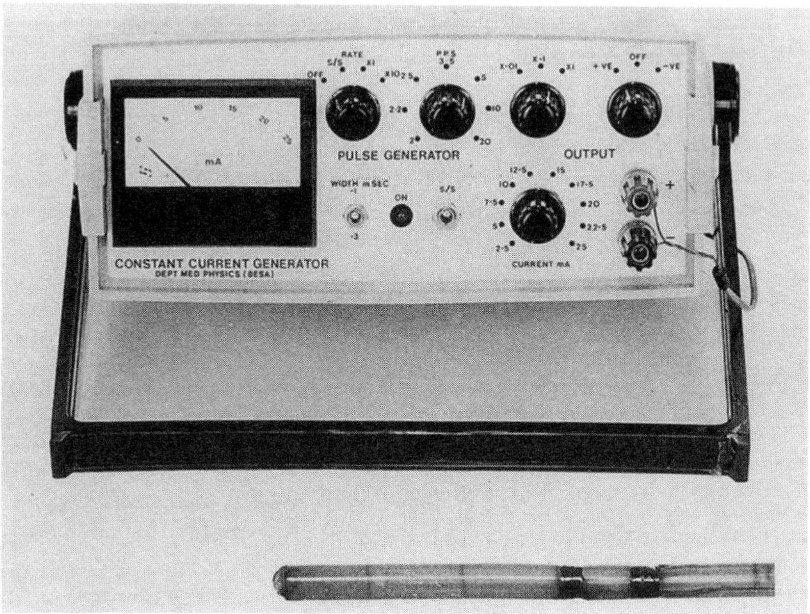

FIGURE 17.1 The constant current generator and the probe for measuring mucosal electrosensitivity. (From Miller et al., 1988.)

Mucosal Electrosensitivity

Sigel (1951) used a square-wave electrical current with a fixed impulse duration and frequency to study cutaneous sensation. Roe et al. (1986) first used this technique to study anal sensation. They used a probe consisting of a 10 FG Dover catheter with two platinum wire electrodes, 1 cm apart near the tip (Department of Clinical Measurement, Royal Devon & Exetor Hospital, Devon, UK). The probe was connected to a battery-powered constant current generator which produced a square-wave stimulus with a frequency of 5 Hz and 100 μsec (Department of Medical Physics, Bristol Royal Infirmary, Bristol, UK) (Fig. 17.1). Anal sensation is assessed in the upper, middle, and lower anal canal. The catheter is well lubricated with a conductive jelly and introduced into the anal canal so that the electrode lies in the upper anal canal. The current across the electrodes is increased in 1-mA increments until the subject feels a tingling or prickling sensation. The voltage at which sensation is felt is then recorded. The procedure is repeated three to five times and the mean of these readings is documented as the threshold of sensation at that particular level in the anal canal. The same process is repeated for the other two levels and the results are documented. In our laboratory we use a custom-made constant current generator connected to a probe and a reference electrode which is placed on the subject's thigh. Anal sensation is recorded as the current strength at which the patient complains of a prickling sensation.

TEMPERATURE SENSATION

Solids, liquids, and gases have different thermal conductivities (Hyndman & Wolkin, 1943). Miller et al. (1987) measured thermal thresholds to investigate whether temperature sensation could play a role in determining the presence and nature of rectal contents. A hot and cold stimulus is provided by a water-perfused thermode (Fig. 17.2). It consists of a 1 cm long bullet-shaped probe through which water of varying temperature can be pumped. The water is supplied from three thermostatically controlled baths, the temperatures of which are set so that the thermode can be held at 37° C and then rapidly increased or decreased by 4.5° C (Miller, 1991).

The temperature of the thermode–mucosa interface is measured by a small thermocouple and continuously recorded on a chart recorder. The subject is asked to indicate when a temperature change is felt and this point is marked on the chart recorder. The thermal threshold is assessed for four temperature ranges, normal to hot, hot to normal, normal to cold, and cold to normal in the same zones as the anal canal as tested for mucosal electrosensitivity. The median value of these four thresholds represents the minimum detectable temperature change for that zone. Miller et al. (1987) showed that the anal canal is extremely sensitive to thermal stimuli and that this thermal sensitivity is diminished in patients with idiopathic fecal incontinence.

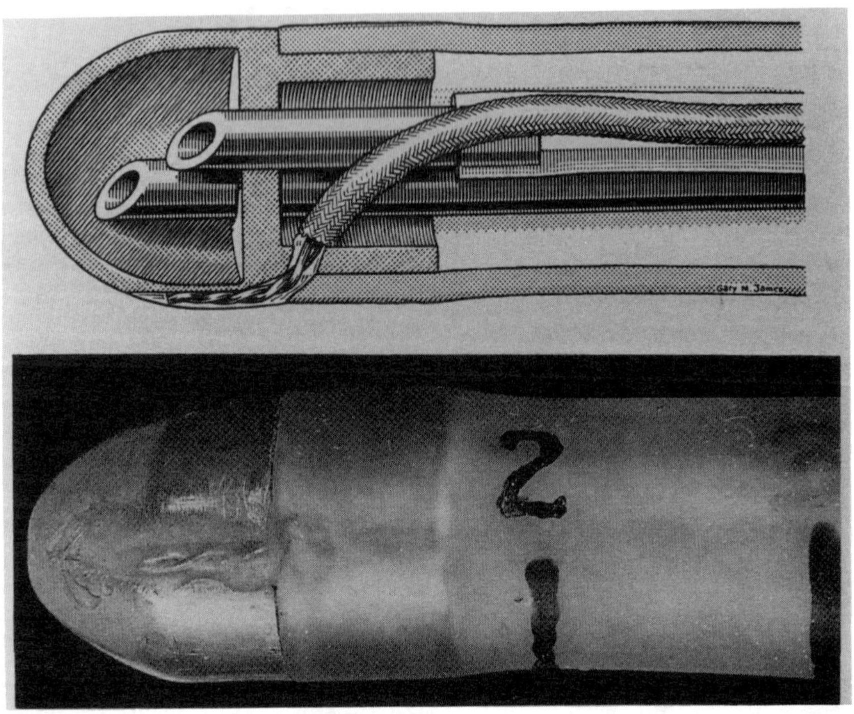

FIGURE 17.2 The internal design and photograph of the thermode used to determine thermal thresholds in the anorectum. (From Miller et al., 1987.)

MEASUREMENT OF RECTAL SENSATION

There is no standard method for the assessment of rectal sensation. The method commonly used is to insert a collapsed balloon connected to a catheter into the rectum. It is ensured that the lower margin of the balloon is well clear of the anal canal. The balloon is then inflated with progressively larger volumes of air from a hand-held syringe (Buser & Miner, 1986; Latimer et al., 1984; Wald et al., 1986). The volume at which first sensation is felt is the *threshold rectal distension volume*. However, this is dependent on the rate of inflation and position of the balloon and should be taken into account when interpreting the results. As the volume of air in the balloon increases, a point is reached when the subject is aware of a constant sensation and this is termed the *volume at constant sensation*. With further increases in the balloon volume, a stage is reached when it becomes uncomfortable and this is termed the *maximum tolerated volume* (Read et al., 1985). This provides an indication of rectal capacity and is strictly speaking not a sensory parameter. Alternatively, air or water can be pumped into the balloon at a constant rate (Varma et al., 1985). If water is used, it must be ensured that it is at 37° C otherwise the feeling of temperature can be interpreted as the threshold volume. This method is also used to measure rectal compliance when a manometric device is incorporated into the balloon so that pressure change can be monitored simultaneously. The pressure is plotted against volume and it provides an estimation of the compliance of the rectum.

CLINICAL VALUE OF ANORECTAL SENSATION

Continence

It is unclear whether the integrity of sensory function in the anal canal plays a role in the maintenance of continence. Keighley et al. (1987) showed that there was no impairment of function following the excision of anal mucosa during proctocolectomy in patients with ulcerative colitis. However, there was sensory impairment in the upper anal canal when they tested their patients objectively for anal sensation. One possible explanation may be that for continence to be impaired, it is necessary to have impairment of both motor as well as sensory function in the anorectum. Fecal incontinence in the absence of impairment of motor function has been reported in patients with higher sensory thresholds to balloon distension (Lubowski & Nicholls, 1988). Similarly, it is possible to have impairment of anorectal function without any objective abnormality of sensation. It is possible that minor degrees of sensory impairment do not by themselves cause impairment of function but motor dysfunction associated with sensory abnormalities result in a more severe disorder. This is often seen in patients with chronic idiopathic constipation who have sensory abnormality of the upper anal canal and impairment of rectal sensation. These patients are not aware of the presence of stool in their rectum and as a result have incomplete or no rectal evacuation. Similarly, in patients with fecal incontinence and sensory impairment of the anal canal, it is possible that the incontinence is due to malfunction of the sphincters, but the sensory abnormality makes the patient unaware of the seepage of fecal material through the anal canal.

The sensory function of the anorectum is also involved in discrimination between flatus, liquid and solid stool. The exact mechanism by which this discrimination takes place is not known. One of the mechanisms suggested is the sensitivity to temperature change (Miller et al., 1987). In their study, normal subjects could detect changes in temperature from as little as 0.6° C in the lower third of the anal canal to 1.1° C in the upper third of the anal canal. In patients with fecal incontinence there was a significantly reduced sensitivity to temperature change in the anal canal. This hypothesis of the role of temperature sensation in the discrimination of flatus, liquid and solid stools was challenged by Rogers and colleagues (1988) who showed that the largest temperature gradient between the rectum and the upper part of the anal canal was only 0.13° C which is four times less than the temperature threshold necessary to produce a conscious appreciation of temperature change in the anal canal of normal subjects. They suggested that the discriminatory function is dependent upon the integrity of all sensory modalities in the anal canal. Sensory abnormalities in isolation therefore do not result in impairment of anorectal function but can contribute to the severity of impairment of function when present in combination with motor dysfunction.

SUGGESTED READINGS

Buser WD, Miner PB: Delayed rectal sensation with faecal incontinence. Successful treatment using anorectal manometry. *Gastroenterology* 91:1186–1191, 1986.

Duthie HL, Gairns FW: Sensory nerves and sensation in the anal region of man. *Br J Surg* 47:585–595, 1960.

Gask GE, Ross JP: *The Surgery of the Sympathetic Nervous System,* ed 2. London, Bailliere Tindall, 1937.

Goligher JD, Hughes ESR: Sensibility of the rectum and colon: its role in the mechanism of anal continence. *Lancet* 543–548, 1951.

Hyndman OR, Wolkin J: Anterior chordotomy. *Arch Neurol Psychiatry* 50:129–148, 1943.

Keighley MRB, Winslet M, Yoshioka K, et al: Discrimination is not impaired by excision of anal transition zone after restorative proctocolectomy. *Br J Surg* 74:1118–1121, 1987.

Lane RHS, Parks AG: Function of the anal sphincters following colo-anal anastomosii. *Br J Surg* 64:596–599, 1977.

Latimer PR, Campbell D, Kasperski: A component analysis of biofeedback in the treatment of faecal incontinence. *Biofeedback Self Regul* 9:311–324, 1984.

Lubowski DJ, Nicholls RJ: Faecal incontinence associated with reduced pelvic sensation *Br J Surg* 75:1086–1088, 1988.

Miller R: The measurement of anorectal sensation. In Kumar D, Waldron D, Williams NS (eds): *Clinical Measurement in Coloproctology*. Springer Verlag U.K., 1991, pp 60–66.

Miller R, Bartolo DCC, Cervero F, et al: Anorectal temperature sensation: a comparison of normal and incontinent patients. *Br J Surg* 74:511–515, 1987.

Read NW, Abouzekry L, Read MG, et al: Anorectal function in elderly patients with faecal impaction. *Gastroenterology* 89:959–966, 1985.

Roe AM, Bartolo DC, Nortensen NJ McC: New method for assessment of anal sensation in various anorectal disorders. *Br J Surg* 73:310–312, 1986.

Rogers J: Rectal and anal sensation. In Swash M, Henry M (eds): *Coloproctology and the Pelvic Floor,* ed 2. Oxford, Butterworth Heinemann, 1992, VII, pp 54–60.

Rogers J, Hayward M, Henry M, et al: Temperature gradient between the rectum and anal canal: evidence against the role of temperature sensation as a sensory modality in the anal canal of normal subjects. *Br J Surg* 75:1083–1085, 1988.

Scharli A, Kieswetter WB: Defaecation and continence: some new concepts. *Dis Colon Rectum* 13:81–107, 1970.

Sigel H: Cutaneous sensory threshold stimulation with high frequency square wave current. *J Invest Dermatol* 18:441–445, 1951.

Varma JS, Smith AN, Busutil A: Correlation of clinical and manometric abnormalities of rectal function following chronic radiation injury. *Br J Surg* 72:875–878, 1985.

Wald A, Chandra R, Chiponis D, et al: Anorectal function and continence mechanisms in childhood encopresis. *J Pediatr Gastroenterol Nutr* 5:346–351, 1986.

CHAPTER 18

The Role of the Coordinator

Linda L. Jensen

THE ROLE OF THE COORDINATOR

The coordinator in the anorectal physiology laboratory should ideally be a nurse with a background of anorectal anatomy, physiology, and defecation disorders. He/she should understand the test protocol(s) and the aim of testing and should be able to improvise and alter protocol to suit individual patient needs. A working knowledge of the laboratory equipment is essential. The coordinator should be empathetic to the patients' anxieties about their condition, the tests, and the possible subsequent therapy.

ESTABLISHING THE LABORATORY

The coordinator plays a central role in the establishment of the anorectal laboratory.

Site Requirements

1. Private office area for interview, consultations, and reviewing results.
2. Private exam room for studies.
3. Easy access to x-ray department. The x-ray room should have an adacent bathroom.
4. Ancillary staff willing to learn about defecation disorders and care for patients with these disorders.

Equipment

The coordinator works with the facility and physician in evaluating and purchasing equipment for specific studies to be done. (See related sections of text for each of the following.)

1. Manometry
2. Defecating proctogram
3. Electromyography
4. Transit time studies
5. Ultrasonography

Inservice Education to Ancillary Staff

A key factor for a smooth-running anorectal laboratory is the support of the ancillary staff within the hospital. An initial and ongoing inservice to the staff is essential. The initial inservice should include a brief review of the pelvic floor anatomy and physiology, an explanation of the principles and methods of the procedures to be performed, and a discussion of the disorders that will be evaluated, such as incontinence, constipation, and rectal prolapse or intussusception. Because of the anxiety of the patients and the nature of the test(s), emphasis should be placed on the importance of patient support during the evaluation process. Establishing the laboratory scheduling procedures and discussion of the charges can be done at this time. Ideally, 1 hr should be allotted per patient, thereby allowing two to three evaluations per morning or afternoon. Interpretation and dictation of the results is done at a separate time. Ongoing education keeps the staff aware of changes in the protocols of existing procedures or new procedures being done.

Inservice to Lay Community

Function as liaison between laboratory and community, giving educational presentations to appropriate groups. The goal would be both as a marketing tool and patient education.

PATIENT-PHYSICIAN-HOSPITAL LIAISON

1. Schedule patients for procedure(s) after referral from primary doctor.
2. Inform patient of the purpose and nature of test(s), and the required preparation. (A few extra minutes spent at this time with the patient in giving a thorough explanation will begin to establish the rapport that will then be carried over to the time of the evaluation.) Follow-up with pamphlet and map (Appendix 1, page 247).
3. Follow-up to physician.

4. Work with patient, hospital, and insurance company regarding explanation of tests, coding, and fees (Appendix 2, page 248).

INTERVIEW AND ADMINISTRATION OF TESTS

Interview

1. Interview patient regarding symptoms, bowel habits, personal medical history (Appendix 3, page 248).
2. Discuss basic sphincter anatomy, using a diagram.
3. Review test procedures, including instructions the patient will be required to follow. Assure the patient that these will be explained again as test(s) proceed. Address any questions or misunderstanding the patient might have. A common concern is that the evaluation will not be relevant if the patient cannot comply with instructions (i.e., squeeze sphincter muscles).

Anal Manometry

1. Check equipment to ensure that it is functioning properly.
2. Do digital rectal exam: have patient squeeze and use Valsalva maneuver for clinical assessment. Verify patients' comprehension of instructions.
3. Remove all air from balloon on catheter and calibrate to the level of the anal canal. Insert well-lubricated catheter into anal canal past the desired level and withdraw to straighten balloon. Administer test in accordance with established protocol.
4. Clean and sterilize catheter according to hospital policy.

Defecatogram

1. Prepare contrast media (either commercial or mixture made in laboratory).
2. With patient in right lateral position, insert or supervise insertion of contrast media (we use a standard barium enema tip and insert our mixture with two 60-cc catheter tip syringes).
3. With the patient positioned to include the pubis and coccyx, take three still shots with patient at rest, squeezing, and pushing.
4. Position commode. (We use the Lahr defecography chair attached to the x-ray table footboard).
5. Assist in positioning patient comfortably on chair while reassuring patient. (Emphasize the need for patient to hold contrast media until everything is lined up.)
6. Oversee video taping of pelvis during defecation to ensure proper visualization of suspected disorder.

EMG-Pudendal Nerve Latency or Recruitment

1. Check and prepare equipment.
2. Review procedure with patient.
3. Position the patient in left lateral position with knees pulled toward chest.
4. Ground patient, if doing recruitment, or physician if doing pudendal nerve latency.
5. Assist physician with procedure.

Transit Time Studies

1. Provide the patient with capsule(s) containing radiopaque markers.
2. Review protocol and restrictions with patient (Appendix 4, page 258).
3. Schedule times with x-ray at patient's convenience.

Endorectal Ultrasound

1. Check and prepare equipment.
2. Review procedure with patient.
3. Position the patient in left lateral position with knees pulled toward chest.
4. Assist physician with procedure.

POSTPROCEDURAL CARE

1. Answer any postprocedural questions the patient might have and send them home with a completed postevaluation form. (Appendix 5, page 258).
2. Complete data on each patient.
3. Work with staff surgeon in forwarding test results (copy of pp 248–257 of Appendix 3 with a cover letter) to the referring physician and be sure patient gets feedback regarding results.
4. Input data into retrieval system.
5. Follow patient's treatment course and recall patient to lab for post-operative studies when indicated.

APPENDIX 1: ANORECTAL PHYSIOLOGY LABORATORY PATIENT TEACHING PAMPHLET

What is Anorectal Physiology?
Anorectal physiology is the study of the function of the anus and rectum. Muscle strength and pelvic floor motion are evaluated to help your physician recommend appropriate medical or surgical treatment for you.
What Can I Expect?
You will have a brief interview by a physician prior to any testing. The physician will explain the purpose of the tests performed at the laboratory, and you will have an opportunity to ask questions.
What Tests are Performed?
Many investigations can be performed. You may be scheduled for only one or several. The physician will explain the investigations you are scheduled for during the interview. Some are explained below.
How Long Does It Take?
To conduct the interview and perform all tests takes about 60 min. If you are not scheduled for all tests, it will take less time. No medications are given. You can leave immediately after the tests have been performed.
When Will I Know The Test Results?
It takes about 10 days for your referring physician to get the results. He will discuss the results on a later date after he has had a chance to review them.
What Is an Anal Manometry?
Anal manometry is an evaluation of the strength of the muscles that control your bowel movements. The test is performed by placing a small tube (the size of a drinking straw) into the rectum. Pressure monitors inside the tube transmit the muscle impulses to a graph similar to that of an electrocardiogram. It is a painless procedure that takes about 15 min to perform.
What Is Electromyography?
If your doctor wishes, we will also perform EMG or electromyographic testing of the muscles around the anus. These tests allow us to determine if the nerves that supply your sphincter muscles are intact and that your muscles relax and contract as they should. These test are performed by placing a small electrode on the nerve or muscle, and measuring the electrical activity. This is not painful.
What is a Defecating Proctogram?
A defecating proctogram is a test of the motion of the pelvic floor, the muscles that control a bowel movement, and the motion of the anus and rectum during evacuation. A small amount of barium is placed in the rectum, and a recording is made during evacuation of the barium. It takes about 20 min to perform this painless test.
How Do I Prepare for the Examination?
You will need to take two Fleet enemas. Take the first enema 2 hr prior to the test and the second 30 min later. These enemas are available at any pharmacy. There are no dietary restrictions.
Please register 15 min prior to your appointment in the Outpatient Registration in the Emergency Room.
Your appointment is ______________________________ at __________.

APPENDIX 2: ANORECTAL PHYSIOLOGY LABORATORY CHARGES

Hospital Charges		Code Number
Anal manometry	$143.00	4099034-2
Defecating proctogram	100.00	4099036-8
EMG	148.00	4099040-0
Doctors' Charges		**Code Number**
Manometry	$200.00	9122
Defecating proctogram	75.00	45999
Interpretation	50.00	90506

APPENDIX 3: ANORECTAL PHYSIOLOGY DATA SHEET

Date: M____ D____ Y____

Patient Information

Name____
Last First M

Address______________________________________

____

Phone ( )____________

Account #____________

Hospital #____________

Age: ____ DOB: M____ D____ Y____

Sex: Male Female

Referring Physician: Name______________________

Address______________________

Phone ( )____________

Previous Sphincter Series: Yes No Date: M____ D____ Y____

ELECTROMYOGRAPHY

Electromyography	____Done	____Not done	
Pudendal Nerve Latency	____Done	____Not done	
right	____ms.	____Normal	____Prolonged
left	____ms.	____Normal	____Prolonged

APPENDIX 3: CONTINUED

Recruitment ____Done ____Not done
____Normal ____Absent ____Paradoxical

Sphincter Mapping ____Done ____Not done
right ____present ____diminished ____not present
left ____present ____diminished ____not present
anterior ____present ____diminished ____not present
posterior ____present ____diminished ____not present

Single Fiber Density ____Done ____Not done
____

MANOMETRY

Anal Rectal Manometry ____Done ____Not done
Reflex present ____Yes ____No ____Unknown
Balloon ____cc air at ____cm

First sensation ____cc
Sensation of fullness ____cc

Vector symmetry index ____

PROCTOMETROGRAM/DEFECATOGRAM

Proctometrogram ____Done ____Not done

Anal canal length rest____cm
push____cm
squeeze____cm

Anal rectal angle rest____degrees
push____degrees
squeeze____degrees

Perineal pubocox distance rest____cm
push____cm
squeeze____cm

Perineal descent with pushing ____cm

Puborectalis length rest____cm
push____cm
squeeze____cm
shift w/squeeze____cm

Defecatogram ____Done ____Not done

Rectocele ____No ____Ant ____Post ____Other
when present ____at rest ____straining ____NA
size ____small ____moderate ____large
principal pathology ____Yes ____No

APPENDIX 3: CONTINUED

Enterocele	____Yes	____No	
Intussusception	____Yes	____No	
prolapse	____No	____mucosal	____complete
rectal emptying	____complete	____partial	____none
opening of anal canal	____complete	____partial	____none
relaxation of puborect	____complete	____partial	____none
	____paradoxical		
straightening of ARA	____complete	____partial	____none

Anal Manometry Pressure

	Resting Tone Trough Pressure				Maximum Voluntary Contraction				Squeeze Pressure			
cm	post	right	ant	left	post	right	ant	left	post	right	ant	left
6												
5												
4												
3												
2												
1												

IMPRESSION

Manometry ____

____

____

Proctometrogram ____

____

____

Defecatogram ____

____

____

EMG ____

____

____

APPENDIX 3: CONTINUED

Conclusion____

____

____

____

Requested follow-up study _____Yes _____No

Recommended Rx

_____Not state
_____biofeedback
_____further evaluation
_____endoanal ant wall plication
_____prolapse-perineal repair
_____total pelvic floor repair
_____prolapse--abd repair
_____subtotal colectomy
_____sphicteroplasty
_____closure colostomy
_____RVF repair
_____normal results
_____post anal repair
_____perineal support device
_____artificial sphincter
_____electrogalvanic stim

DX Class

_____incontinence
_____prolapse
_____ulcerative colitis
_____injury
_____postanal repair
_____anal stenosis
_____fissure
_____normal control
_____RVF (post-op)
_____other
_____nonspec rectal pain
_____incont w/prolapse
_____constipation
_____sphincteroplasty
_____RV fistula
_____pouch post op
_____proctopexy (post op)
_____Altmeier
_____fistula in ano
_____encopresis
_____spastic puborect
_____anal stim therapy

Bowel Habits—Functional Review

Stool Consistency: _____liquid _____semiliquid _____formed/soft
_____formed/hard _____pellet

Sensation of incomplete evacuation _____Yes _____No
Frequent attempts to evacuate _____Yes _____No
attempts/day _____
time _____minutes
Pruritus _____Yes _____No
Tenesmus _____Yes _____No

Pelvic Pain _____constant _____intermittent _____none
standing _____better _____worse _____same _____none
sitting _____better _____worse _____same _____none

APPENDIX 3: CONTINUED

sleeping	____better	____worse	____same	____none
lying	____better	____worse	____same	____none
w/defecation	____Yes	____No		

Mucous discharge ____No ____between BM ____with BM

Rectal bleeding	____Yes	____No			
at defecation	____Yes	____No	bright red	____Yes	____No
on paper	____Yes	____No	dark red	____Yes	____No
in toilet	____Yes	____No	clots	____Yes	____No
mixed w/stool	____Yes	____No	intermittent	____Yes	____No
between stools	____Yes	____No	continuous	____Yes	____No

Urinary stress incontinence ____Yes ____No

Sensation of Prolapse ____Yes ____No

Prolapse type ____occult ____spontaneous
____manual ____irreducible

Bowel Urgency ____Yes ____No

Bowel Habits—Incontinence

Incontinence	____Yes	____No	
frequency	____always	____rarely	____sometimes
incont gas	____none	____active	____rest
incont liq	____none	____active	____rest
incont solid	____none	____active	____rest
type	____air	____liquid	____solid
severity	____soil underwear	____use pad	
duration:	____________		
every	____days		

Incontinence Scoring System

Incontinence gas	____none	<1/mo (1)	>1/mo (2)	>1/wk (3)
Incontinence liq	____none	<1/mo (4)	>1/mo (5)	>1/wk (6)
Incontinence solid	____none	<1/mo (7)	>1/mo (8)	>1/wk (9)
Significantly affects lifestyle	____none	<1/mo (10)	>1/mo (11)	>1/wk (12)

(max. score 30 pts.)

Bowel Habits—Constipation

Constipation	____Yes	____No		
frequency	____rarely	____sometimes	____always	
BM every	____day(s)	spontaneous	____Yes	____No
Mechanical intervention		____Yes	____No	
Enema	____never	____rarely	____sometimes	____always

use enemas since ____ / ____ / ____

APPENDIX 3: CONTINUED

Disimpaction ____never ____rarely ____sometimes ____always
hospitalization required ____Yes ____No
Digital interven ____never ____rarely ____sometimes ____always
Digital type ____none ____rectal ____vaginal ____both
Laxative use ____Yes ____No
Use since ____ / ____ / ____
Frequency every ____ days
Type ____bulk ____stimulant ____softner
____lubricant ____combination

Transit Study

Transit study ____Done ____Not done
markers remaining ____ ____Normal ____abnormal
Location ____ascending ____transverse ____descending
____sigmoid ____rectosigmoid

Operative History—Abdominal

Abdominal Surgery ____Yes ____No ____Unknown

small intestine ____Yes ____No ____Unknown
site ____stomach ____duodenum ____jejunum
____ileum ____other ____unknown
date ____ / ____ / ____
colon ____Yes ____No ____Unknown
site ____appendix ____segmental ____right
____left ____sigmoid ____ant resect
____subtotal ____total ____unknown
date ____ / ____ / ____

Relation oper. to dysfunction ____none ____some ____directly
Operative Repair—Prolapse (Abdominal)
Prolapse ____Yes ____No ____Unknown
Date ____ / ____ / ____
Type ____occult ____spontaneous ____manual
____irreducible ____unknown
Technique ____unknown ____proctopexy ____Frykman/Gold
____Ripstein ____ant. resection
Relation oper. to dysfunction ____none ____some ____directly

Operative History—Constipation
Constipation ____Yes ____No ____Unknown
Date ____ / ____ / ____
Type ____spincterotomy ____TAC & IAA/IRA
____subtotal ____sigmoidectomy
____other
Relation oper. to dysfunction ____none ____some ____directly

APPENDIX 3: CONTINUED

Operative History—Gynecological

Gynecological ____Yes ____No ____Unknown
Date ____ / ____ / ____
Type ____TAH BSO ____TAH ____SO ____VagHyster
____vag prolapse ____rectocele ____cystocele
____other ____unknown
Relation oper. to dysfunction ____none ____some ____directly

Operative History—Anorectal

Prior A/R	____Yes	____No	____Unknown
a/r abscess	____Yes	____No	____Unknown
fistula in ano	____Yes	____No	____Unknown
R/V fistula	____Yes	____No	____Unknown
fissure	____Yes	____No	____Unknown
hemorrhoids	____Yes	____No	____Unknown
incontinence	____Yes	____No	____Unknown
prolapse/rectal	____Yes	____No	____Unknown

Operative History—Abscess

a/r abscess ____Yes ____No ____Unknown
abscess date ____ / ____ / ____
abscess type ____acute ____chronic ____recurrent
____atypical ____unknown
abscess drainage ____spontaneous ____I&D ____neither
relation of operation to dysfunction ____none ____some
____directly

Operative History—Fistula in ano

fistula in ano ____Yes ____No ____Unknown
date ____ / ____ / ____
type ____unknown ____subcutaneous
____low intersphincteric ____transph
____transinfralevator ____transupralev
____extrasphincteric ____high intersph
____other
technique ____unknown ____I&D ____fistulotomy
____ectomy ____seton ____marsupialization
____core out ____flap ____colostomy
____other
relation of operation to dysfunction ____none ____some
____directly

Operative History—Rectal Vaginal Fistula

R/V fistula ____Yes ____No ____Unknown
date ____ / ____ / ____
site ____unknown ____low ____mid ____high

APPENDIX 3: CONTINUED

technique ____unknown ____ostomy ____excision
____invagination ____flap ____s'plasty
____endorectal ____gracilis ____other
relation of operation to dysfunction ____none ____some
____directly

Operative History—Fissure
Fissure ____Yes ____No ____Unknown
date ____ / ____ / ____
type ____unknown ____acute ____chronic
____recurrent ____atypical ____other
technique ____unknown ____dilate ____excision
____sphincterotomy lat ____post
____other
relation of operation to dysfunction ____none ____some
____directly

Operative History—Hemorrhoids
Hemorrhoids ____Yes ____No ____Unknown
date ____ / ____ / ____
type ____internal ____external ____unknown
degree ____1st ____2nd ____3rd ____4th
____unknown
technique ____unknown ____med ____dilation
____band ____sclerosis ____cryo ____coag
____open ____closed
relation of operation to dysfunction ____none ____some
____directly

Operative History—Incontinence
Incontinence ____Yes ____No ____Unknown
date ____ / ____ / ____
pre-op grade ____0 ____I ____II ____III ____Unknown
technique ____unknown ____postanal ____gracilis
____Thiersch ____s'plasty ____art/neo sph
relation of operation to dysfunction ____none ____some
____directly

Operative History—Prolapse—Rectal Repair
Prolapse ____Yes ____No ____Unknown
date ____ / ____ / ____
type ____occult ____spontaneous ____manual
____irreducible ____unknown
technique ____unknown ____Delorme ____Thiersch
____Altmeier
relation of operation to dysfunction ____none ____some
____directly

APPENDIX 3: CONTINUED

Traumatic Anal Injuries

History of trauma	____Yes	____No	____Unknown
date	____ / ____ / ____		
pelvic fracture	____Yes	____No	____Unknown
soft tissue injury	____Yes	____No	____Unknown
impalement	____Yes	____No	____Unknown
relation of operation to dysfunction		____none	____some
	____directly		

Pregnancy

C-section	____Yes	____No		____Unknown	
C-section number	____				
vaginal deliveries	____Yes	____No		____Unknown	
vag. delivery #	____				
traumatic	____Yes	____No		____Unknown	
traumatic #	____				
technique	____primary	____secondary		____unknown	
grade of tear	____0	____I	____II	____III	____IV
	____unknown				

Neurological/Medical History

spinal trauma	____Yes	____No	____Unknown
meningocele	____Yes	____No	____Unknown
sacral surgery	____Yes	____No	____Unknown
degenerative dis	____Yes	____No	____Unknown
tumor/metastasis	____Yes	____No	____Unknown
diabetes mellitus	____Yes	____No	____Unknown
multiple strokes	____Yes	____No	____Unknown
multiple sclerosis	____Yes	____No	____Unknown
urinary incontinence	____Yes	____No	____Unknown
dementia	____Yes	____No	____Unknown

Previous Investigations

UGI	____Yes	____No	____Unknown
barium enema	____Yes	____No	____Unknown
transit study	____Yes	____No	____Unknown
fistulogram	____Yes	____No	____Unknown
sinogram	____Yes	____No	____Unknown
ct abd/pelvis	____Yes	____No	____Unknown
proctogram	____Yes	____No	____Unknown
defecography	____Yes	____No	____Unknown
proctoscopy	____Yes	____No	____Unknown
colonoscopy	____Yes	____No	____Unknown
manometry	____Yes	____No	____Unknown
EMG	____Yes	____No	____Unknown
RUS	____Yes	____No	____Unknown

APPENDIX 3: CONTINUED

Physical Exam

Physical exam	____done	____not done		
Visual inspection				
excoriation	____Yes	____No		
deformity	____none	____minimal	____mod.	____severe
patulous anus	____Yes	____No		
anal wink	____Yes	____No		
Visible pathology				
ext. hemorrhoid	____Present	____Absent		
int. hemorrhoid	____Present	____Absent		
RMP	____Present	____Absent		
fissure	____Present	____Absent		
fistula	____Present	____Absent		

Digital Exam

Tone	____normal	____diminished		
anal stenosis	____none	____mild	____mod.	____severe
squeeze	____normal	____fair	____poor	
puborectalis				
with strain	____normal	____equivocal	____paradoxical	
prolapse defect	____none	____anterior	____right	____left
	____posterior			
overt prolapse	____Yes	____No		
if yes	____cm			
cystocele	____Yes	____No		
rectocele	____Yes	____No		

APR Summary

____
____
____
____
____
____
____
____
____
____
____
____
____
____
____

APPENDIX 4: ANORECTAL PHYSIOLOGY LABORATORY TRANSIT TIME STUDY

Your doctor would like you to have a transit time study of the colon. This study is done to evaluate the amount of time it takes ingested food particles to travel through the GI system.

The study is done by taking a series of simple abdominal x-rays after you have ingested radiopaque markers. There will be no barium or air introduced into the colon.

Preparation for the study is as follows:

1. Take the gelatin capsule(s) (which contain radiopaque markers) 24 hr before the first x-ray.
2. No fasting is required; no dietary restrictions are necessary.
3. If you are on a high-fiber diet, you may continue that regimen (including bran).
4. If you are taking a bulk laxative agent (Metamucil, Effersylium, Hydrocil, Perdiem Plain), you should continue to do so. DO NOT take any stimulant laxatives such as Citrate of Magnesium®, Dulcolax®, Milk of Magnesia®, Ex Lax®, etc.

The series of x-rays should take place at the same time each day for 5 consecutive days, or until all markers have been passed. In order to get a true evaluation of your GI system, it is important that you DO NOT TAKE LAXATIVES (except bulk agents), ENEMAS, OR SUPPOSITORIES until the entire series has been completed.

Your test is scheduled to begin on ______________________________ .
After the series of x-rays is completed, they will be reviewed by your doctor, who will contact you with the results.

APPENDIX 5: ANORECTAL PHYSIOLOGY LABORATORY POSTEVALUATION INSTRUCTIONS

Date____________________

You have just completed:

______Anal Manometry	______Rectal Capacity Study
______Defecating Proctogram	______Evaluation Efficiency
______Transit Study	______EMG
______MMPI	______Saline Infusion
______Other (specify)	

APPENDIX 5: CONTINUED

There are generally no adverse side effects from these procedures. Notify your doctor if you have questions or concerns.

If barium was instilled into your rectum, drink extra fluids (water or juice) for the next 24 hr to prevent constipation from the barium.

Your doctor will contact you when all the test results have been interpreted.

I have received and understand these follow-up instructions.

________________________ Patient Signature

________________________RN/MD MD Office Phone ________________________

CHAPTER 19

Biofeedback for Constipation

Steve Heymen
Steven D. Wexner

INTRODUCTION

A standardized profile of diagnostic tests (described in Chapters 2 and 22) is used to determine the cause of constipation. Occasionally, the result of this evaluation demonstrates that the patient is actually not constipated but merely unsatisfied with their bowel function. This is "treated" simply by reassuring the patient and by educating them as to normal bowel function and the quantity or frequency of bowel movements that they should expect. If the patient's concerns are persistent and seem unreasonable, a referral for psychotherapy may be indicated.

When the test results show the cause of the constipation to be physiological, it is categorized as colonic inertia or an outlet obstruction such as paradoxical puborectalis contraction (PPC).

PPC occurs when an individual incorrectly contracts the puborectalis and external anal sphincter muscles during attempts to defecate, thereby obstructing their own intention to evacuate the rectum. These muscles must be relaxed during attempted defecation to allow the passage of stool through the rectum and the anal canal.

ETIOLOGIES OF PPC

There appear to be many routes toward developing PPC. Anything causing pain during defecation can cause a tensing of the pelvic floor. Such precipitating pain can be initiated by surgery, injury, fissures, or hemorrhoids.

Many people's beliefs and habits learned from childhood have predisposed them to develop PPC. Although these beliefs may seem bizarre to the health care professional, the patient usually strongly adheres to them. Perhaps the most common misconception is patients' fear that they must defecate every day. Some feel that fecal matter is toxic and must be eliminated as soon as possible. The fear is that if they don't eliminate daily, something will rupture, they will become impacted, or some other dangerous effect will occur. Many of these individuals started using laxatives or enemas at a very early age and have become dependent on them. They report that one or both of their parents suffered from constipation and that discussions in the home, concerning bowel function, were very tense. Others feel that if they don't use a laxative "nothing will come out." Having succeeded with this strategy in the past, they are reinforced to continue this behavior, but with diminishing results.

In addition to these misconceptions about bowel function, many patients have adopted poor defecation habits. Patients will often be insistent about when they defecate. They have rigid schedules and will use a laxative or enema in the morning every day so that they are free to resume their schedule and not have to deal with bowel function for the rest of the day. The elderly often become constipated because of difficulty getting to a toilet. This may be due to physical handicaps or unavailability of a facility. Some individuals are just "tuned out" to this area of their body. They may feel it is disgusting to talk about bowel function. Histories of sexual or emotional trauma may accompany this finding.

Often stress and general tension can lead to pelvic floor tension much the same as a muscle tension headache a patient suffers from stress. It is important that the therapist not assume, in these cases, that effectively reducing the stress will sufficiently deal with the problem. If the patient has had difficulty with constipation for any length of time, they may have begun straining with excessive effort to defecate. Although this maneuver may effectively evacuate the rectum, at least initially, it contributes to the development of PPC. The more intense the effort, the more likely the patient is to tense the entire region, including the pelvic floor muscles.

Often physiological and psychological problems coexist in patients with constipation. This fact is evidenced by the results of several studies of constipated patients using the Minnesota Multiphasic Personality Inventory (MMPI) or Hopkins Sx Checklist (HSC) to assess their psychological functioning.

The studies reveal personality profiles that show a somaticizing defense mechanism at work for many of these constipated patients (Devroede et al., 1989; Heymen et al., 1993). This phenomenon describes individuals who unconsciously redirect psychological distress into physical symptoms. There has been ongoing debate as to whether this kind of psychotherapy causes constipation and irritable bowel syndrome (IBS) or is the result of protracted suffering from this condition (Whitehead & Crowell, 1991).

Some psychological disorders that can influence constipation include personality disorders, obsessive compulsive, psychotic, anxiety, eating disorders, and some affective disorders such as depression. Mental retardation and dementias may also play a role in the development of constipation (Strickland & Heymen, 1995).

Finally, it is important to acknowledge the discomfort and disruption that this disorder can cause in these people's lives and that the consequences of having to deal with this chronic problem can create physiological changes that exacerbate the symptoms. Such disorders can include, but are not limited to, changes in eating behaviors and activity levels, depression, laxative abuse, and the development of PPC.

TREATMENT

A conservative form of treatment for pelvic floor muscle disorders involves biofeedback training. There are many studies reporting the use of biofeedback for retraining and strengthening of the pelvic floor muscles to successfully eliminate or greatly reduce the incidence of fecal incontinence (Cerulli et al, 1979; Engel at al, 1974; MacLeod, 1987) with success rates ranging from 75% to 100%.

Since 1979, there have been several studies reporting success using biofeedback for the treatment of chronic constipation and childhood encopresis thought to be a result of chronic constipation. In the studies listed in Table 19.1, the subjects were found to have abnormal defecation dynamics, either paradoxically contracting or nonrelaxing pelvic floor muscles. The biofeedback treatment strategies described involved intra-anal EMG, perianal EMG, manometry, or some combination of these therapies. While there may be advantages to each, it appears that the intra-anal EMG sensor provides the most accurate feedback of the muscle activity of the pelvic floor. In some cases, intrarectal balloon sensitivity training may be an advantageous adjunctive therapy for those patients lacking in perception of rectal distension.

One important issue that has been consistent throughout all of the cited (Table 19.1) cases of biofeedback treatment for constipation is the absence of any risk factors or medical complications as a result of the biofeedback treatment. Although not all of the patients who received biofeedback for constipation improved, none of them got any worse, nor did pursuit of this approach to treatment hinder any other efforts to treat the patient.

TABLE 19.1 CASES OF BIOFEEDBACK TREATMENT FOR CONSTIPATION

Author	Date	N	Age	DX*	TX**	#TX	%
Bennings	1993	29	5–16	enc	man	5	55
Wexner	1992	18	67	PPC	EMG	9	89
Turnbull	1992	7	29–42	PPC	man	4.5	71
Dahl	1991	14	6–60	PPC	EMG/bal	5	93
Kawimba	1991	15	45	PPC	EMG	7	87
Lestar	1991	16	42	PPC	man/bal	1	44
Loening-Baucke	1991	38	6–15	enc	EMG	6	37
Loening-Baucke	1990	22	5–16	enc	EMG	6	77
Keren	1988	12	8.3	PPC	man	4.1	100
Bleijenberg	1987	10	19–48	PPC	EMG	in-pt	70
Wald	1987	9	6–15	PPC	man	4	67

DX* enc = encopresis; PPC = paradoxical puborectalis contraction;
TX** man = manometry; EMG = electromyography; bal = balloon.

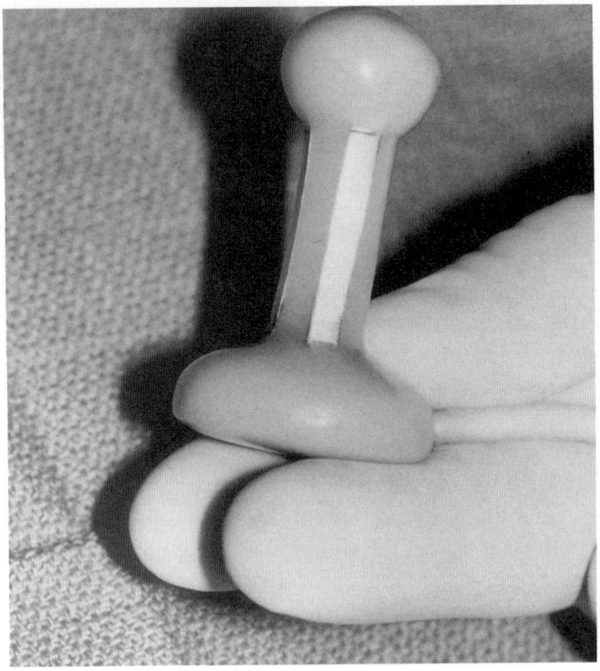

FIGURE 19.1 Intra-anal EMG sensor (Biotechnical PerryMeter Systems EPS-21).

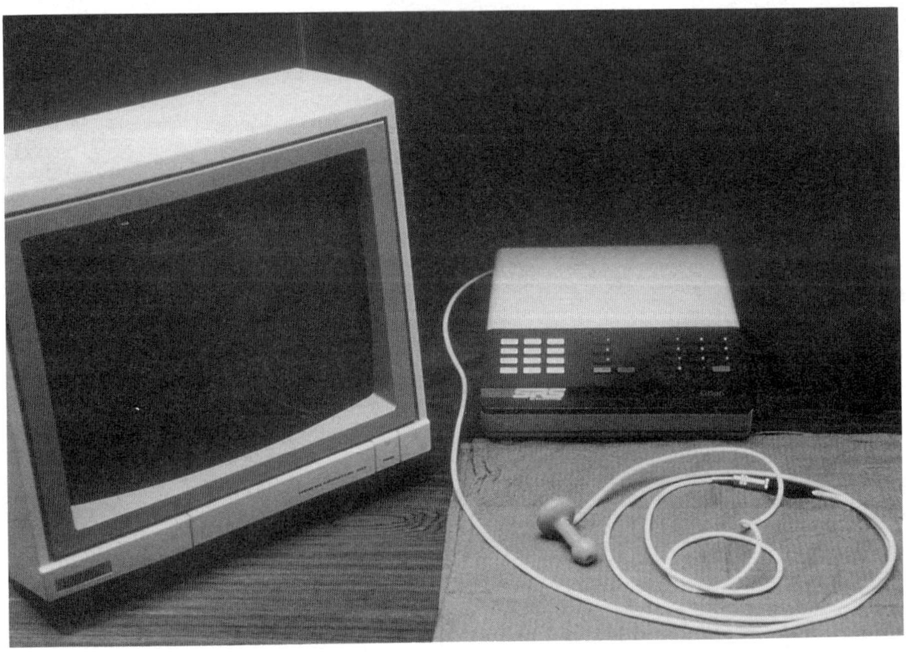

FIGURE 19.2 Computerized biofeedback instrument (SRS Orion 8600).

METHODOLOGY

Biofeedback retraining of the pelvic floor muscles is done at Cleveland Clinic Florida using an intra-anal EMG sensor (Biotechnologies PerryMeter Systems EPS-21)(Fig. 19.1) on a 100–200 Hz bandwidth. Feedback is presented to the patient using the SRS Orion 8600 (Fig. 19.2).

EMG BIOFEEDBACK TRAINING

Patients receive weekly 1 hr long biofeedback sessions. These sessions include the feedback display of EMG activity of pelvic floor muscles (Fig. 19.3), education as to proper bowel and pelvic floor physiological functions, and operant conditioning techniques to retrain these functions.

To begin training patients to "tune in" to the pelvic floor muscles, diagrams of the anatomy and a video of a cinedefogram are utilized to explain the correct dynamics and incorrect or paradoxical dynamics of the pelvic floor. The patient's ability to perceive muscle activity in the anal canal begins with an understanding of *what to look for*. By starting to educate them about this body function, the patient is included as part of the treatment team.

Patients are then trained using EMG biofeedback to control pelvic floor muscles and to discriminate among three events: rest, squeeze, and push in order to

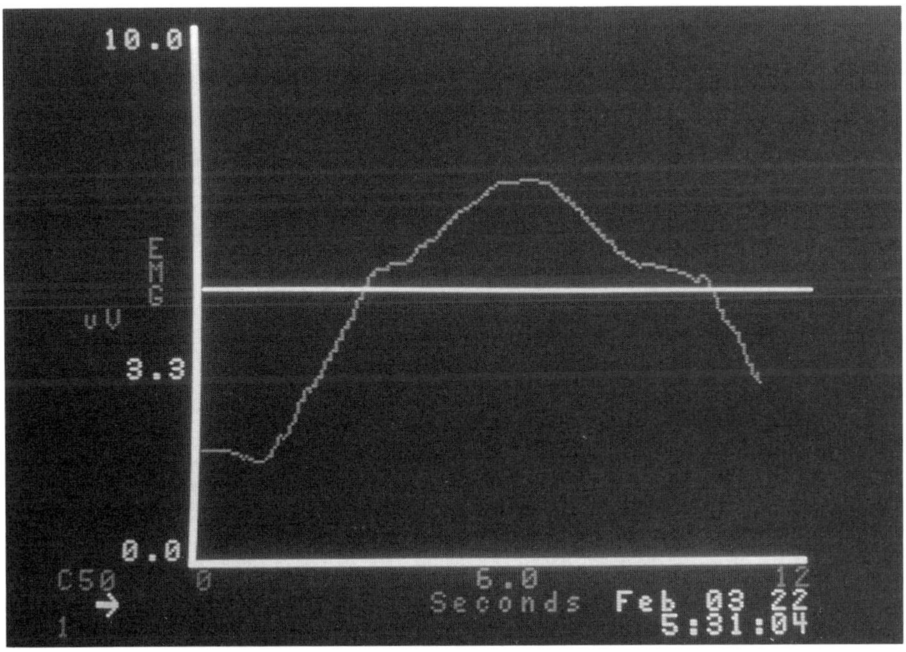

FIGURE 19.3 EMG feedback display (SRS Orion 8600).

eliminate paradoxical puborectalis contractions (PPC). *Rest* is defined as the basal muscular activity of the pelvic floor during the inactive state (EMG < 2.0 Uv). *Squeeze* is defined as appropriate contraction of the pelvic floor muscles (EMG values may vary considerably but should reach at least 5.0 Uv for a 10-sec average). *Push* is defined as appropriately simulating attempted defecation without contraction of the pelvic floor muscles (EMG < 2.0 Uv or ideally < resting values).

Patients are asked to practice the squeeze/relax (Kegel) exercise at home. The Kegel exercise is practiced five sets per day. A set is accomplished by 20 cycles of 10 sec of squeezing the sphincter and puborectalis muscles, followed by 10-sec rest periods. These exercises should be done, at least initially, in a distraction-free environment.

Constipation patients with PPC must learn how *not* to contract these muscles during attempts to defecate. This exercise is called push. It is a simulated attempt to have a bowel movement (Valsalva maneuver) and must be done without any paradoxical contractions of the pelvic floor muscles. The push exercise is done only in session and when the patient is attempting to have a bowel movement. It is not practiced in the same sense as the Kegel exercise.

Patients are instructed to keep a daily log (Fig. 19.4) of the home practice of pelvic floor exercises, relaxation techniques, and general physical exercises, in addition to recording the occurrence of bowel movements, the use of cathartics, and the use of other medications. The log is carefully reviewed with the patient at the beginning of each session as part of the training and educational experience.

Physical exercise is required of all constipated patients, but is especially important for those with a stress-related feature to their problem. Physical exercise is helpful by increasing motility and is a very effective tool for stress reduction. Some constipated patients also receive a more global, total body relaxation type of biofeedback training and/or psychotherapy when indicated.

During subsequent sessions, once home practice of biofeedback exercises and charting have been reviewed, baseline EMG values at rest, squeeze, and push are taken. During the training portion of each session, standard biofeedback techniques such as shaping, motor copy, "coaching," generalization, and weaning from feedback will be employed as the patient learns to correctly discriminate among rest, squeeze, and push events. In addition to learning proper coordination of the pelvic floor muscles, patients may require coaching in a variety of related areas. These areas include proper physical posturing during defecation, reduced dependence on laxatives, digitation, and enemas, the need to reduce their preoccupation with bowel functioning, toileting schedules, stress management education and general relaxation training, physical exercise, and most importantly the cessation of straining with extreme intensity to defecate.

As patients begin to demonstrate improved control of pelvic floor dynamics, they are given support and encouragement to wean themselves off the use of laxatives and enemas. This step is often a difficult process and should be broached with gradually increasing persistence by the therapist. However, it is important that the patient have control of when and how fast this actually occurs. The patients are told that they will not be forced to give up what is working for them until it is replaced with something more effective—their biofeedback skills.

FIGURE 19.4 Weekly constipation record.

PATIENT NAME: ______________________ CCF #: ______________

DATE & TIME	UNASSIST BM	ENEMA ASST BM	LAXATIVE ASST BM		KEGEL X #/DAY	PHYS X #/DAY	RELAX X #/DAY	OTHER MEDICATIONS	OTHER COMMENTS
1)									
2)									
3)									
4)									
5)									
6)									
7)									
WEEKLY TOTALS									
PRE TX/ WEEK									

B.M DESCRIPTORS:

1) CONSISTENCY: H = HARD, A = AVERAGE, L = LOOSE
2) EVACUATION: C = COMPLETE, I = INCOMPLETE
3) DISCOMFORT: Y = YES, N = NO, S = SOMEWHAT

10 sec EMG values – Narrow (bp) DATE: __________

	rest	push	squeeze
BL	____	____	____
W/FB	____	____	____

Occasionally, it becomes evident that a patient will be unable to attend to instruction or they may have memory deficits that make learning new skills through biofeedback unlikely. Still other patients may be so anxious or depressed that pursuing biofeedback seems impractical. Some of these patients may benefit from individual psychotherapy or stress management biofeedback before proceeding with pelvic floor EMG biofeedback. In many cases, the MMPI has been helpful in identifying these patients.

Discharge from therapy will be determined by continued success and control of pelvic floor muscles as reflected by EMG and by reduction and resolution of constipation symptoms, as indicated by the patients' home charting. If patients demonstrate no improvement in EMG values or in reported bowel function, they are considered a treatment failure.

Patients are asked to return after 3 months from discharge for reevaluation to ensure that they continue to successfully control pelvic floor muscles and have unassisted bowel movements. Further training should not be necessary, however a few patients may want to continue meeting with the therapist once per year or every 6 months for reassurance.

SUGGESTED READINGS

Barnes P, Hawley P, Preston D, et al: Experience of posterior division of the puborectalis muscle in the management of chronic constipation. *Br J Surg* 72:475–477, 1985.

Beck DE, Jagelman DG, Fazio VW: The surgery of idiopathic constipation. *Gastroenterol Clin North Am* 16:143–156, 1987.

Bennings MA, Buler HA, Taminiau JA: Biofeedback training in chronic constipation. *Arch Dis Childhood* 68(1):126–129, 1993.

Bleijenberg G, Kuijpers H: Treatment of the spastic pelvic floor syndrome with biofeedback. *Dis Colon Rectum* 30(2):108–111, 1987.

Cerulli M, Nikoomanesh P, Shuster M: Progress in biofeedback conditioning for fecal incontinence. *Gastroenterol* 76:742–746, 1979.

Dahl J, Lindquist BL, Tysk C, et al: Behavioral medicine treatment in chronic constipation with paradoxical anal sphincter contraction. *Dis Colon Rectum* 34(9):769–776, 1991.

Devroede G, Gilles G, Bouchoucha M, et al: Idiopathic constipation by colonic dysfunction: relationship with personality and anxiety. *Dig Dis Sci* 34(9):1428–1433, 1989.

Engel B, Nikoomanesh P, Shuster M: Operant conditioning of rectosphincteric response in the treatment of fecal incontinence. *N Engl J Med* 290:646–649, 1974.

Halan R, Melling J, Womack N, et al: Treatment of anismus in intractable constipation with Botilium A toxin. *Lancet* 1:714–717, 1988.

Heymen JS, Wexner SD, Gulledge HD: MMPI assessment of patients with functional bowel disorders. *Dis Colon Rectum* 36(6):593–596, 1993.

Kawimba BM, Papachrysostomou M, Binnie NR, et al: Outlet obstruction (anismus) managed by biofeedback. *Gut* 32(10):1175–1179, 1991.

Kegel AH: Progressive exercise in the functional conditioning incontinence. *N Engl J Med* 290:646–649, 1948.

Keren S, Wagner Y, Heldenberg D, et al: Studies of manometric abnormalities of the rectoanal region during defecation in constipated and soiling children: modification through biofeedback therapy. *Am J Gastroenterol* 83(8):827–831, 1988.

Lestar B, Penninckx F, Kerremans R: Biofeedback defecation training for anismus. *Int J Colorect Dis* 6(4):202–207, 1991.

Loening-Baucke V: Persistence of chronic constipation in children after biofeedback treatment. *Dig Dis Sci* 36(2):153–160, 1991.

Loening-Baucke V: Modulation of abnormal defecation dynamics of biofeedback treatment in chronically constipated children with encopresis. *J Pediatrics* 116(2):214–221, 1990.

MacLeod JH: Management of anal incontinence by biofeedback. *Gastroenterol* 93:291–294, 1987.

Preston DM, Lennard-Jones JE: Anismus in chronic constipation. *Dig Dis Sci* 30:413–418, 1985.

Turnbull GK, Ritvo PG: Anal sphincter biofeedback relaxation treatment for women with intractable constipation symptoms. *Dis Colon Rectum* 35(6):530–536, 1992.

Wald A, Chandra R, Gabel S, et al: Evaluation of biofeedback in childhood encopresis. *J Pediatr Gastroenterol Nutr* 6:554–558, 1987.

Wasserman IF: Puborectalis syndrome. *Dis Colon Rectum* 7:87–98, 1964.

Wexner SD, Cheape JD, Jorge JM, et al: A prospective assessment of biofeedback for the treatment of paradoxical puborectalis contraction. *Dis Colon Rectum* 35(2):145–150, 1992.

Wexner SD, Daniel N, Jagelman DG: Colectomy for constipation: physiologic investigation is the key to success. *Dis Colon Rectum* 34:851–856, 1991.

Wexner SD, Jagelman DG: Chronic constipation. *Postgrad Adv Colorect Surg* 1(12):1–22, 1989.

CHAPTER 20

Urinary Incontinence: Evaluation and Diagnosis

Lindsey A. Kerr

No discussion of disorders of the anus and rectum is complete without reviewing lower urinary tract disorders. The function of both of these systems is similar, that is, the storage and complete expulsion of the body's waste products. Both systems receive autonomic as well as somatic innervation. This innervation arises from the same region of the spinal cord. Pathologic processes that have an effect on one of these organ systems have profound effects on the other. Understanding the relationship and similarities between the two leads to superior patient management and better clinical outcomes.

NORMAL URINARY TRACT FUNCTION

The bladder and outlet (also referred to as the vesicosphincteric unit) has two modes of operation. It is responsible for the storage and efficient release of urine. For adequate urinary storage to occur, urine must be accommodated in a sterile manner at low pressure (to protect the kidneys) in the presence of an outlet that remains closed during filling (to protect the skin). The outlet must be able to resist increases in abdominal pressure (e.g., coughing or lifting) by increasing its tone. The bladder must not contract prematurely and sensation must be intact so that one knows when the bladder is full and needs to be emptied. For efficient emptying to occur, the bladder must maintain a contraction of sufficient magnitude and duration to empty itself completely. The outlet must fully relax so that it does not interfere with the release of urine. There can be no anatomic obstruction at any point that impedes the flow of urine. Any alteration in this course of events will lead to storage failure or emptying failure.

The vesicosphincteric unit receives its innervation from sensory afferent as well as autonomic and somatic efferent. Both parasympathetic and sympathetic innervation is present. Parasympathetic innervation is derived from spinal segments S2 through S4 which reaches the vesicosphincteric unit primarily through the pelvic nerve. Parasympathetic preganglionic nicotinic receptors are in close proximity to the bladder and postganglionic muscarinic receptors are found within the bladder wall itself. Sympathetic innervation is derived from the thoracolumbar chain and reaches the vesicosphincteric unit via the inferior hypogastric plexus and hypogastric nerve. Adrenergic receptors are located within the bladder wall and smooth muscle sphincter as well at the level of the parasympathetic ganglia. Adrenergic innervation to the bladder body is primarily β in nature and facilitates bladder relaxation and urine storage during the filling phase. Innervation to the bladder base and smooth muscle sphincter is primarily α_1 and serves to increase tone, thus preventing untimely urinary loss. Adrenergic innervation to the parasympathetic ganglia is α_2 in nature and can be thought of as providing negative feedback to the parasympathetic ganglionic cells. Somatic innervation is provided to the striated sphincter via the pudendal nerve and results in sphincteric contractions.

Although the exact details of bladder filling and emptying have yet to be fully worked out, the following will serve as a model for discussing bladder testing and therapeutic intervention. During physiologic bladder filling there is accommodation of large volumes of urine with only a small increase in intravesical pressure. At the beginning of the storage phase this takes place in the absence of neuronal input and is thought to be secondary to the viscoelastic properties of the bladder wall itself (smooth muscle and connective tissue). Subsequently, there is sympathetic discharge to the bladder body to induce relaxation and to the smooth muscle sphincter to increase its tone as well as somatic discharge to the striated sphincter to increase its activity. Sympathetic discharge is also seen at the level of the parasympathetic ganglia, preventing premature discharge of the parasympathetics and bladder contraction. Other nonadrenergic, noncholinergic neurotransmitters are thought to be involved but are beyond the scope of discussion. The net result is accommodation of a large volume of urine at low pressure. When the bladder is full, intravesical pressure begins to rise and this results in the sensation of fullness. Cortical input helps delay bladder contraction and emptying until a socially acceptable place to do so is located. Subsequent bladder emptying is the result of coordinated activity at the level of the pons whereby sympathetic and somatic activity decreases while coordinated parasympathetic discharge is initiated. In the absence of outlet resistance, and in the presence of a coordinated bladder contraction, the bladder empties to completion and the cycle begins again.

The above discussion is a cursory overview of bladder dynamics, but will serve as a framework to discuss vesico/sphincteric dysfunction. By dividing the pathologic processes into two groups, based on emptying failure or storage failure, voiding dysfunction can be further simplified and readily understood.

URODYNAMIC TESTING

Urodynamic testing is used to evaluate bladder/sphincter function. There are a number of different tests and the choice of which ones to perform should be based on the patient's history and physical examination. In the ideal situation the testing itself should reproduce the patient's symptoms, although this is not always the case. Familiarity on the part of the operator with urodynamic techniques and findings aids in diagnostic accuracy and appropriate treatment plans. It is imperative that the operator perform these tests on a regular basis to remain facile as there is great latitude for alternative interpretations by the uninitiated. The following tests make up a urodynamic evaluation although all are not required in every patient:

(1) Cystometrogram (CMG)
(2) Electromyography (EMG)
(3) Uroflowmetry
(4) Urethral pressure profilometry (UPP)
(5) Leak point pressure (LPP)
(6) Cystography/voiding cystourethrography (VCUG)

All findings need to be interpreted in light of the patient history and physical.

EQUIPMENT

Most urodynamic laboratories are equipped with sophisticated multichannel urodynamic equipment that also has fluroscopic capability (videourodynamics) (Fig. 20.1). Certainly less expensive and less complicated equipment can provide useful information for treatment planning. The key is knowing what to choose when. Filling studies may be done with gas or liquid. The former is "cleaner" (fewer spills, etc.) the latter is more physiologic. Emptying studies require liquid. When video studies are done, radiopaque contrast is used.

CYSTOMETRY

Cystometry measures the change in bladder pressure for a given volume of infusate. It is used to quantitate storage parameters and helps to define the problems associated with storage failure. A small (10F or smaller) urodynamics catheter is placed in the bladder, the bladder is emptied of all urine and appropriate urine cultures are sent. For accuracy the bladder is filled via a constant rate infusion pump with or without the use of a weighted transducer to monitor fluid delivery. Gas infusion is done at a standard volume/minute as well. Typically for a fluid study this catheter has two ports (one sensing and one filling). For a gas study only one port is needed (fills and senses). A third port, located along the urethra may be used to monitor urethral pressure during the study. The bladder can be considered the "first channel" and the urethra the "third." A "second channel" may be added by monitoring intra-abdominal pressure via a rectal pressure sensing balloon. Because the vesical channel senses all pressure changes within the bladder it cannot differentiate between a pressure increase secondary to increased total abdominal pressure which presses on the bladder (i.e., laughing, coughing, straining, changing position) and that due to an intravesical event (i.e., a bladder contraction). If the abdominal channel reading is subtracted from the intravesical channel only true detrusor activity remains. This is referred to as a *subtracted detrusor pressure* and represents only bladder phenomena.

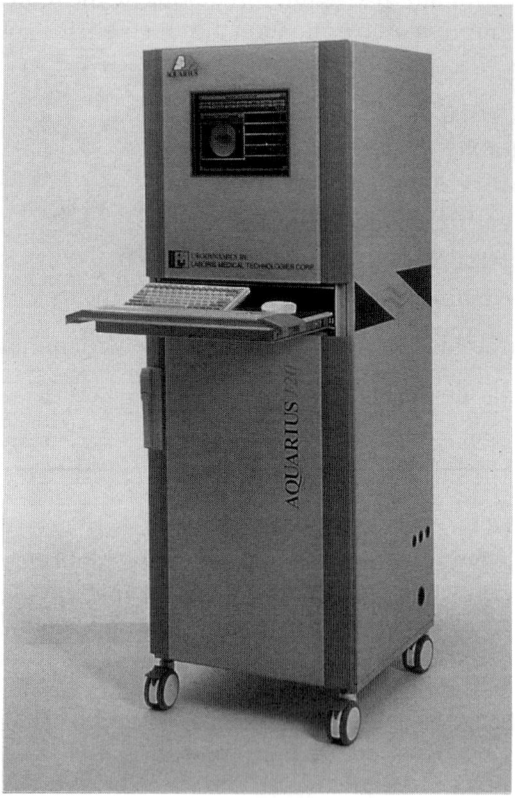

FIGURE 20.1 Example of a multichannel Urodynamics machine.

A normal filling cystometrogram is divided into three phases (Fig. 20.2). In the first phase intravesical pressure rises as filling ensues until resting detrusor pressure is reached. Thereafter intravesical pressure rises only slightly as bladder volume increases (phase 2). In the third phase of filling the pressure once again starts to rise, as the end of the bladder compliance curve is reached and the bladder can no longer stretch to accommodate volume. Contractions at this point in time can still be suppressed. Normal bladder capacity in the adult is 400–750 cc. During filling, subtracted detrusor pressure should rise less than 15 cm H_2O. If the filling rate is fast (e.g., 100–150 cc/min), higher intravesical volumes may not be tolerated and intravesical pressure may rise erroneously. Filling at physiologic rates (2–3 cc/min) would be far too time-consuming and so a compromise is reached by using inflow rates of $\geqslant$ 50 cc/min. It must be remembered that if gas is used, it is a compressible "fluid" and small changes in intravesical pressure may not be detected.

Increasing detrusor pressure greater than 15 cm H_2O is seen in fibrotic or contracted bladders with low compliance (Fig. 20.3). These patients often relate a history of outlet obstruction with detrusor hypertrophy, spinal cord injury or other suprasacral neurologic lesions, recurrent urinary tract infections, or radiation therapy. A rapid increase in intravesical pressure during filling associated with the urge to urinate is referred to as an *unstable bladder contraction* (Fig. 20.4).

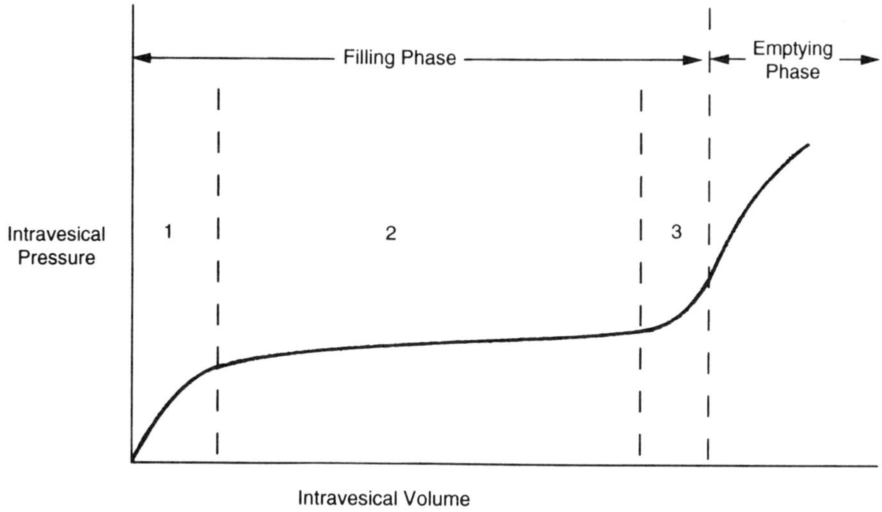

FIGURE 20.2 Normal filling cystometrogram plotting increase in intravesical pressure as a function of increasing intravesical volume. See text for details.

Patients exhibiting this pattern but with no known neurologic lesion are diagnosed with *detrusor instability*. The same phenomenon in those with neurologic deficits is called *detrusor hyperreflexia*. Increased compliance may be seen in certain pathologic states (diabetic cystopathy, infrasacral lesions) where detrusor decompensation has occurred and hyporeflexia or areflexia exists. The measured variables during testing are volume infused, recorded intravesical, abdominal, and subtracted detrusor pressure and bladder capacity. Compliance can be calculated at any given volume or for the whole filling phase from this information (change in volume/change in pressure in cc/cm H_2O). Contractility, the volume and pressure of the first sensation, and any sensation of urgency can be observed.

The fourth phase of the normal cystometrogram is really the emptying phase where a detrusor contraction is generated at the end of intravesical filling (Fig 20.2). This may be difficult to demonstrate in the supine position and may be voluntarily inhibited in any position. Usually a contraction can be initiated in the standing position in men and in the sitting position by use of a urodynamics commode in women. Its absence however does not reflect abnormal function as cortical suppression of detrusor contractions in the laboratory situation is common.

ELECTROMYOGRAPHY

Electromyography (EMG) measures the activity of the skeletal muscles of the pelvic floor. It is usually done in conjunction with CMG testing and yields information about urinary storage as well as emptying activity. When needle electrodes are used, monitoring of urethral sphincteric activity can be done directly. Unfortunately these are painful to place in most patients and so are usually reserved for

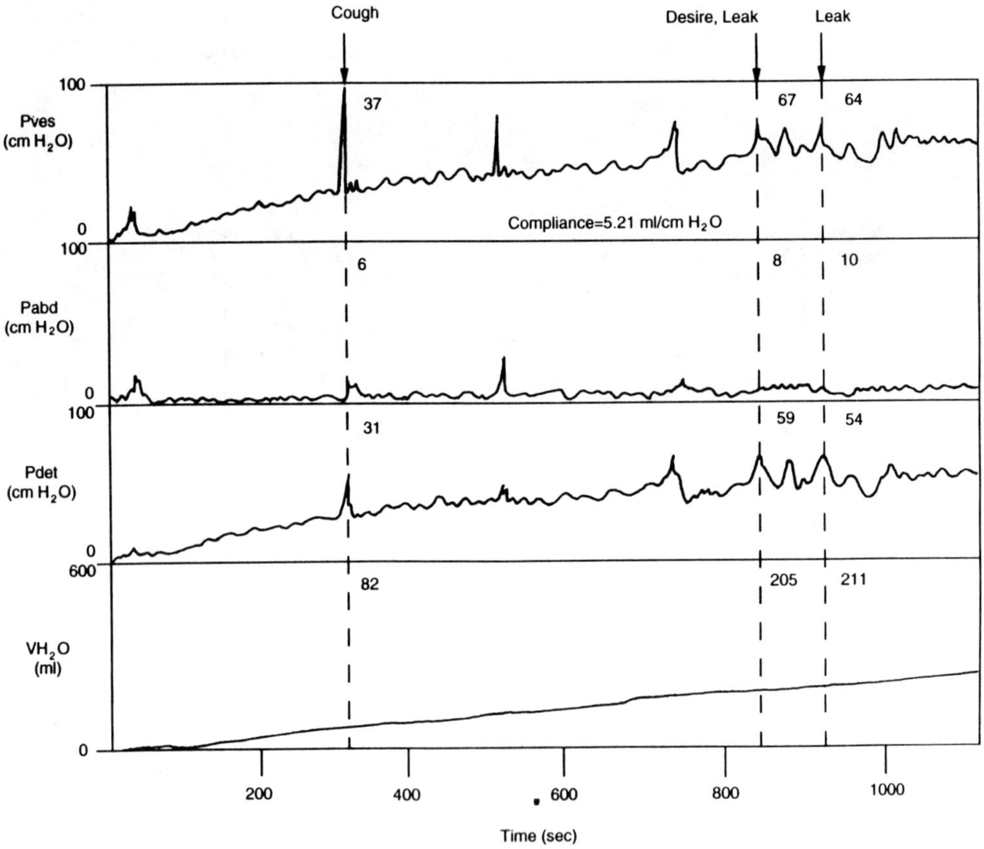

FIGURE 20.3 Filling cystometrogram from a patient with decreased bladder compliance. Pves – intravesical pressure in cm H_2O, Pabd = [intraabdominal pressure in cm H_2O. Pdet – subtracted detrusor pressure in cm H_2O (Pves – Pabd) reflecting true detrusor pressure. VH_2O – volume infusate in ml.] Note rapid increase in detrusor pressure with small increases in infused volume (= decreased compliance).

those with neurologic lesions and sensory deficits (e.g., spinal cord injury or spina bifida patients). Monitoring of neurologically intact patients is done with surface electrodes and it is inferred that their activity reflects that of the urethral sphincter. Sophisticated needle EMG testing requires an oscilloscope and neurophysiologist's interpretation. It is extraordinarily useful in neurologic patients as the deficits can be defined and denervation/renervation monitored. Motor unit action potentials can be recorded as well as fibrillation potentials (indicative of denervation) and positive sharp waves. Concentric needle electrodes are used where the outer needle is the reference electrode for the inner needle. When surface electrodes are used, they are placed just lateral to the anus for recording purposes with a reference electrode placed on an extremity. A vaginal sponge electrode or rectal sponge electrode are also options. EMG activity should be flat in the supine position with the exception of patient movement. A cough should increase EMG activity as sphincter tone rises to prevent urinary loss and is often used to check proper connections. A change to the upright position also results in increased EMG

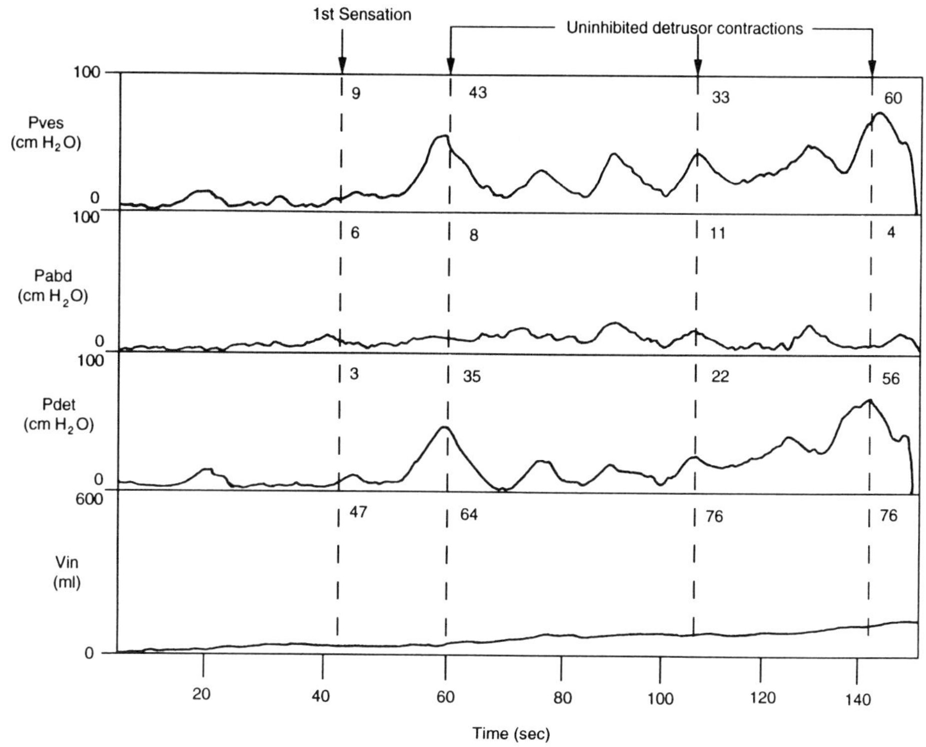

FIGURE 20.4 Filling cystometrogram from a patient with unstable detrusor contractions. Pves = intravesical pressure in cm H_2O Pabd = etc. see [above copy here]

Note spike of Pdet with increase in detrusor pressure up to 56 cm H_2O at a volume infused = 76 ml. These were associated with the urge to void.

activity. As filling increases, especially near capacity, EMG activity should correspondingly increase (guarding reflex). Just before a spontaneous detrusor contraction ensues, EMG activity should become silent again if the normal neuronal reflex loops are intact. In spinal cord injury patients, EMG activity may actually rise with a detrusor contraction. This is called *detrusor-striated sphincter dyssynergia* and can significantly impair bladder emptying (Fig. 20.5). *Pseudodyssynergia,* which resembles dyssynergia to the untrained eye, can also occur. It is seen in patients with detrusor instability or supraspinal lesions. The difference between pseudodyssynergia and dyssynergia is that EMG in pseudodyssynergia activity actually does silence just before the detrusor contraction and the subsequent increase in activity is an attempt on the part of the patient to voluntarily close the sphincter to prevent urinary loss. If one does not examine the CMG/EMG tracing closely, this subtle difference may be missed.

UROFLOW

Uroflow records the volume of urine expelled per unit time and is expressed in graph form plotting flow rate per elapsed time. It should be recorded electron-

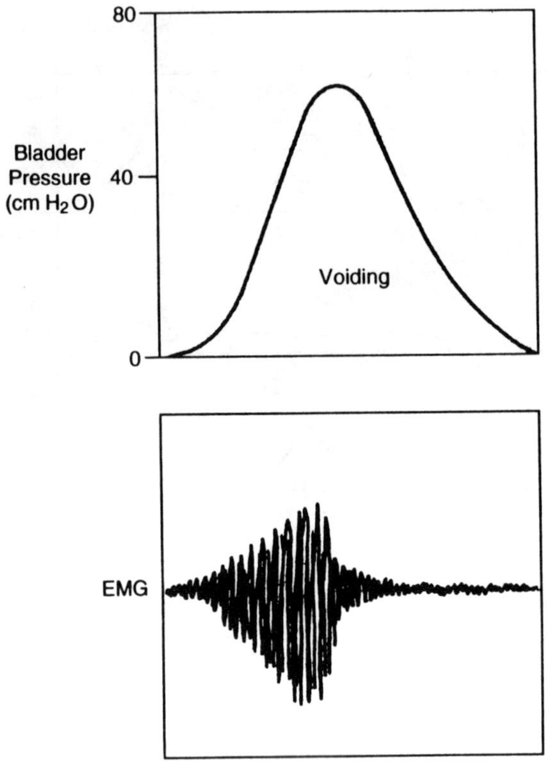

FIGURE 20.5 Detrusor Striated Sphincter Dyssynergia – Plot of Bladder pressure during diary voiding (top plot, in cm H_2O) and EMG activity of striated sphincter (bottom plot). Note increased EMG activity during first half of voiding attempt, reflecting Detrusor striated Sphincter dyssynergia.

ically and the following parameters measured or calculated: maximal flow rate, average flow rate, time to maximal flow, and flow time (Fig. 20.6). The time to maximal flow should be approximately one-third of the total voiding time and slightly less than one-half the volume of urine should be expelled during this time. Observation of the flow pattern is also important. For completeness, residual urine volume should be measured at the end of the study, either by straight catheterization or by bladder ultrasound. This value should be less than 25 cc. Flow rates are dependent on voided volume and a minimum of 150 cc should be expelled if the data is to be interpreted. Nomograms are available for flow rates based on sex, age, and voided volume. A normal flow rate and pattern is consistent with a normally functioning bladder and urethra (Fig. 20.6A). Mild benign prostatic enlargement or urethral stricture disease in the presence of a hypertrophied bladder will result in a normal peak flow rate, but prolonged flow time and decreased average flow. Patients with sphincteric incontinence (no anatomic obstruction) have short flow times and elevated flow rates (Fig. 20.6B). When patients use abdominal muscles (the so-called strain pattern), a seesaw pattern is produced (Fig. 20.6C). One cannot differentiate between poor flow due to anatomic obstruction and poor flow secondary to a hypocontractile bladder (e.g., diabetic cystopathy). In this situation the combination of cystometry and uroflow, a "pressure/flow study," is useful.

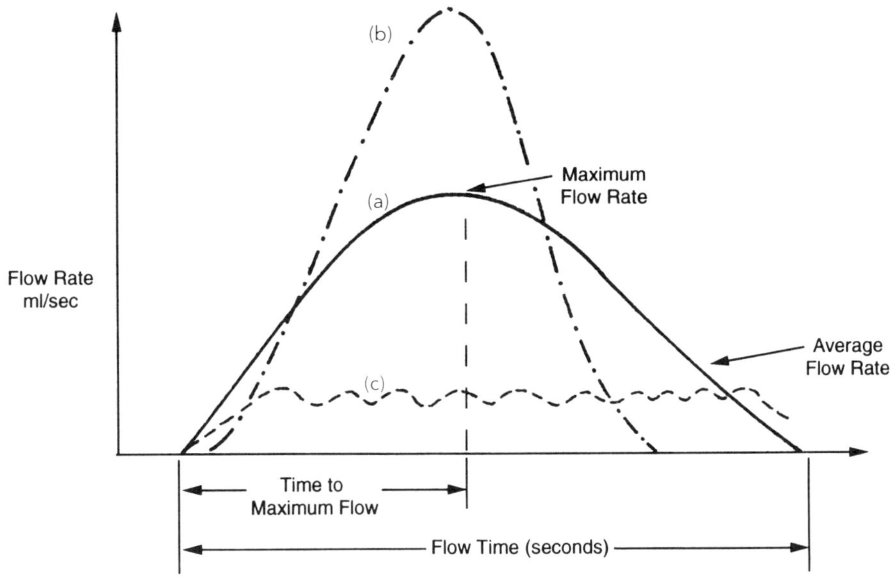

FIGURE 20.6 Uroflow Graph plotting flow time (x-axis) vs. flow rate (ml) (y-axis). Calculated parameters include time to maximum flow, (see), total flow time (in see), maximal flow rate, average flow rate. 6a: – (---) normal uroflow graph. 6b. (--.--.) plot from patient with sphincteric incontinence, with high peak and average flow, short maximal and total flow rates. c. (---) plot from patient with outlet obstruction with low peak and average flow, long maximal and total flow rates.

URETHRAL PRESSURE PROFILE

The urethral pressure profile (UPP) measures the passive and active tone of the urethra. Several technical options are available to record a UPP. A urodynamics catheter with two ports can be used for this test, one to monitor the bladder/urethral pressure and one for filling. Beginning in the bladder, the catheter is pulled at a constant rate through the urethra and the urethral pressure is recorded. A graph of urethral pressure versus length is generated. For infusion profilometry, the pressure generated represents the resistance to flow of the infusate as the urethra is distended. A second option for monitoring is a catheter tip transducer. These are infusion independent and may be more accurate but are fragile and costly. Urethral function itself and the mechanisms for continence are complicated and hotly debated topics. The UPP measures only limited aspects of this activity. Because the UPP is done in the static mode (neither during bladder filling or emptying) with the patient lying still on the table, it does not give any information as to urethral function during bladder cycling. The test cannot separate out contributions to continence from the striated versus the smooth muscle urethral sphincter versus the viscoelastic properties of the urethra. Without patient cooperation, the examiner cannot differentiate between active sphincter contraction and a sphincter at rest. Unfortunately, with little regard for its pitfalls, the urethral pressure profile is routinely used to describe urethral function and predict clinical outcome. Parameters measured include total urethral length, functional urethral

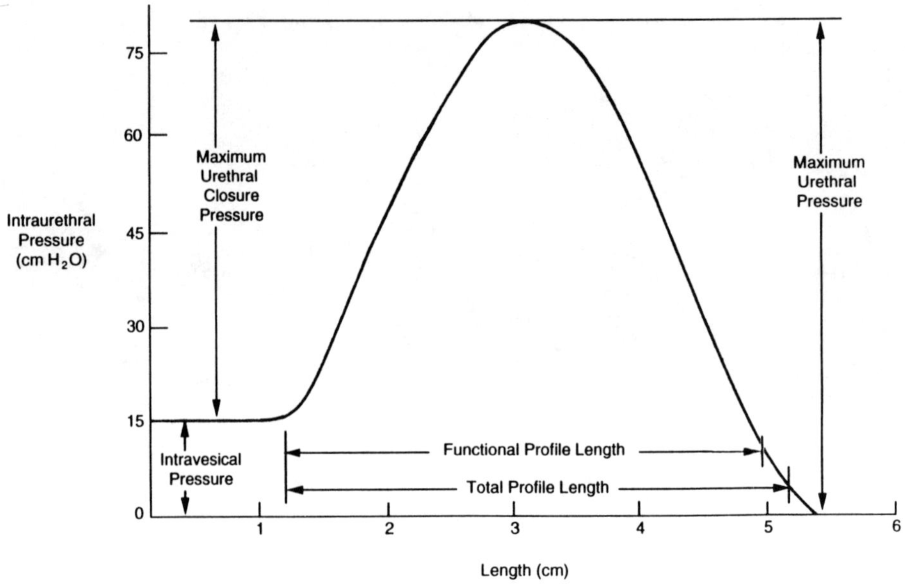

FIGURE 20.7 Urethral Pressure Profile from female patient. Plot of intraurethral pressure (cm H_2O) and urethral length (cm). Functional profile length of urethra where pressure is equal to or exceeds intravesical pressure. Maximal Urethral Closure Pressure = maximal urethral pressure − intravesical pressure.

length (the distance over which urethral pressure exceeds bladder pressure), maximal urethral pressure (the maximal pressure reached within the urethra), and maximal urethral closure pressure (the difference between the maximal urethral pressure and intravesical pressure). Representative curves of a female urethra and a male urethra are shown in Figures 20.7 and 20.8. The UPP is useful to compare pre- and postoperative changes in patients who have undergone surgical procedures for incontinence. In general, maximal urethral pressure decreases with age in females. High maximal closure pressure does not preclude incontinence and a significant number of patients with low closure pressure are dry. In males, functional length increases with age and reflects prostatic growth. The first peak in the male profile is secondary to the bladder neck and prostate, the second represents the external sphincter.

There are several variations on this test including the stress profile and the dynamic profile. Briefly, the stress profile requires a catheter tip transducer with two sensors, one of which remains in the bladder during the test. As the catheter is withdrawn at a constant rate, the patient is asked to cough in a rhythmic fashion. This cough pressure is transmitted equally to the bladder and urethra in female patients who are dry but not those with stress incontinence. The dynamic profile also requires microtip transducers and measures urethral response to filling, voiding, and various stress maneuvers. Its setup and interpretation are beyond the scope of the discussion here, but may be useful in diagnosing various dyssynergic states.

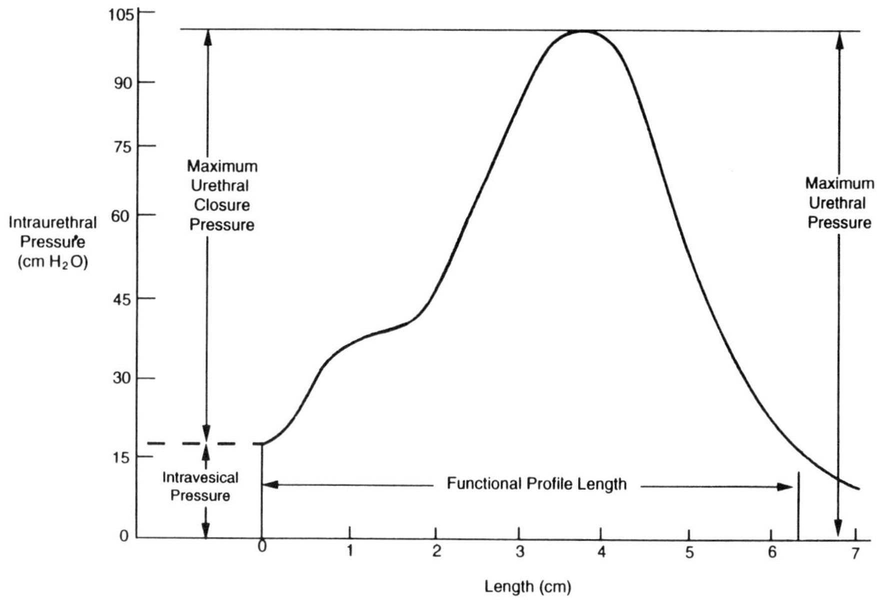

FIGURE 20.8 Urethral Pressure Profile for male patient. Plot of intraurethral pressure (cm H_2O) and urethral length (cm). Functional profile length is length of urethra where pressure is = to or exceeds intravesical pressure.

LEAK POINT PRESSURE

Leak point pressure (LPP) has been recently proposed as another measurement to define urethral function. It is most easily performed with the use of fluoroscopy and the recording of total vesical pressure by CMG. With the patient in the oblique position and the bladder filled to a specified volume (250 cc is suggested), the patient is asked to bear down and strain as if passing flatus. The pressure at which urine loss is visualized is recorded as the LPP. In the absence of urethral mobility or cystocele, a low leak point pressure reflects the inability of the urethra to coapt and prevent urinary loss at the time of increased total bladder pressure. In the spina bifida population, a variation of this test (using subtracted detrusor pressure) is used to predict upper tract deterioration. For this group of patients, bladder emptying only occurs by "leakage" in the absence of a normal sustained bladder contraction and urethral relaxation. A high subtracted detrusor LPP ($\geq$ 40 cm H_2O) can lead to renal failure secondary to reflux or upper tract obstruction. For the subtracted detrusor test, the patient is filled to capacity and the pressure at which leakage occurs is recorded. These two values as discussed above may be different. For non-neurogenic incontinent females, a leak point pressure that is less than 60 cm H_2O indicates poor urethral closure and the need to consider alternative therapy to bladder neck suspension, such as sling surgery, periurethral collagen, or artifical genitourinary sphincter placement. There is an equivocal range of 60 to 90 cm H_2O over which the diagnosis of urethral dysfunction needs to be entertained but where a bladder neck suspension may suffice. Male patients with urinary loss secondary to urethral sphincteric dysfunction (postprostatectomy being the most common cause) will also have a low leak point pressure and benefit from similar surgical considerations as female patients do. In patients with low leak point pressures and detrusor instability/hyperreflexia, the latter needs to be brought under control before treatment of the sphincteric insufficiency. If this is not done, intravesical pressures will be abnormally elevated at the time of an unstable contraction (leakage is prevented by the surgery) and this can lead to upper tract obstruction and deterioration.

VOIDING CYSTOURETHROGRAPHY

Voiding cystourethrography (VCUG) is an extraordinarily useful exam, especially in conjunction with CMG/EMG studies. Although this is an emptying study, it is very useful to observe the bladder flouroscopically during filling and stress maneuvers and record this information on videotape. Even static films of filling, strain maneuvers, and voiding can provide information of use to the urodynamicist.

Abnormal bladder configuration in the AP and oblique position can be noted and any bladder contractions can be observed. In female patients, urethral and bladder hypermobility with coughing or increases in intra-abdominal pressure can be recorded. This is useful in making the diagnosis of genuine stress urinary incontinence and planning surgical repair. In males, the observation of incontinence during stress maneuvers leads one to the diagnosis of sphincteric insufficiency. Conversely, detrusor/sphincter dyssynergic patients will fill their posterior urethra with no passage of contrast material during a bladder contraction because of simultaneous contraction of the sphincter and this can be noted. Fistulas and diverticula can be diagnosed as can vesicoureteral reflux. The fluoroscopic equipment required for this procedure is expensive and often these studies are done in conjunction with the radiology department. If standard nomenclature is used and the urologist and radiologist come to an agreement on the interpretation of the films, this arrangement is very reasonable.

SUGGESTED READINGS

McGuire EJ, Fitzpatrick CC, Wan J, et al: Clinical assessment of urethral sphincter function. *J Urol* 150:1452, 1993.

Siroky MB, Olsson CA, Krane RJ: The flow rate nomogram. 1. Development. *J Urol* 122:665, 1979.

Siroky MB, Olsson CA, Krane RJ: The flow rate nomogram. 2. Clinical correlation. *J Urol* 123:208, 1980.

Wein AJ, Barrett DM: *Voiding Function and Dysfunction*. Year Book Medical Publishers, 1988.

CHAPTER 21

Anorectal Ultrasound

Jeffrey Milsom

Endoluminal ultrasonography (ELUS) has rapidly become a popular technique for imaging the low rectum, anal sphincters, and pelvic floor in patients with a variety of anorectal diseases. In contrast to conventional transcutaneous ultrasonography, which uses externally placed transducers to image structures within the body cavities, ELUS places the transducer directly into a body cavity, within millimeters of the region of interest, thus allowing high levels of resolution and imaging quality with minimal patient discomfort. Although first utilized in the 1950s by Reid and Wild, this technique was not described again for anorectal imaging until the early 1980s, when it was primarily used for the staging of rectal cancers. Since then, it has emerged as a valuable test for evaluating the anatomical condition of the anal sphincters and pelvic floor. Current indications for anorectal ultrasonography include the following: (1) incontinence, both traumatic and idiopathic; (2) evaluation of complex perianal fistulae/abscesses; (3) staging of anal malignancies.

EQUIPMENT REQUIREMENTS

This examination can be performed in any standard patient examination room, or in the operating room as necessary. Currently, the Brüel & Kjær scanner type 3535 (Nærum, Denmark) with a rotating hand-held endoprobe (type 1850) is the most popular instrument in our clinic for endoluminal ultrasonography of the anal canal. Although different transducers are available, the 10-MHz transducer offers the highest resolution of the anal canal structures because its focal zone (the area of maximal resolution) is between 1 and 4 cm. The transducer itself should be covered with a hard plastic cone, thus allowing some distention of the anal canal around the transducer.

Preparation involves only a cleansing enema (phosphosoda, 45 ml immediately prior to the exam) if the patient does not have a tender anal canal. The examination takes only about 10 to 15 min, and if a comfortable digital anal examination can be done in the office, no analgesic medication or sedation is required. It is important that the hard plastic cone be completely purged of all air, because air will block sound waves and lead to aberrant images on the ultrasound screen. During the examination, the patient is placed in the left lateral decubitus position and the probe is passed blindly into the lower rectum for 6 to 8 cm, then the probe is slowly withdrawn into the anal canal. It may be necessary to pass the probe in and out of the anal canal several times during the examination, and images are recorded at the upper, mid, and lower anal canal for purposes of mapping the sphincters.

ULTRASOUND ANATOMY

There are six ultrasonographic layers of the anal canal starting from superficial to deep that have been described by Bartram: (1) a hyperechoic layer that is the interface of the cone or latex balloon with the tissues; (2) a hypoechoic layer that represents the mucosa; (3) a hyperechoic layer that represents the subepithelial tissues; (4) a hypoechoic layer that is the internal anal sphincter; (5) a hyperechoic layer that represents the intersphincteric plane and the longitudinal muscle of the sphincters; and (6) a layer of mixed echogenicity representing the external anal sphincter (striated muscle) (Fig. 21.1).

The upper, mid, and lower anal canal in many patients have distinguishing characteristics. In the upper anal canal, the external anal sphincter merges with the pelvic floor muscles, which may look U-shaped and hypoechoic. The vagina may also be seen at this point. In the mid anal canal, the external and internal anal sphincters are well visualized. The lower anal canal contains the subcutaneous portion of the external anal sphincter, and it is in this area where the intersphincteric plane may be most easily seen. By convention, each of these areas should be imaged when performing anal ultrasonography. When performing ultrasonography for anal fistulous disease, highlighting of the fistulous tract may be achieved by injection of the external opening of the fistula with a small amount of hydrogen peroxide. This may be accomplished by placement of a small mushroom catheter into the external opening of the fistula, or by placing a blunt tipped needle into the sinus tract. The fistulous tract appears as a bright or hyperechoic streak during anal endoluminal ultrasound imaging.

Further highlighting of the boundaries of the anal sphincter in a woman may be achieved by placement of the index finger into the vagina and pressing on the posterior wall. The phalanx of the examiner is then highlighted as a hyperechoic U-shaped ridge, which can be used to delineate the posterior vaginal wall. This may otherwise not be highlighted ultrasonographically because the vagina may be poorly visualized secondary to air entrapped within it.

Finally, in considering appropriate equipment for endoluminal ultrasonography, there may be an advantage to obtaining some longitudinal images, particularly in instances of a complex sphincteric injury, fistulous tract, or malignancy. The Brüel & Kjær sector probe 8551 provides this ability, and additionally allows for multiplanar imaging by simply turning a switch on the probe handle. We have used this with great success in performing longitudinal ultrasounds of the anal

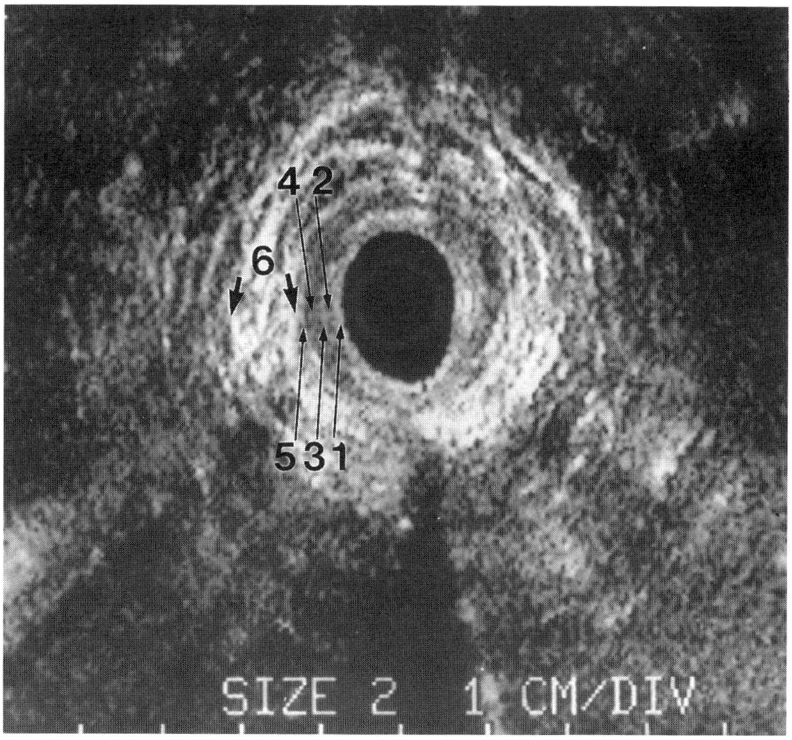

FIGURE 21.1 The six ultrasonographic layers of the anal canal are depicted: *1.* Hyperechoic (*white*) interface of the plastic cone or latex balloon of the ultrasound instrument with the tissues. *2.* Hypoechoic (*dark*) layer representing the mucosa. *3.* Hyperechoic layer representing the subepithelial tissues. *4.* Hypoechoic layer representing the internal anal sphincter. *5.* Hyperechoic layer representing the intersphincteric plane and the longitudinal muscle. *6.* A thick layer of mixed echogenicity representing the external anal sphincter.

canal, and the probe itself is equipped with a needle guide if ultrasound-guided biopsies are deemed advisable. The needle used is an 18-gauge spring-loaded core biopsy needle (Microvasive, Watertown, Mass.).

RESULTS

Use of endoluminal ultrasound for incontinence has been highly satisfactory, and, in a study performed at the Cleveland Clinic, 11 patients undergoing both electromyography (EMG) and anal ELUS felt ELUS was considerably less painful, and the examination by ELUS led to equal if not better accuracy in mapping sphincteric defects compared with EMG. Unsuspected anal sphincteric damage has been noted in a significant number of patients considered to have idiopathic incontinence. Multiple sphincteric defects may also be readily demonstrated using endoluminal ultrasonography (Fig. 21.2).

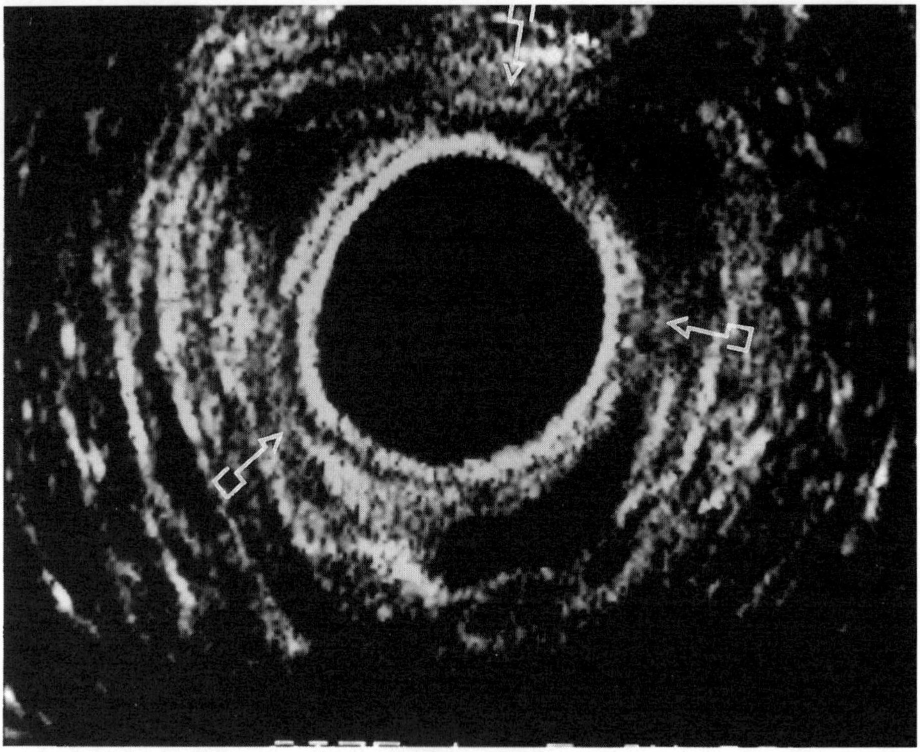

FIGURE 21.2 This anal ultrasound image depicts multiple defects of the internal anal sphincter (IAS) secondary to previous hemorrhoid surgery (*arrows* point to markedly thinned IAS)

ELUS may be useful in assessing complex and recurrent fistulae, in part because of the useful information that anal ultrasonography provides regarding the relationship of the tract to the anal sphincters.

Squamous cell cancers of the anus have also been evaluated using anal ultrasonography, and anal ultrasonography can accurately assess tumor penetration beyond the muscular wall of the anus, as well as invasion into adjacent organs. Enlarged lymph nodes in the pelvis may also be visualized using endoluminal ultrasound.

Finally, anal ultrasonography may play a role in the evaluation of patients with congenital abnormalities, particularly in identifying the sphincteric mechanism following operations for imperforate anus.

CONCLUSIONS

The use of ELUS in the anal region is primarily to evaluate patients with incontinence, either traumatic or idiopathic. Anal ultrasonography is appealing for a number of reasons: (1) it is noninvasive and involves no irradiation; (2) it is usually a procedure performed in the office setting, but can be used in concert with the surgical procedure in the operating room; (3) the ultrasound test is relatively economical and well-tolerated by most patients.

It has gained an important position as a diagnostic test in the evaluation of the anatomical condition of the anal sphincters. It appears to be less painful than electromyography, and is superior to electromyography in identifying defects in the external anal sphincter. Endosonography may complement nerve conduction studies, and it has been proposed to be the only other test needed besides physical examination to evaluate incontinence. It is the only test currently available to evaluate the status of the internal anal sphincter.

Its ultimate role in the evaluation of certain anal conditions is likely to improve with improvements in ultrasound technology, which are on the horizon. This will especially hold true as clinicians and ultrasonographers become more familiar with the performance of ELUS studies.

SUGGESTED READINGS

Bartram CI, Burnett SJD: *Atlas of Anal Endosonography*. Oxford, Butterworth-Heinemann, 1991, p 1.

Burnett SJ, Spence-Jones C, Spearman CT, et al: Unsuspected sphincter damage following childbirth revealed by anal endosonography. *Br J Radiol* 64:225–227, 1991.

Cheong DM, Nogueras JJ, Wexner SD, et al: Anal endosonography for recurrent anal fistulas: image enhancement with hydrogen peroxide. *Dis Colon Rectum* 36:1158–1160, 1993.

Law PJ, Kamm MA, Bartram CI: A comparison between electromyography and anal endosonography in mapping external anal sphincter defects. *Dis Colon Rectum* 33:370–373, 1990.

Law PJ, Talbot RW, Bartram CI, et al: Anal endosonography in the evaluation of perianal sepsis and fistula in ano. *Br J Surg* 76:752–755, 1989.

Nielsen MB, Hauge C, Pedersen JF, et al: Endosonographic evaluation of patients with anal incontinence: findings and influence on surgical management. *AJR* 160:771–775, 1993.

Nielsen MB, Pedersen JF, Hauge C, et al: Endosonography of the anal sphincter: findings in healthy volunteers. *AJR* 157:1199–1202, 1991.

Speakman CT, Burnett SJ, Kamm MA, et al: Sphincter injury after anal dilatation demonstrated by anal endosonography. *Br J Surg* 78:1429–1430, 1991.

Tjandra JJ, Milsom JW, Schroeder T, et al: Endoluminal ultrasound is preferable to electromyography in mapping anal sphincteric defects. *Dis Colon Rectum* 36:689–692, 1993.

Tjandra JJ, Milsom JW, Stolfi VM, et al: Endoluminal ultrasound defines anatomy of the anal canal and pelvic floor. *Dis Colon Rectum* 35:465–470, 1992.

CHAPTER 22

An Algorithm for Constipation

Lee E. Smith

This chapter is designed to outline an approach to the evaluation of defecation disorders. Our goal is to define the etiology of either difficult evacuation or infrequent stools. Usually these problems are caused by either a motility disorder of the colon or small bowel, or an outlet problem due to a pelvic floor disorder. An orderly series of steps will be provided to help define the appropriate physiological tests needed to define the etiology of the defecation disorder.

Many of these patients have problems with quality of life and are anxious to have treatment without going through the proper steps. It is important to go through the process until a possible answer is evident. In general the series is begun with easy, noninvasive investigations and becomes more complicated and costly as the process proceeds. The protocol should be conducted over an extended period of time so that the stability of symptoms and the patient's emotions may be evaluated. By embarking upon less invasive tests and treatments first, time may be gained. Emotional disorders merit psychological evaluation.

Normal is not completely understood. Continence and defecation represent a complex series of integrated neural and muscular activities in which both the autonomic and central nervous systems act upon a combination of smooth and striated muscles. One or more parts of this complex series of activities may be dysfunctional. Sometimes the abnormality is simple and management can be directed easily (Example: An inadequate fluid intake merits an increased fluid intake). At other times the abnormality is more complex and involves more than one element of dysfunction (Example: An inadequate fluid intake plus a pelvic floor disorder). The percentage of improvement can be expected to be related to the percentage of the corrected abnormality. Often, an emotional component overlies a physical abnormality and despite correction of the physical problem, the emotional problem if not identified and corrected, will cause dysfunction to persist. Sometimes both a motility and an outlet obstruction exist together and again both may need to be corrected to achieve good functional results.

The approach consists of four steps.

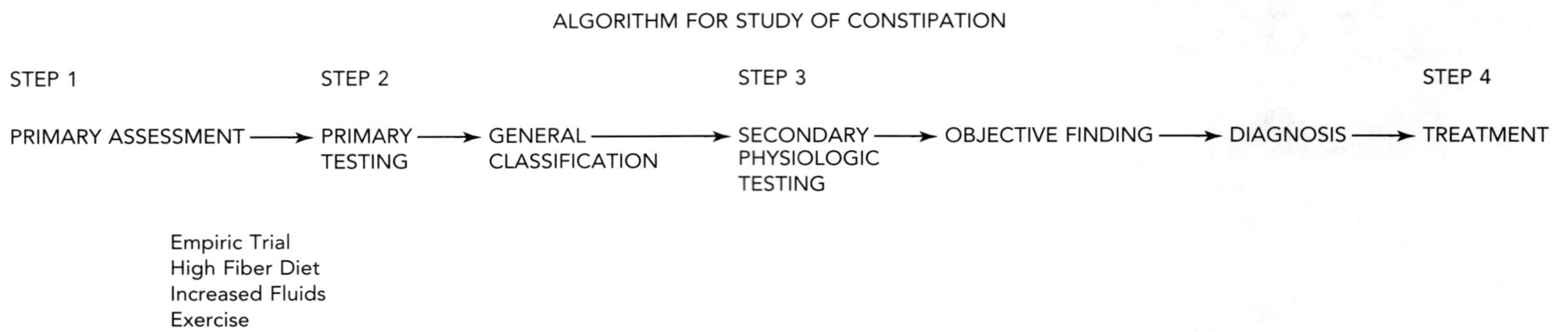

FIGURE 22.1 General steps for categories

In Figure 22.1 the general steps and categories are shown. In Step 1 the primary assessment is performed, which includes the history, physical, endoscopy, barium enema, and selected laboratory studies. Step 1 leads to Step 2, Primary Testing. Primary Testing is the series of basic, noninvasive physiological tests used to sort patients into a General Classification. The two broad classifications are evacuation and motility disorders. These classifications are further sorted at Step 3, where more invasive physiological tests reveal Objective Findings. Findings, in turn, lead to a Diagnosis. Finally, the Diagnosis directs Treatment, Step 4. Some of the history, physical, endoscopy, roentgenogram, and laboratory studies in Step 1 lead directly to a Finding and Diagnosis (see Fig. 22.2).

Observe that Psychological Evaluation is listed under Primary Assessment. Many patients have psychological problems and if these are detected early an extensive workup may be avoided. Most patients will deny anxiety, stress, and emotional disorders. Through psychological testing, personality and emotional profiles may point out aberrant characteristics that are important to correct before proceeding to a more extensive workup.

Step 1, the Primary Assessment, can be performed by any primary care physician who has patients presenting with constipation. Often by taking a history and performing a physical examination, a working diagnosis can be sorted out as to whether an outlet obstruction or a motility problem is the basic disorder. Certain conditions associated with constipation can be revealed by careful interview: For example, some drugs (such as narcotics, anticonvulsants, calcium channel blockers, anticholinergics, and antidepressants) are constipating. These drugs should be substituted or discontinued. Endocrine, neurologic, metabolic, and psychologic disorders may already be known. These may be the sole source of the constipation. Calcium and thyroid function tests may give clues to disorders that cause secondary constipation.

The key findings of the physical examination include determining whether there are neurological disorders and whether the colon, rectum, and anus are free of organic disease. Specific clues must be sought by inspection, digital examination, anoscopy, sigmoidoscopy, barium enema, and/or colonoscopy. These examinations may have already been performed during the patient's pilgrimage through other doctors to reach you (see Chapter 2 for details). If there is not an obvious disease or disorder, outline a management regimen to include dietary fiber (30 gm or more per day), increase fluids (8 oz every 2 hr while awake), and exercise to tolerance. A small enema or glycerin suppository may be advised to promote the bowel movement. Most patients should go through this management routine prior to proceeding to Step 2, at which point physiological tests are used.

Figure 22.3 isolates the steps and categories that apply to evacuation disorders and motility disorders. Step 2 entails a panel of physiological tests that generally categorize the type of constipation. Three tests are included: balloon evacuation, transit time, and manometry. These three relative noninvasive tests determine the general classification, i.e., whether there is a motility disorder or an evacuation disorder. Biofeedback might be enlisted at this point if the diagnosis is subdivided into the outlet group. In an elderly or poor risk patient this may be all that is necessary and appropriate. See Chapters 18 and 19 for the method.

Balloon evacuation is a method for grossly determining whether there is difficulty evacuating. A 50-cc Foley balloon is filled within the rectum and the patient is asked to evacuate it. Failure to achieve this suggests an outlet disorder.

ALGORITHM FOR STUDY OF CONSTIPATION

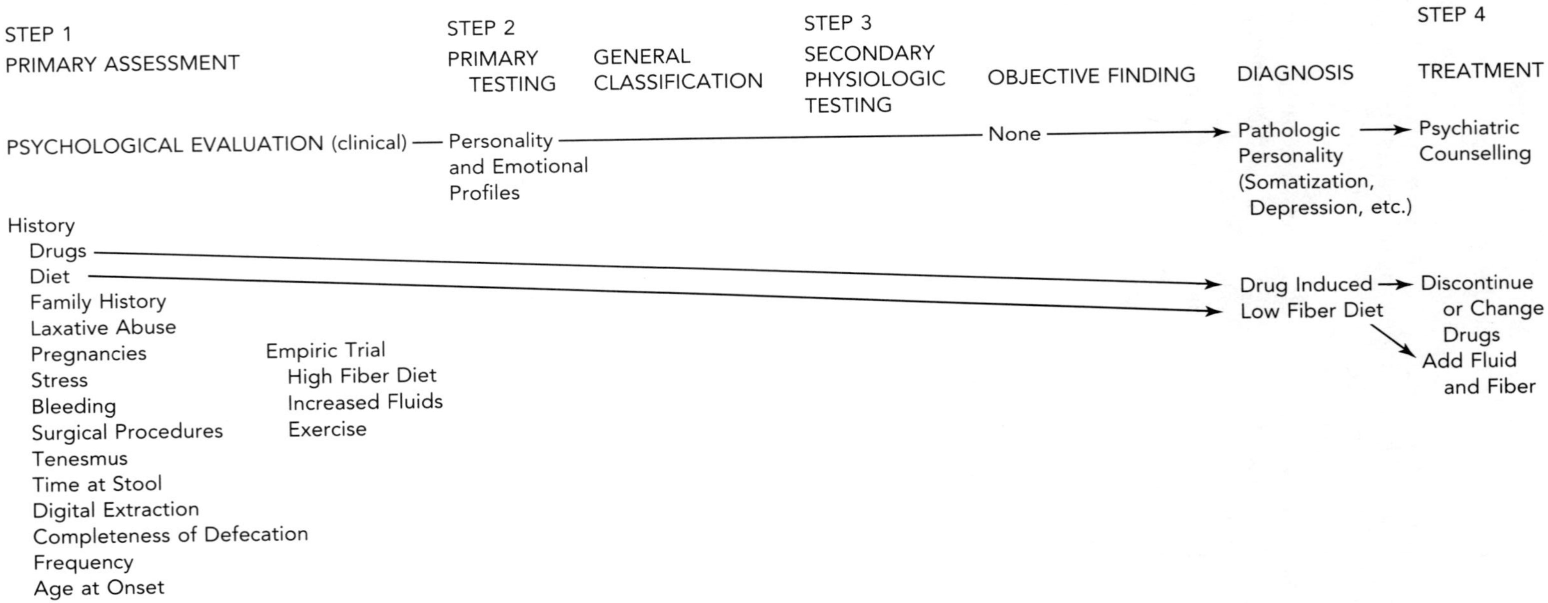

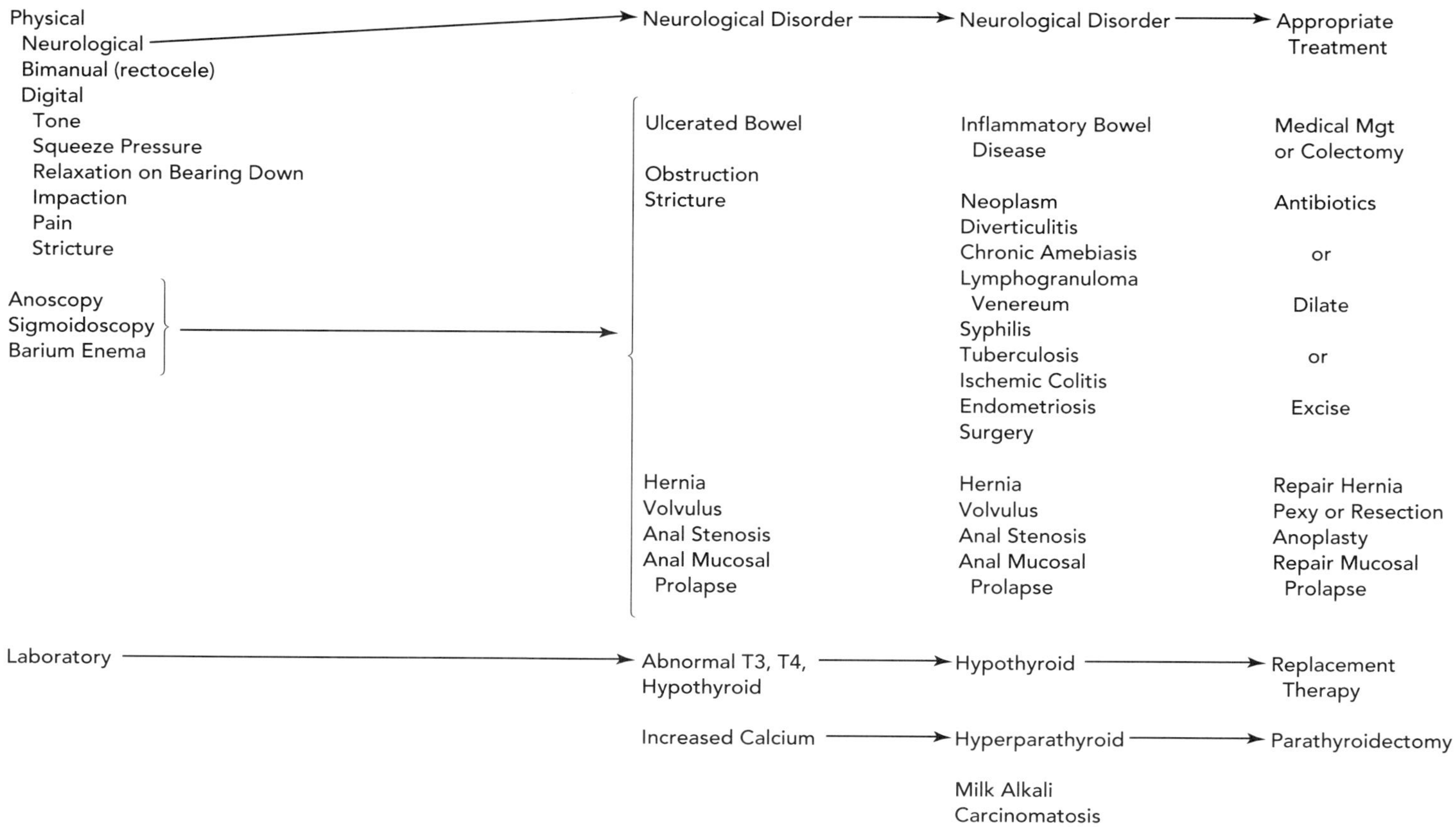

FIGURE 22.2 Findings and diagnosis leading directly from primary assessment.

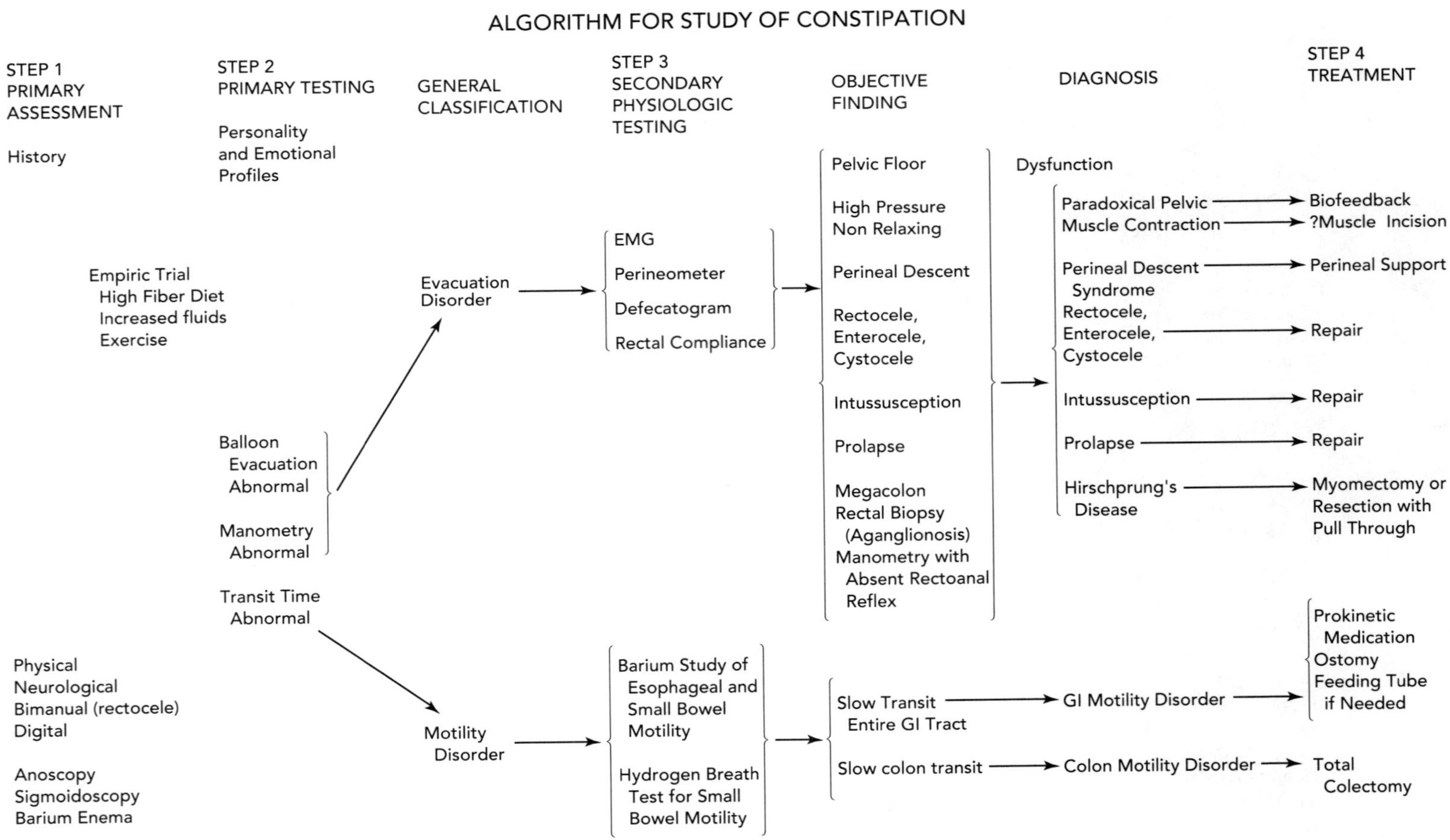

FIGURE 22.3 Disorders defined by physiological testing.

Having classified the disorder, secondary physiological tests may be used. If hypomotility is diagnosed, testing must be directed to determine the segment of the intestinal tract responsible. Hypomotility may be confined to the colon, the upper intestinal tract, or both. A simple upper intestinal barium study might provide a clue as to an esophageal or gastric motility abnormality. A hydrogen breath test might help determine motility from the mouth to the cecum. Of course, total gastrointestinal hypomotility precludes surgical intervention.

The electromyelogram verifies the nonrelaxing sphincter, which is consistent with paradoxical pelvic muscle contraction (see Chapter 13). This is also referred to as anismus. The standard EMG, pudenal nerve terminal motor latency, or the single-fiber EMG points out a neuropathy which is often associated with pelvic floor descent (see Chapter 13). If the patient has an obvious mechanical obstruction problem, the approach may be surgical. If it is not obviously mechanical, reconsider psychiatric counseling, continue dietary management, and biofeedback (see Chapter 19). In patients who have symptoms of an outlet obstruction, the diagnosis may be reached by defecography. This test may better define a mechanical disorder such as intussusception, rectocele, perineal descent, or a nonrelaxing puborectalis muscle.

Step 4 is the treatment of the diagnosed disorder or disease. However, medical management or surgical techniques for the management of disorders that are diagnosed are beyond the scope of this manual. The exception is biofeedback, which is a physiologic technique applied to the anorectum. The algorithm is given in its entirety in Figure 22.4.

The algorithm is designed to guide the physician to a more precise diagnosis and treatment. In recent years better diagnosis has minimized the errors and directed an appropriate therapy. Most patients will respond to the dietary, exercise, fluid, biofeedback, perineal support, and/or prokinetic agent regimen. However, surgery such as local anorectal procedures, rectocele repair, prolapse repair, perineal support procedures, colectomy, subtotal colectomy, anorectal myomectomy, and total colectomy with pull-throughs have a proper place in the treatment scheme.

Three examples will be followed through: (1) prolapse; (2) paradoxical pelvic muscle contraction (anismus); and (3) colonic hypomotility.

PROLAPSE IN A 55-YEAR-OLD FEMALE

Step 1: Primary Assessment

The history reveals inability to empty the rectum. The patient sits at length on the toilet and strains. Laxatives are sometimes helpful, and many laxatives have been tried without success. Manual extraction is sometimes attempted. Physical examination and laboratory studies are unrevealing. A trial of high-fiber diet, exercise, and fluid intake improved but did not resolve the problem.

Step 2: Primary Testing

The failed balloon evacuation is abnormal. Manometry and the transit time are normal. An outlet obstruction is the working diagnosis, (The General Classification in Evacuation Disorder).

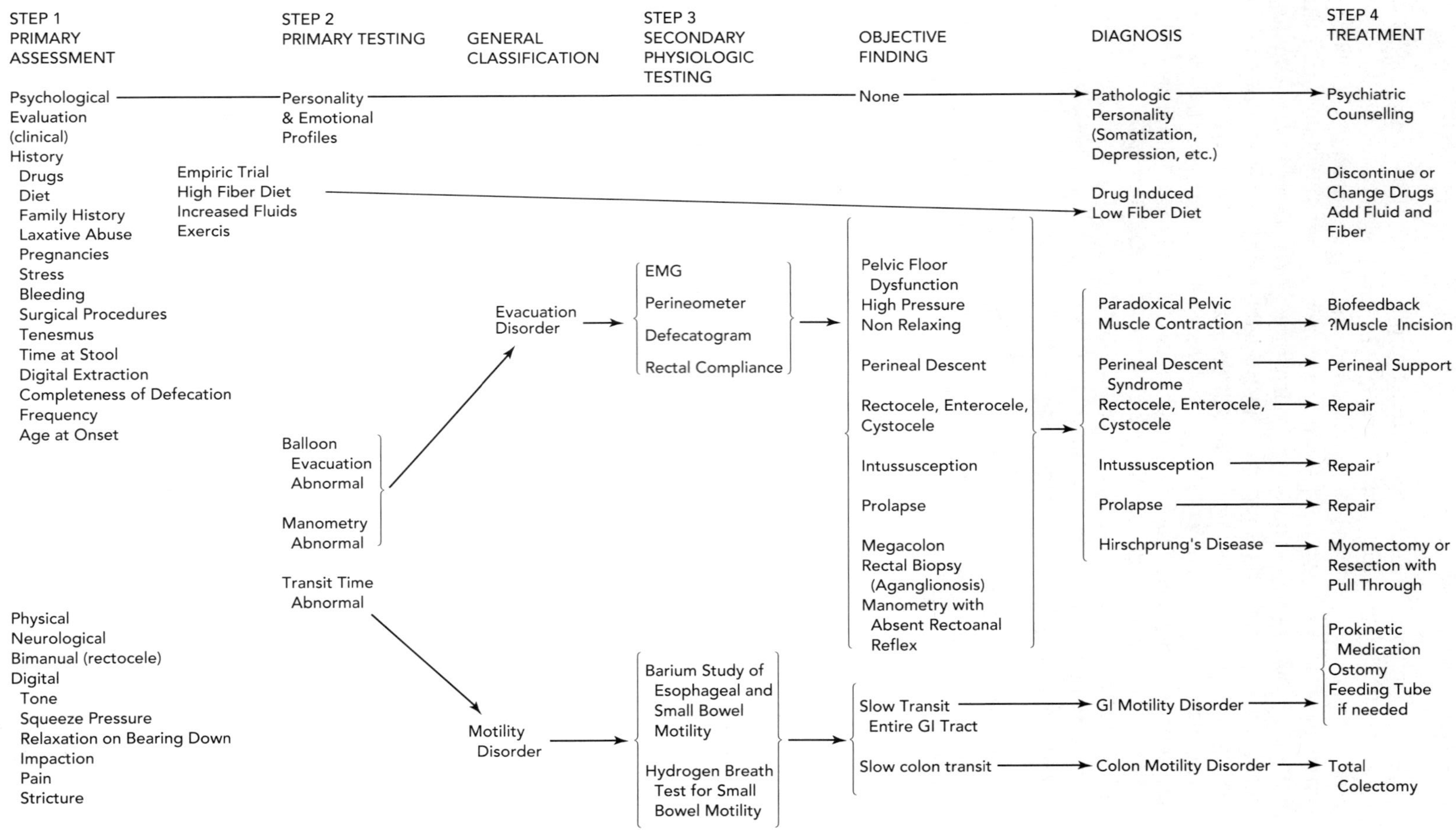
STEP 1
PRIMARY
ASSESSMENT
STEP 2
PRIMARY TESTING
GENERAL
CLASSIFICATION
STEP 3
SECONDARY
PHYSIOLOGIC
TESTING
OBJECTIVE
FINDING
DIAGNOSIS
STEP 4
TREATMENT
Psychological
Evaluation
(clinical)
Personality
& Emotional
Profiles
None
Pathologic
Personality
(Somatization,
Depression, etc.)
Psychiatric
Counselling
History
Drugs
Diet
Family History
Laxative Abuse
Pregnancies
Stress
Bleeding
Surgical Procedures
Tenesmus
Time at Stool
Digital Extraction
Completeness of Defecation
Frequency
Age at Onset
Empiric Trial
High Fiber Diet
Increased Fluids
Exercis
Drug Induced
Low Fiber Diet
Discontinue or
Change Drugs
Add Fluid and
Fiber
Balloon
Evacuation
Abnormal
Manometry
Abnormal
Evacuation
Disorder
EMG
Perineometer
Defecatogram
Rectal Compliance
Pelvic Floor
Dysfunction
High Pressure
Non Relaxing
Perineal Descent
Rectocele, Enterocele,
Cystocele
Intussusception
Prolapse
Megacolon
Rectal Biopsy
(Aganglionosis)
Manometry with
Absent Rectoanal
Reflex
Paradoxical Pelvic
Muscle Contraction
Biofeedback
?Muscle Incision
Perineal Descent
Syndrome
Perineal Support
Rectocele, Enterocele,
Cystocele
Repair
Intussusception
Repair
Prolapse
Repair
Hirschprung's Disease
Myomectomy or
Resection with
Pull Through
Transit Time
Abnormal
Physical
Neurological
Bimanual (rectocele)
Digital
Tone
Squeeze Pressure
Relaxation on Bearing Down
Impaction
Pain
Stricture
Motility
Disorder
Barium Study of
Esophageal and
Small Bowel
Motility
Hydrogen Breath
Test for Small
Bowel Motility
Slow Transit
Entire GI Tract
GI Motility Disorder
Prokinetic
Medication
Ostomy
Feeding Tube
if needed
Slow colon transit
Colon Motility Disorder
Total
Colectomy

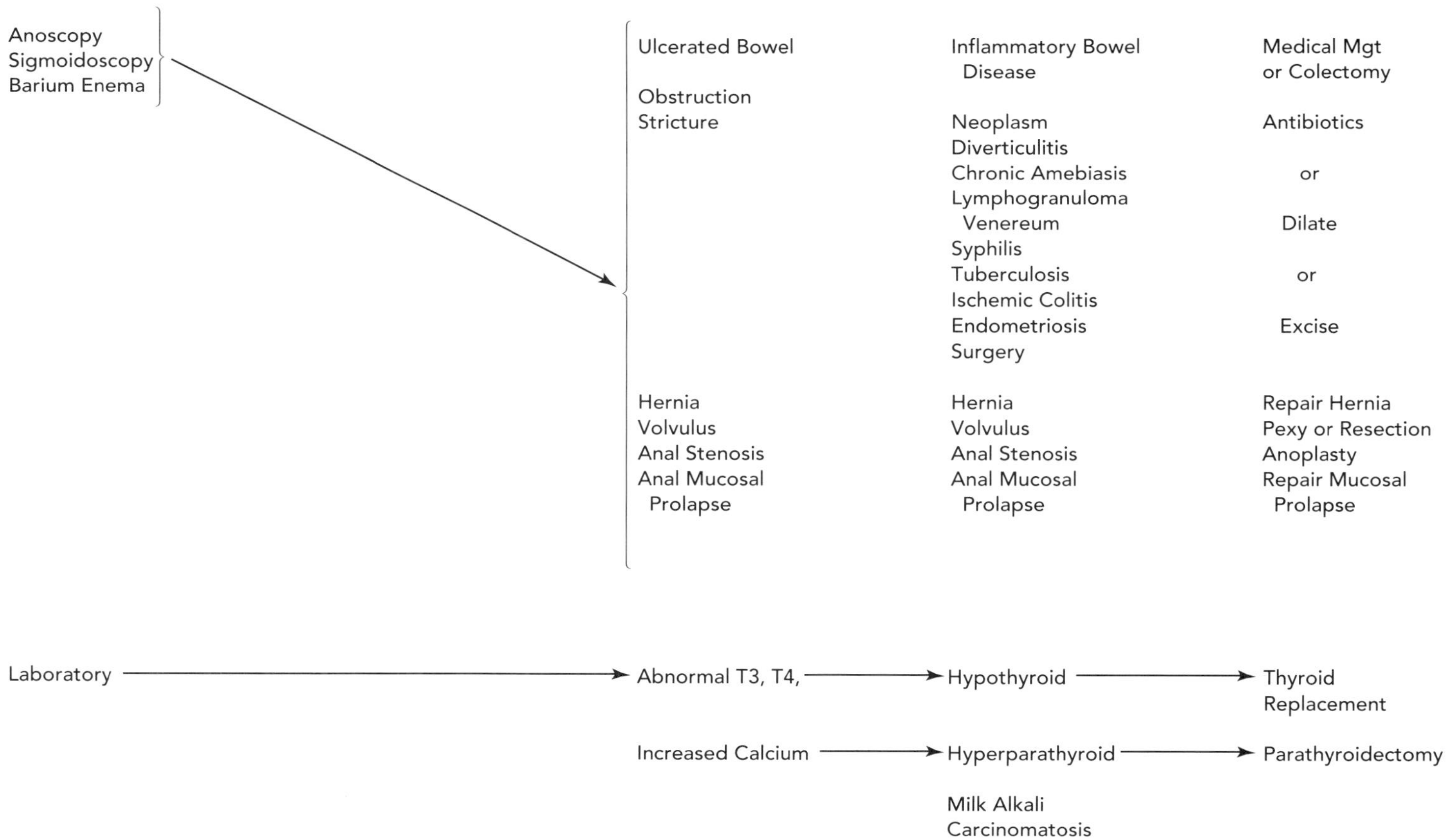

FIGURE 22.4 Algorithm for study of constipation.

Step 3: Secondary Physiological Testing

The defecatogram is abnormal, showing the internal prolapse and rectocele plus inability to empty completely. Yet, the anal canal opens appropriately. The electromyogram may be skipped if the sphincter is manometrically normal.

Step 4: Treatment

Repair the diagnosed prolapse and rectocele.

PARADOXICAL PELVIC MUSCLE CONTRACTION (ANISMUS) IN A 39-YEAR-OLD MALE

Step 1: Primary Assessment

The history reveals a feeling of incomplete emptying, long times on the toilet with straining, and attempts to manually remove the stool. Laxatives and enemas are tried often. Physical examination reveals a very tightly contracted anal sphincter. Barium enema sigmoidoscopy and laboratory studies are normal.

Step 2: Primary Testing

Manometry reveals increased resting pressure and a high voluntary squeeze pressure. Spiking slow waves and large ultra slow waves can be seen. The transit time is normal. Failure at balloon evacuation signaled an evacuation disorder (General Classification).

Step 3: Secondary Physiological Testing

The defecatogram shows no relaxation of the puborectalis muscle or external sphincter while straining to evacuate. In fact, it appears that the anorectal angle becomes more acute. Most of the barium is retained. The working diagnosis, paradoxical pelvic muscle contraction, can be confirmed by electromyogram. This EMG will not show the external sphincter to be electrically quiet when the attempt to strain as if to defecate is made.

Step 4: Treatment

Biofeedback may be used to attempt reeducation of the sphincter mechanism toward relaxation and promotion of proper defecation.

HYPOTONIA (INERTIA) OF THE COLON IN A 25-YEAR-OLD WOMAN

Step 1: Primary Assessment

The chief complaint is hard stools coming only once every week. Laxatives and enemas are required to have a bowel movement. The physical and laboratory examination are normal. The barium enema shows a long redundant colon.

Step 2: Primary Testing

The manometry and balloon evacuation are normal. The transit time is prolonged; thus the General Classification is a motility disorder.

Step 3: Secondary Physiological Testing

The barium swallow and the small bowel follow-through reveal a normal upper gastrointestinal transit time, hence, the diagnosis is a colonic motility disorder.

Step 4: Treatment

A total colectomy with an ileoproctostomy cures the problem.

CHAPTER 23

Fecal Incontinence: Evaluation

Bruce A. Orkin

INTRODUCTION

The goal of this chapter is to suggest how the physiological tests described in this manual may be used to clarify the pathogenesis of fecal incontinence and, in so doing, how they may help to direct therapy. As with constipation, incontinence is really a symptom, not a disease. The actual causes of fecal incontinence are quite varied and include direct injuries to the muscular structures, congenital disorders, systemic and metabolic diseases, acquired neurological deficits, and diseases of the colon and rectum (Table 23.1). Congenital disorders that present in early childhood will not be discussed in this chapter; however, Hirschsprung's disease, which may present in later childhood or even in adulthood, will be alluded to.

The normal mechanisms of fecal continence have been discussed in a previous chapter. These include the motor function of the anal sphincters and pelvic floor muscles, the role of the rectum and sigmoid colon as a fecal reservoir with capacitance, compliance and intrinsic motor activity, the effects of stool consistency, volume and delivery rate, the anorectal angle, and anorectal sensation. It is the coordinated integration of these factors that confers continence. When one of these contributing factors is compromised, the others may be able to compensate. However, their ability to do so varies considerably among individuals, and dysfunction in a single component of this complex mechanism may be enough to cause incontinence. The clinician must attempt to define the major and minor contributing factors to the individual's incontinence and design a treatment program to address them. To obtain a satisfactory result it may be necessary to correct only one of these factors. Also, simple additions to an intervention, such as a bowel management program or constipating agents, may convert a poor result into a good one.

INCIDENCE/PREVALENCE

Incontinence is probably a much more common problem than realized. Because of the social and professional stigmata associated with this condition, most individuals are reluctant to discuss it, even with their physician. In a recent study of patients presenting to a medical office, the prevalence of fecal incontinence was 13.6% for those seeing a primary care physician and 29.3% for those seeing a gastroenterologist. There was a progressive rise from 12.3% for those patients under 30 years of age to 19.4% after age 70. Only one-third had ever discussed this problem with a physician, yet 17% used pads or diapers, 12% used various medications, and 10% avoided leaving home for fear of an accident. Undoubtedly, many persons suffer for years without relief, and adoption of a reclusive lifestyle is more common than recognized.

Although the true incidence of fecal incontinence is unknown, one study estimated the prevalence to be 4.2/1000. Analysis of data from the Wisconsin Family Health Survey of 1993 revealed an incontinence rate of 2.2%. The population groups at particular risk seem to be the elderly and institutionalized persons, women (especially after multiple or traumatic deliveries), and patients with neurological disorders. In the over 65-year age group the known prevalence is 5/1000 but may actually approach 10/1000. In one study the incidence in geriatric and psychiatric hospital wards was 26% and 31%, respectively. A 43% rate of fecal incontinence in Wisconsin nursing home residents has been reported with the rate increasing with increasing age. Another study estimates the incidence in the elderly to be up to 60%. In a review of vaginal deliveries in 20,500 women, the incidence of third or fourth degree tears was 5%. Forty-one women (0.002%) experienced major fecal incontinence during short-term follow-up. In an ultrasonographic study of 62 women complaining of incontinence of flatus or stool following obstetric trauma, 90% had defects in the external sphincter, 65% in the internal sphincter, and 44% had disruption of the perineal body. Although these studies demonstrate different rates of incontinence, the message is clear—fecal incontinence is a very common problem which is often not identified unless sought.

PATHOGENESIS

The reason for a patient's fecal incontinence may be quite apparent or very elusive. Minor incontinence, defined as soiling or occasional incontinence to flatus or to loose or watery stools, is quite common and is often transitory. This may be seen with self-limited diarrheal syndromes, with poor hygiene, or with prolapsing hemorrhoids. Chronic minor incontinence may be seen with almost any of the disorders listed in Table 23.1, including prolapsing hemorrhoids, a persistent fistula, or a chronically draining abscess cavity. It is also a frequent result of anal anastomotic procedures, presumably due to injury of the internal sphincter muscle and loss of reservoir capacity. This type of incontinence is particularly problematic at night. Internal anal sphincter dysfunction alone, often due to stretching

TABLE 23.1 CLASSIFICATION OF FECAL INCONTINENCE BY ETIOLOGY

- I. Primary
  - A. Congenital
    - 1. Muscular/anatomical
    - 2. Neurological—Hirschsprung's disease
    - 3. Lumbar meningomyelocele
  - B. Traumatic
    - 1. Accidental
    - 2. Obstetrical
    - 3. Sexual
    - 4. Operative
      - a. Sphincterotomy
      - b. Fistulotomy
      - c. Mucosectomy
      - d. Stretch—transanal procedures or Lord's procedure
  - C. Acquired
    - 1. Rectal prolapse
    - 2. Mucosal prolapse
    - 3. Hemorrhoidal prolapse
    - 4. Anorectal infection—herpes, lymphogranuloma venereum
  - D. Neurological
    - 1. Idiopathic (primary neurogenic fecal incontinence)
    - 2. Upper motor neuron lesion
      - a. Cerebral
        - (i) Multiple strokes
        - (ii) Metastases and other tumors
        - (iii) Dementia and other degenerative disorders
        - (iv) Trauma
      - b. Spinal
        - (i) Multiple sclerosis
        - (ii) Metastases and other tumors
        - (iii) Degenerative diseases (e.g., vitamin B_{12} deficiency)
    - 3. Lower motor neuron lesion
      - a. Cauda equina (tumor or trauma)
      - b. Peripheral neuropathy (diabetes mellitus, multiple sclerosis)
      - c. Tabes dorsalis
      - d. Lumbar meningomyelocele (spina bifida)
- II. Secondary
  - A. Diarrhea
  - B. Metabolic (diabetes mellitus)
  - C. Laxative abuse
  - D. Drug intoxication (esp. in the elderly)
  - E. Fecal impaction
  - F. Colorectal disease
    - 1. Malignancy, inflammatory bowel disease, irritable bowel disease, villous tumor
  - G. Postoperative
    - 1. Sphincter-saving procedures
    - 2. Intestinal resection

(manual dilatation, rectal prolapse, post-transanal surgery) or to cutting (sphincterotomy, myomectomy, trauma) may cause minor fecal incontinence. Poor rectal sensation may also play a role in minor incontinence and seepage.

Major incontinence, defined as deficient control of stool of normal consistency with frequent and unheralded evacuations of formed bowel movements, is a very distressing problem for the patient. Whereas minor incontinence may often be fairly well tolerated, major fecal incontinence demands evaluation and treatment. Direct sphincter injury without neurological compromise, usually due to obstetrical mishap or trauma, may be repaired with the anticipation of a good result. Patients with incontinence due to neurological impairment are much less likely to regain normal function after local procedures; nevertheless, some patients benefit from biofeedback, or, rarely, Parks' postanal repair.

Secondary incontinence, or incontinence associated with normal sphincter and pelvic floor function, is most often due to a diarrheal syndrome or fecal impaction. With diarrhea, the normal mechanisms are overwhelmed by the sudden challenge of copious liquid stool. This may occur in virtually anyone; however, it may also uncover an underlying weakness of the anal sphincter mechanism. Treatment is directed at the underlying problem. Fecal impaction, principally diagnosed by digital examination, causes persistent rectal distention and inhibition of the internal sphincter muscle. Liquid stool builds up behind the fecolith and overflows around the impaction. This is called encopresis in children and may be an acquired problem if the child withholds stool to avoid evacuation. It is also commonly seen in the elderly, in institutionalized or immobilized patients, and in patients with central neurological disorders such as multiple sclerosis or stroke. Treatment involves disimpaction and bowel cleansing followed by a rigorous bowel management program.

Neurological deficits may involve afferent nerve fibers, efferent fibers or both. Afferent nerve injury results in decreased or absent anorectal sensation with impaired ability to detect rectal filling or a late or absent urge to evacuate. Efferent damage results in poor pelvic floor or external sphincter function and may also affect rectal capacity and compliance.

Lower motor neuron lesions may cause denervation of the pelvic floor striated muscles. This may occur anywhere from the level of the sacral foramina to the motor endplates within the muscle. Cauda equina syndrome may result from lumbar or sacral spondylosis and spinal canal narrowing, from disc prolapse or other intraspinal space-occupying lesions. Trauma may also injure the nerve roots in this region. Pelvic lesions and disorders may injure the nerves in the lumbosacral plexus and in the retroperitoneum. Other generalized lower motor neuron disorders may cause incontinence along with a host of other related symptoms.

In these neurological disorders, the level of the injury may be localized using the EMG techniques discussed in earlier chapters and below. Lesions of the pelvis and lumbosacral region may be visualized using x-ray, CT and MRI scanning techniques.

Pudendal neuropathy is the most common cause of fecal incontinence after diarrhea and direct obstetrical injury to the muscle. This entity has been referred to as idiopathic incontinence. It is now felt that the majority of these cases are due to primary injury of the nerves supplying the striated muscles of the pelvic floor and sphincter mechanism. Although some skeletal muscle denervation is a normal consequence of aging, it does not usually become apparent until the seventh or eighth decade of life. The currently accepted explanation for pudendal neuropathy is that the distal pudendal nerve is injured when it is stretched. The nerve bundle descends from the sacrum laterally, through Alcock's canal along the pelvic wall and around the ischial spine as it passes through the sacrospinous ligament. At this point the nerve is tethered. The bundle then crosses the fat-filled ischiorectal space and inserts into the external sphincter muscle on either side. Excessive descent of the perineum may stretch the distal pudendal nerve, causing injury. This may occur during severe straining to have a bowel movement or with childbirth. Associated disorders include the descending perineum syndrome, pelvic outlet constipation (nonrelaxing puborectalis), solitary rectal ulcer syndrome (internal intussusception), and complete rectal procidentia. In the latter, chronic or repeated dilatation of the anal canal by the prolapsing rectum may cause concomitant internal sphincter damage. The amount of descent of the pelvic floor measured in incontinent patients with the descending perineum syndrome could result in a 20% increase in the length of the pudendal nerves, more than enough to cause injury. Vaginal delivery has been implicated as a cause of pelvic nerve injury, particularly in multiparous women with a prolonged second stage of labor, with a large child, with breech presentation, or with the use of forceps. Electromyography studies reveal increased fiber density on single-fiber EMG, prolonged pudendal nerve terminal motor latency, polyphasic potentials using concentric probes, and prolonged motor latency detected in the external and sphincter with stimulation of the spinal cord at L1 or the cauda equina at L4 with no difference in calculated L1-L4 conduction.

Upper motor neuron disorders, such as spinal cord trauma, multiple sclerosis, or multifocal vascular disease, may also cause fecal and/or urinary incontinence. Disorders involving the orbitofrontal cerebral cortex are likely to present with incontinence since the central nervous system representation of sphincter control is contained in this region. In addition, diffuse diseases of the brain such as the various dementias are often accompanied by incontinence since the conscious response to the call to stool may not be recognized or may be ignored.

EVALUATION

Clinical Evaluation

History

The patient should be asked about the onset, degree, and duration of incontinence, associated problems such as urinary incontinence or other anorectal disorders, bowel habits, regional injury, prior surgery, obstetrical history, concomitant disease (e.g., neuromuscular, diabetes mellitus), medications, radiation treatment, recent gastroenteritis, and foreign travel. A complaint of diarrhea may, on further questioning, really be one of incontinence.

Questioning about sexual practices, although potentially embarrassing, is important, especially in younger patients. Anoreceptive intercourse, penile or otherwise, may be a major contributing factor in certain individuals. Any patient at risk for harboring the human immunodeficiency virus should be strongly encouraged to undergo serological testing since this information may be pivotal in making therapeutic decisions and for general care of the individual.

A neurological lesion may be suspected if the history is short, includes perineal or low back pain, or if there are associated motor and/or sensory symptoms in the legs or buttocks.

Examination

The physical examination should include a general review as well as directed scrutiny of the anorectum. Examination of the abdomen and the central and peripheral nervous system may give clues as to the etiology of incontinence and associated dissorders. Inspection of the perineum may reveal soiling, pruritic changes, scars, a patulous anus, or ectropion. Straining, especially while squatting or sitting, may reveal significant perineal descent or hemorrhoidal or rectal prolapse. Perineal sensation should be tested for skin prick (sharp) and cottontip (dull). The anocutaneous reflex is checked by stroking the skin at the anal verge and watching for sphincter contraction. The absence of this reflex may indicate the presence of a pudendal neuropathy or cauda equina lesion. The anal verge should be gently separated, exposing the lower anal canal for direct scrutiny, looking for ease of separation, fissures, and scars. The canal may be well opposed or patulous at rest or with separation. Each quadrant should be viewed at this time and during anoscopy.

Digital examination is fundamental and may reveal anatomical defects in the anal muscular ring or the posterior ridge and anorectal angle formed by the levators and the puborectalis (PR). Strictures or scars, gross resting and squeeze pressures, the presence of a fecal impaction, and low rectal tumors may also be detected.

Colorectal Studies

Anoscopy and proctosigmoidoscopy will provide additional information, including the presence of neoplasms, fistulas, hemorrhoids, internal intussusception, solitary rectal ulcers, and other colorectal disorders. Colonoscopy and/or barium enema studies will help to identify infectious disorders, inflammatory bowel diseases, and benign or malignant colorectal tumors. Visualization of the entire colon is not always necessary but is often helpful and is performed at the discretion of the treating physican.

Laboratory evaluation of the stool and blood, although usually not helpful, may be necessary to rule out many systemic and infectious disorders.

Physiological Evaluation

Although most of the reasons for incontinence will be discovered with clinical evaluation, physiological testing of the anorectum is of use in defining etiologies that remain unclear and in documenting the specific deficits. Subsequently, these tests may also help in monitoring progress and to determine objectively what has been altered by therapeutic intervention. Figure 23.1 outlines the steps in evaluation of the patient with fecal incontinence. All of these tests do not need to be done in every patient; rather, the physician's clinical evaluation and judgment will determine which tests are desirable.

Anorectal Manometry

Manometry generally includes assessment of the resting and squeeze pressures of the anal canal and the rectal inhibitory reflex. Manometric evaluation of the anal canal may be performed in a variety of ways well described in the preceding chapters. Today, most workers are using methods that generate a profile of the anal canal in the longitudinal axis and in four or eight quadrants. The information derived from this data includes the functional length of the anal canal and the level of maximal resting and squeeze pressures.

The internal anal sphincter muscle contributes about 80–90% of the anal canal resting pressure in healthy individuals, since paralysis of the striated muscles produces about a 10–20% drop in resting pressure. However, with injury of the internal anal sphincter, the external sphincter is able to compensate and may contribute much more than 20% of resting tone. Although experimental studies of this phenomenon are lacking in humans, therapeutic division of the internal sphincter usually does not usually result in incontinence when the external sphincter is intact.

Voluntary squeeze pressure is produced by contraction of the striated muscles surrounding the anal canal, specifically the external anal sphincter and the puborectalis. If these muscles are completely divided then incontinence will likely ensue, since there is no force left to compensate for the reflex relaxation of the internal sphincter with rectal filling.

Incontinent patients have lower resting pressures than age-matched continent subjects. In addition, the maximal squeeze pressures attainable are also lower but more so in patients incontinent to both liquids and solids as opposed to those incontinent to liquids only. The difference between patients incontinent to liquids only versus those incontinent to both liquids and solids is that although both may have internal sphincter dysfunction, it is the poor function of the external sphincter that is critical in maintaining continence to solids. The radial distribution of pressures within the anal canal may identify the zone of weakness; however, the presence of a rigid scar in one area may give rise to a falsely high reading in that quadrant. More commonly, diffusely low pressures will be observed even when the defect is in one quadrant only. Therefore, as with all tests, manometry must be interpreted with knowledge of the history, physical examination, and any other tests already performed.

Neuromuscular Testing

Electromyographic evaluation is the most accurate and direct method of assessing neuromuscular function of the perianal striated muscles and the pelvic floor. Together, the following tests allow localization of the level and extent of a neuromuscular deficit contributing to fecal incontinence. The major disadvantage

FIGURE 23.1. Steps in the evaluation of fecal incontinence.

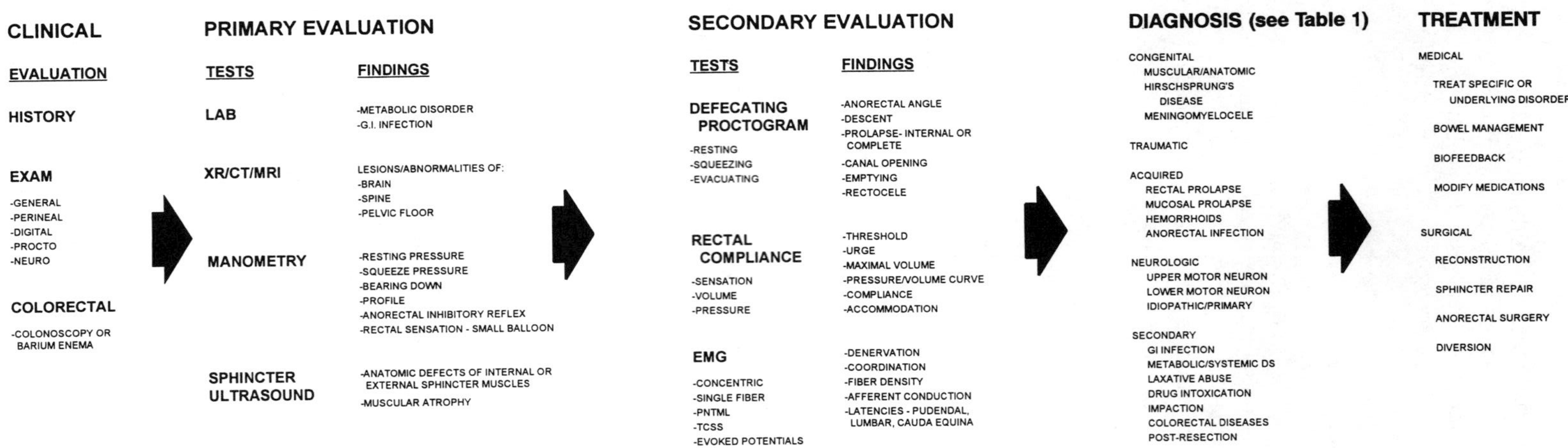

of these tests is that some require placement of a needle electrode directly into the muscle which may be poorly tolerated.

Monopolar EMG. Monopolar measurements of intramuscular electrical activity tend to be qualitative only. They will record activity from a fairly large area since the reference electrode is placed on the skin, some distance away from the active electrode (the needle). Resting activity and a percentage of normal recruitment with squeezing may be estimated, along with some gross evaluation of spike potential morphology. The results will vary, depending on the exposed surface area of the needle and its location in the muscle. This technique may be useful for mapping of the sphincter prior to repair of an injury or before a pull-through procedure in a child with imperforate anus. Although monopolar EMG is useful, most laboratories rely on concentric needle and single-fiber density studies.

Concentric needle EMG. Concentric needle EMG is widely used for testing of skeletal muscle. Since the active and reference leads are close together and both are placed in the muscle body, the activity recorded can be confidently attributed to the muscle in which the needle is placed. Generally, several nerve fibers are recorded at each location, although occasionally a single fiber will be sampled. Much of the data obtained from concentric needle recordings is qualitative; nevertheless, much may be learned and, outside of strict research protocols, enough information may be obtained so that single-fiber studies are not necessary. Concentric needle studies only require one or two sites in each quadrant.

Attempts have been made to accurately quantify concentric needle studies but most workers now comment on the resting activity and gross morphology of the waveforms, estimate percent recruitment with squeezing, and determine whether there is decreased or increased activity with bearing down. Measurements of the duration of the motor unit potentials (MUPD) in both the external anal sphincter and the puborectalis have been performed and demonstrate that the means were longer in patients with the descending perineum syndrome and incontinence versus controls. The mean of the integrated activity during 1 sec of maximal contraction has been calculated from the external sphincter and the puborectalis and was almost one-third lower in incontinent patients than in controls.

In practice, we study the sphincter in four quadrants and in the puborectalis posteriorly. Comments are made on the quality and quantity of activity in each quadrant at rest, during squeezing, and with bearing down. At rest, the muscle may be mildly, moderately, or very active or not active at all. With squeezing the screen should be filled with action potentials and this activity is assigned a percentage with from 80 to 100% being normal. Muscle activity should be inhibited with bearing down. Individual potentials are examined and the amount of polyphasic activity is estimated. An occasional polyphasic potential when most are normal is not pathological. Many polyphasic potentials are an indication of denervation. If there are few potentials at rest, the patient is asked to squeeze gently to induce potentials that may be examined sequentially.

Single-fiber EMG. Single-fiber EMG needles have a very small exposed active lead surface which permits recording of action potentials from single muscle fibers. A quantitative assessment of fiber density may be derived by measuring the number of times the individual potential crosses the baseline. One time crossing the baseline within the complex is normal; more than one is polyphasic. Phases are counted in 10 to 20 different potentials in each area and the mean is calculated. Occasional polyphasic potentials are normal so that normal values average up to 1.5. Some increases in the fiber density are common after age 60. It is thought that denervated muscle that has been reinnervated gives rise to larger and broader potentials, representing more muscle fibers in a single motor unit. Supportive studies show that fiber density in the external anal sphincter is higher in many incontinent patients than in controls. This is consistent with a denervation-reinnervation pattern. Although this technique is very quantitative, it is less well tolerated than concentric needle studies because of the large number of needle sticks.

Pudendal nerve terminal motor latency. This technique tests the motor function of the distal portion of the pudendal nerve as it crosses the ischiorectal fossa to insert into the external sphincter muscle. This is the portion of this nerve felt to be most at risk for stretch injury during childbirth or with the various pelvic floor syndromes. Transrectal stimulation of the pudendal nerve at the level of the ischial spine results in contraction of the external anal sphincter. Velocity may be calculated as the time lapse between stimulation and contraction. For simplicity this is measured in milliseconds since the distance the impulse has to travel is fixed (3 cm). Normal in most labs is 2.0 ± 0.2 msec. Pudendal nerve terminal motor latency is often prolonged in incontinent patients and indicates that there is a neurological injury. This may be in addition to a sphincter muscular defect.

Transcutaneous spinal stimulation. Transcutaneous electrical stimulation of the spinal cord at L1 or the cauda equina at L4 will evoke a muscle response in the external anal sphincter and the puborectalis. The latency time may be calculated for each, and the L4-latency time subtracted from the L1-latency time will equal the L1-L4 or cauda equina conduction velocity. Abnormalities in these measurements may be found in patients with lesions of this region or with demyelinating disorders such as multiple sclerosis.

Stimulation of the pudendal nerve normally results in a measurable response in the external anal sphincter but not in the puborectalis muscle (PR). Transcutaneous stimulation of L1 results in a motor response in both the external and sphincter and the puborectalis, supporting the notion that the puborectalis muscle is primarily innervated by branches that run above the levator muscles and not through fibers in the pudendal nerve. Therefore, injury to the innervation of the PR would not be accounted for by pudendal nerve stretch but rather by direct trauma to the nerves that run along the pelvic floor above the levators. This may well occur with fetal descent during delivery or with relaxation of the suspension of the rectum and the uterus in patients with straining or prolapse.

Sensory evoked potentials. This modality evaluates the ascending or sensory neural pathways to the cerebral cortex by stimulating the sphincter and other locations and, by means of computer averaging, by isolating the cortical EEG response. It may be helpful in assessing sensory deficits and other neurological disorders involving the central nervous system. However, this test requires a full set of control values for each laboratory and dedicated equipment and a technician. It may be most significant when there are side-to-side asymmetries.

Defecating Proctography

Dynamic radiography of the rectum and pelvic floor while at rest, with squeezing and with straining or bearing down to evacuate may reveal many anatomic abnormalities often not seen by endoscopic or passive radiological exams. Intussusception, rectoceles, perineal hernias, pelvic floor descensus, inadequate emptying, small or large capacity, and the changes in the anorectal angle with each maneuver may all be demonstrated with this technique. In a study of incontinent patients, the anorectal angle measured at rest, during straining, and during voluntary contraction of the sphincter was significantly more obtuse in incontinent patients versus controls.

Rectal Balloon/Compliance

This test assesses rectal volume and pressure, sensation, compliance, and accommodation. The threshold of sensation, the urge to defecate, and the maximal tolerated volumes may be measured. Poor compliance, low capacity or volume, high contractility, poor rectal sensation, and rectal irritability (e.g., with proctitis) may all contribute to fecal incontinence. Poor rectal capacity and accommodation and a low tolerated volume may be seen in patients who have an inflammatory bowel disease involving the rectum or those who have had patients with disorders with neurological manifestations such as diabetes mellitus and cerebral palsy and after cerebral vascular accidents. These disorders, along with fecal impaction as a consequence of them or for any other reason, may result in a dilated, flabby rectum with little contractility, a large volume, and low compliance. Overflow incontinence may then ensue.

Transit Studies

Transit studies, using radiopaque markers, scintigraphic techniques, and/or the hydrogen breath test, may be used to quantify intestinal transit. Rapid transit associated with a motility disorder, with an infectious etiology, or with an inflammatory bowel disease, may result in urgency and diarrhea, which may present with incontinence. This test is rarely used in the evaluation of patients with incontinence. However, it is very useful in the workup of the constipated patient.

Anal Sphincter Ultrasound

Endorectal ultrasound using a commercially available probe with a distensible balloon on the end has become a standard method for the evaluation of rectal lesions. The need to distend the balloon made it difficult to use in the anal canal. A newly designed tip using a narrow, rigid cover has made it much easier to image the anal canal and its surrounding structures. With this system the anal sphincters and a portion of the puborectalis may be imaged in horizontal cross sections. There is a significant learning curve in the use of this technique. However, if an examiner experienced in anal canal imaging performs the exam, specific defects and generalized thinning of the sphincters may be detected with fairly good reliability. The internal and external sphincters may be seen separately. As the examiner proceeds cephalad an apparent defect in the upper external sphincter may be observed. One must differentiate between a real defect and the separation of the puborectalis muscle fibers as they head toward the pubic bone. This study generates reliable information about anatomic defects of the sphincter. Some authors feel that this test will replace sphincter EMG. Certainly, it is better tolerated and gives as much or more information about anatomic defects. Therefore, mapping EMG will not be necessary when the information needed only concerns a muscular injury. However, ultrasound tells us nothing about the neurological integrity and function of the sphincter mechanism. When this is of concern, particularly in the presence of a prolonged pudendal nerve terminal motor latency, then EMG is still indicated.

TREATMENT

Based on the evaluation described, rational decisions about treatment should be easier to make (Table 23.2). Nonsurgical treatment may be the initial approach selected in most patients, except in those with a recent or obvious muscular defect.

NONSURGICAL TREATMENT

Bowel Management

A well-regulated bowel management program is the first mode of treatment for most patients with fecal incontinence and may be the only treatment necessary for many of them. It is particularly helpful in patients with fecal impaction, neurological disorders, and sphincter compromise. Patients with minor incontinence often note a marked improvement in their symptoms. This program may be the only option available in certain situations, including the patient who refuses an operative alternative or who has failed operative repairs and does not want or is too poor a risk for colostomy. Patients with soiling due to fecal impaction may often be best treated by an aggressive bowel management program. This would include initial disimpaction and education, followed by regulation of habits using the methods noted below.

Depending on the patient and their underlying problem, a bowel management program may consist of any or all of the following components: (1) a well-balanced diet including fiber and fluids eaten at a routine time; (2) sitting to evacuate 20 to 30 min after eating at the same time each day (taking advantage of the gastrocolic reflex); (3) cautious and well-controlled usage of suppositories, laxatives, and/or enemas; (4) bulking agents and/or stool softeners; (5) motility-altering medications; and (6) careful perineal care.

Diarrheal Disorders

Many patients with diarrhea and incontinence, even with some pelvic floor dysfunction, may be restored to an acceptable functional level simply by controlling their diarrhea. A large, formed fecal bolus is much easier to hold and to voluntarily evacuate than is a large volume of liquid stool. Infectious causes may be self-limited or, if persistent, treated medically after identifying the agent. Neoplasms such as villous adenomas or carcinomas should be resected, using an appropriate method. Inflammatory bowel disease may be treated medically or may require surgery to control the associated diarrhea.

TABLE 23.2 TREATMENT OPTIONS FOR PATIENTS WITH FECAL INCONTINENCE

I. Nonsurgical
  A. Bowel management
    1. Fiber/bulking agents
    2. Disimpaction
    3. Motility-altering agents
    4. Alteration of laxative/enema use
  B. Treatment of diarrheal disorders
  C. Treatment of other underlying medical disorders
  D. Biofeedback

II. Surgical
  A. Repair of prolapse
  B. Direct sphincter repair
    1. Wrapping—overlapping sphincteroplasty
    2. Plication
  C. Park's postanal repair
  D. Sphincter supplementation
    1. Thiersch loop
    2. Gracilis muscle transposition/electrical stimulation
    3. Free muscle graft
    4. Artificial sphincter
  E. Treatment of colonic disease (e.g., inflammatory bowel disease, neoplasm)
    1. Colectomy with ileorectal anastomosis
    2. Colectomy with ileostomy
    3. Colectomy with ileal pouch—anal anastomosis
    4. Colectomy with Kock's continent ileostomy
    5. Resection of neoplasm (transanal, transabdominal)
    6. Treatment of neoplasm (chemotherapy, radiation therapy, local ablation)
  F. Diversion
    1. Ileostomy
    2. Colostomy

Underlying Medical Disorders

Metabolic and medication-induced incontinence is best treated by addressing the underlying problem. Brief usage of bulking agents and motility-altering medications may be of help. Laxative abuse, once diagnosed, is treated by discontinuing these medications and placing the patient on a strict bowel management program to encourage the development of spontaneous regular movements. Many of these patients will need concurrent psychiatric therapy.

Biofeedback

Biofeedback may be very effective in a majority of carefully selected patients, including some with varying degrees of neurological impairment of the pelvic floor. It may be used to enhance sensation and discrimination in patients with a sensory deficit, to strengthen and improve control of the external anal sphincter and puborectalis muscles, and to better coordinate both muscle contraction in response to rectal distention and attempts at defecation. The technique of biofeedback is described in Chapter 19.

Thus far, direct electrical stimulation of the striated muscles of the pelvic floor has not proved to be of great benefit.

Surgical Treatment

Rectal Prolapse

Resuspension and repair of rectal procidentia may be accomplished by a variety of methods, all of which give fairly good results and prevent further dilation of and injury to the anal sphincters by the prolapsing segment. With these methods, up to 88% of patients with incontinence due to the prolapse may regain significant function. The remainder may have suffered internal sphincter injury and/or pudendal nerve injury. Their respective contributions to the problem may be clarified by manometry and EMG studies. If incontinence persists, the internal sphincter may be plicated, resulting in improved anal canal resting pressure, or external sphincter and puborectalis function may be improved by either biofeedback or by one of the operative reconstructions described below.

Direct Sphincter Repair

Incontinence due to a discrete muscular injury in the presence of normal innervation is the most amendable to repair and is the most likely to be successfully treated.

Wrapping. Overlapping sphincteroplasty works best when there is a definable and isolated anatomical defect in the muscular ring with an asssociated scar. This is the preferred method of treatment in patients who have had an obstetrical laceration or direct trauma. Although rarely indicated, some improvement may be seen in patients with neurological injury but some retained function. This may be because of the improved mechanical advantage conferred by closer apposition of the sphincters, allowing the functioning fibers to generate a higher anal canal pressure by not having to shorten as much and by lengthening the functional high pressure zone of the anal canal.

Plication. Plication of the internal sphincter muscle may improve resting anal pressure by reducing the diameter of a patulous canal. This is done from the luminal side of the internal sphincter and may be easily accomplished during the course of other operative procedures involving the anal canal, such as ileal pouch-anal anastomosis, the Delorme repair for prolapse, rectal muscosal advancement flaps, or even hemorrhoidectomy. In general, limited benefit is derived from this procedure.

Parks' Postanal Repair

This operation was considered by many to be the procedure of choice for surgical treatment of neurogenic fecal incontinence. In early studies up to 70% of patients with neurogenic fecal incontinence were improved. Although anal canal resting pressures are not significantly altered, squeeze pressures and the length of the anal canal may be increased. There is also a suggestion that the sensation associated with the urge to defecate may be improved. Correlation between increased squeeze pressures and improved continence is poor. The operation may help to restore the anatomical configuration but not to directly affect neural or muscular activity. Though it was originally thought that the procedure works by restoring the anorectal angle, this has not been demonstrated by follow-up studies. Additional studies of the effectiveness of this procedure and longer follow-up of these patients have been disappointing. Success rates have fallen markedly and most surgeons have abandoned this approach.

Sphincter Supplementation

Thiersch loop. A passive method of tightening a patulous anus, the Thiersch loop was originally made from wire but now is usually constructed from synthetic materials. The loop forms a relative obstruction at the anal outlet. Since it does not function, these patients may become relatively obstructed or continue to be incontinent. The tension on the loop must be carefully set during the procedure so that the anal canal accepts a 1-cm digit. This procedure is appropriate in the occasional elderly or debilitated patient who will not tolerate a more extensive procedure or an ostomy. It is particularly helpful in patients with rectal prolapse and incontinence because it keeps the rectum reduced. A careful bowel management program must be followed including fiber supplements, fluids, and stool softeners. Regular enemas may also be necessary to avoid impaction.

Gracilis muscle transposition. This procedure attempts to replace the function of the anal sphincters with the transposed muscle body and tendon of the gracilis muscle. The end result may be an endogenous Thiersch loop since the anal canal is actually encircled by tendon, not muscle, and the graft has limited muscular activity. This is a complex procedure and has quite a variable success rate in different hands. There is probably a limited role for the technique, perhaps in the patient with normal lower extremity function but complete anal denervation.

In the last few years this procedure has been revived and revised by adding electrical stimulation of the muscle. The goal is to transform the short-acting, fast-twitch muscle fibers of the gracilis muscle into longer-acting, slow-twitch muscles, capable of sustaining anal canal closure for longer periods of time. The technique currently includes the muscle transposition and implantation of an electrical stimulator. The muscle is then trained over a number of months. Several groups are now working on this with some early success. Although the process is long and cumbersome, there may be a wider role for this procedure in the future.

Free muscle transplantation. A variety of procedures have been described, none of which are proven or have been routinely used.

Artificial sphincter. An artificial sphincter has been developed and is being used in investigational protocols in very limited settings. Although it may ultimately become a useful tool, the artificial sphincter is a foreign body and is at risk for infection or erosion that may cause further sphincter destruction. Although further experience is warranted, the device is not currently available.

Treat Colonic Disease

Inflammatory bowel disease. Patients with inflammatory bowel diseases may have severe diarrhea and be unresponsive to medical management. In these patients, incontinence may be a relative indication for a sphincter-sparing operation. Colectomy with ileorectal anastomosis or total proctocolectomy with ileal pouch-anal anastomosis are options that, when used appropriately, may maintain the normal route of elimination, remove the diseased bowel responsible for the diarrhea, and avoid a stoma. However, recommendation of these procedures presupposes a normal sphincter mechanism if continence is to be anticipated. Since a large volume of relatively liquid stool will still be presented to the anal canal, although without the tenesmus and urgency commonly experienced preoperatively, the sphincters must be able to cope. Anorectal manometry should be performed to assess sphincter strength. If a significant deficit is demonstrated, the patient may be counseled to elect another surgical alternative. In selected patients, a sphincter repair or plication may be performed at the time of the colectomy or later. This repair will be protected by the temporary ileostomy commonly constructed with these procedures and may be tested prior to ileostomy closure. Preoperative evaluation of rectal function is advisable in patients undergoing elective ileorectal anastomosis to ensure that the rectum will be able to assume adequate reservoir function in the absence of the colon.

Ileoanal anastomosis and coloanal anastomosis may substitute one cause of incontinence for another. The mucosectomy commonly performed with many of these procedures frequently injures the internal sphincter muscle, either by the prolonged stretch required for the operative approach or by direct injury to the internal sphincter muscle or its nervous supply during the submucosal dissection. Manometrically determined resting pressures are often lower postoperatively. Internal anal sphincter injury may be avoided by using stapled anastomoses whenever possible, avoiding mucosectomy and anal stretching.

Neoplasms. Villous adenomas and malignant tumors of the colon and rectum may contribute to incontinence because of secretions, partial obstruction, or direct invasion of the pelvic floor and sphincter mechanism. Similarly, anal canal neoplasms may be a cause of fecal incontinence. Management is primarily treatment of the lesion.

Diversion

A colostomy or ileostomy may be used as an adjunct to sphincter repair or pelvic floor reconstruction, especially after trauma as a temporary measure. However, it may also be the preferred permanent alternative in the individual with severe pelvic floor atrophy and no hope of regaining function. This may be the elderly patient or one with a severe generalized neurological disorder. Although it is a last resort, a well-constructed ostomy is much easier to care for than a widely patulous anus.

CONCLUSION

There is still much to learn about both the evaluation and the treatment of fecal incontinence. However, a solid scientific foundation has been established on which we may build a more complete understanding.

SUGGESTED READINGS

Bartolo DCC, Jarratt JA, Read MG, et al: The role of partial denervation of the puborectalis in idiopathic fecal incontinence. *Br J Surg* 70:664–667, 1983.

Beersiek F, Parks AG, Swash M: Pathogenesis of ano-rectal incontinence: a histometric study of the anal sphincter musculature. *J Neurol Sci* 42:111–127, 1979.

Brocklehurst JC: Management of anal incontinence. *Clin Gastroenterol* 4:479–487, 1975.

Burnett SJ, Speakman CT, Kamm MA et al: Confirmation of endosonographic detection of external anal sphincter defects by simultaneous electromyographic mapping. *Br J Surg* 78:448–450, 1991.

Burnett SJ, Spence-Jones C, Speakman CT, et al: Unsuspected sphincter damage following childbirth revealed by anal endosonography. *Br J Radiol* 64:225–227, 1991.

Clarke N, Hughes AO, Dodd KJ, et al: The elderly in residential care: patterns of disability. *Health Trends* 11:17, 1979.

Deen KI, Kumar D, Williams JG, et al: Anal sphincter defects. Correlation between endoanal ultrasound and surgery. *Ann Surg* 218:201–205, 1993.

Emblem R, Dhaenens G, Stien R, et al: The importance of anal endosonography in the evaluation of idiopathic fecal incontinence. *Dis Colon Rectum* 37:42–48, 1994.

Henry MM: Pathogenesis and management of fecal incontinence in the adult. *Gastroenterol Clin North Am* 16(1):35–45, 1987.

Henry MM, Parks AG, Swash M: The pelvic floor musculature in the descending perineum syndrome. *Br J Surg* 69:470–472, 1982.

Henry MM, Swash M: Fecal incontinence. B. Pathogenesis and clinical features. In Henry MM, Swash M *Coloproctology and the Pelvic Floor*. London, Butterworths, 1985, pp 222–228.

Johanson JE: Epidemiology of fecal incontinence—the silent affliction. *Gastroenterology* 106:A11, 1994.

Kiff ES, Swash M: Slowed conduction in the pudendal nerves in idiopathic (neurogenic) faecal incontinence. *Br J Surg* 71:614–616, 1984.

Kiff ES, Swash M: *J Neurol Neurosurg Psychiatry* 47:820–823, 1984.

Lubowski DZ, Swash M, Henry MM: Neural mechanisms in disorders of defecation. *Bailliere's Clin Gastroenterol* 2(1):201–223, 1988.

Neill ME, Swash M: Increased motor unit fibre density in the external sphincter muscle in anorectal incontinence: a single fibre EMG study. *J Neurol Neurosurg Psychiatry* 43:343–347, 1980.

Neill ME, Swash M: Physiologic studies of the anal sphincter musculature in faecal incontinence and rectal prolapse. *Br J Surg* 68:531–536, 1981.

Nelson R, Norton N, Cautley E: Fecal incontinence in Wisconsin households. Abstract presented at the 1994 meeting of the American Society of Colon and Rectal Surgeons, Orlando, Florida.

Parks AG: Anorectal incontinence. *Proc R Soc Med* 68:21–30, 1975.

Parks AG, Swash M, Urich H: Sphincter denervation in ano-rectal incontinence and rectal prolapse. *Gut* 18:656–665, 1977.

Read NW, Bartolo DCC, Read MG: Differences in anal function in patients with incontinence to solids and in patients with incontinence to liquids. *Br J Surg* 71:39–42, 1984.

Scheuer M, Kuijpers HC, Jacobs PP: Postanal repair restores anatomy rather than function. *Dis Colon Rectum* 32:960–963, 1989.

Snooks SJ, Henry MM, Swash M: Faecal incontinence due to external and sphincter division in childbirth is associated with damage to the innervation of the pelvic floor musculature: a double pathology. *Br J Obstet Gynecol* 92:824–828, 1985.

Snooks SJ, Nicholls RJ, Henry MM, et al: Electrophysiological and manometric assessment of the pelvic floor in the solitary rectal ulcer syndrome. *Br J Surg* 72:131–133, 1985.

Snooks SJ, Swash M, Henry MM, et al: Injury to the innervation of the pelvic floor musculature in childbirth. *Lancet* 2:546–550, 1985.

Snooks SJ, Swash M, Henry MM, et al: Risk factors in childbirth causing damage to the pelvic floor innervation. *Int J Colorect Dis* 1:20–24, 1986.

Sunderland S: *Nerves and Nerve Injuries*, ed 2. Edinburgh, Churchill-Livingstone, 1978, pp 62–66.

Thomas TM, Egan M, Walgrove A, et al: The prevalence of fecal and double incontinence. *Community Med* 6:216–220, 1984.

Tjandra JJ, Milsom JW, Schroeder T, et al: Endoluminal ultrasound is preferable to electromyography in mapping anal sphincteric defects. *Dis Colon Rectum* 36:689–692, 1993.

Tuckson WB, Fazio VW: Anal incontinence. In Fazio VW (ed): *Current Therapy in Colon and Rectal Surgery*. Philadelphia, BC Decker, 1990.

Venkatesh KS, Ramanujam PS, Larson DM, et al: Anorectal complications of vaginal delivery. *Dis Colon Rectum* 32:1039–1041, 1989.

Womack NR, Morrisson JF, Williams NS: Prospective study of the effects of postanal repair in neurogenic fecal incontinence. *Br J Surg* 75:48–52, 1988.

INDEX

E

F

G

H

I